Communication Disorders
Following Traumatic Brain Injury:
Management of Cognitive, Language, and Motor Impairments

Communication Disorders Following Traumatic Brain Injury:
Management of Cognitive, Language, and Motor Impairments

Edited by

David R. Beukelman, Ph.D.
Department of Special Education and
Communication Disorders,
Meyer Children's Rehabilitation Institute,
University of Nebraska, Lincoln

Kathryn M. Yorkston, Ph.D.
Department of Rehabilitation Medicine,
University of Washington, Seattle

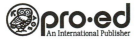
8700 Shoal Creek Boulevard
Austin, Texas 78757

Library of Congress Cataloging-in-Publication Data
Main entry under title:

Communication Disorders Following Traumatic Brain Injury:
Management of Cognitive, Language, and Motor Impairments / edited
by David R. Beukelman, Kathryn M. Yorkston
 p. cm.
  Includes bibliographical references.
  ISBN 0-89079-295-X
  1. Brain—Wounds and injuries—Complications and sequelae.
 2. Communicative disorders. 3. Deglutition disorders.
 I. Beukelman, David R., 1943– . II. Yorkston, Kathryn M., 1948–
.
  [DNLM: 1. Brain Injury—complications. 2. Communicative Disorders—
etiology. 3. Deglutition Disorders—etiology. WL 354 C7335]
  RD594.C65 1990
  617.4'81044—dc20
  DNLM/DLC
  for Library of Congress   89-14560
                                              CIP

Printed in the United States of America

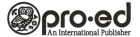
An International Publisher
8700 Shoal Creek Boulevard
Austin, Texas 78757

  5 6 7   98

Contents

Contributing Authors

David R. Beukelman, Ph.D.
Department of Special Education and Communication Disorders, Meyer Children's Rehabilitation Institute, University of Nebraska, Lincoln

Jo Ann Brockway, Ph.D.
Department of Rehabilitation Medicine, University of Washington, Seattle

Marvin Brooke, M.D.
Department of Rehabilitation Medicine, University of Washington, Seattle

Frank DeRuyter, Ph.D.
Communication Disorders Department, Rancho Los Amigos Hospital, Downey, California

David J. Fordyce, Ph.D.
Outpatient Brain Injury and Rehabilitation Program, Virginia Mason Medical Center, Seattle

Robert T. Fraser, Ph.D., C.R.C.
Departments of Neurological Surgery and Rehabilitation Medicine, University of Washington, Seattle

Melissa J. Honsinger, M.A.
Speech Pathology Services, University of Washington Medical Center, Seattle

Mary R. T. Kennedy, M.A.
Communication Disorders Department, Rancho Los Amigos Hospital, Downey, California

Cathy L. Lazarus, M.A.
Department of Communication Sciences and Disorders, Northwestern University, Chicago

Alvin McClean, Jr., Ph.D.
Department of New Medico Community Reentry Service of Washington, Mount Terrace, Washington

Nickola Wolf Nelson, Ph.D.
Department of Speech Pathology and Audiology, Western Michigan University, Kalamazoo

Barbara Schwentor, M.A.
Education and Rehabilitation Services, Western Michigan University,
Kalamazoo

Jay M. Uomoto, Ph.D.
Department of Rehabilitation Medicine, University of Washington, Seattle

Kathryn M. Yorkston, Ph.D.
Department of Rehabilitation Medicine, University of Washington, Seattle

Preface

Communication Disorders Following Traumatic Brain Injury: Management of Cognitive, Language, and Motor Impairments was written for graduate students and practicing professionals interested in the communication and swallowing disorders of persons with traumatic brain injury (TBI). In this text, the authors have written extensive, detailed chapters concerning the communication and swallowing disorders associated with TBI. In areas where the literature is as yet limited, we invited authors who clinically serve individuals with TBI to provide a perspective that reflects current clinical practice.

The consequences of TBI are pervasive, with long-term physical, cognitive, communicative, and social disabilities that profoundly affect these individuals, their families, and society at large. During the past ten years, a variety of services have been developed for survivors of TBI and their families. These service delivery programs vary considerably in mission and scope in an effort to provide emergency care, acute rehabilitation, long-term rehabilitation, long-term care, and community reentry. As programs such as these continue to be developed the need for trained, clinical personnel will continue to expand. In the early years this need was met through retraining professionals from many fields. However, as the number of service programs has increased and the roles of personnel have been clarified, an effort to include detailed information about TBI in preprofessional as well as continuing education programs has become necessary. *Communication Disorders Following Traumatic Brain Injury: Management of Cognitive, Language, and Motor Impairments* is provided as a substantive text to support the preparation of professionals to serve brain-injured persons.

Organizationally, the book is divided into three major divisions: service delivery, cognitive and language, and motor control issues. The range of communication services provided to individuals with TBI is extensive. These services may begin on the neurosurgery unit during acute hospitalization. Almost without exception the need for these services extends through acute rehabilitation into communication integration. The service delivery section of this book is provided to familiarize the reader with the contexts in which TBI survivors receive communication and swallowing services. Because of the traumatic causes of TBI, the survivor usually begins the journey of recovery with a period of extensive medical assistance. Therefore, it is necessary for clinicians at all levels of service delivery to appreciate the nature and extent of the medical support provided to the acutely injured individual. Chapter 2 introduces the reader to much of the medical terminology associated with TBI and with the sequences of medical treatment that many TBI survivors experience. Chapter 2 also outlines the various service delivery models that are available to survivors of TBI depending on their severity and geographic location. The authors bring to this chapter the perspectives of psychology and vocational counseling in the postacute rehabilitation settings. Clinicians serving the communication and swallowing problems of individuals with TBI find themselves working in these environments. Chapter 3 introduces the reader to the psychosocial aspects of TBI. The organic issues (the brain injury) and the adjustment issues to TBI result in extensive psychosocial problems for many survivors, their family members, and close friends. Any services that are provided to individuals with TBI are provided in this psychosocial context.

The second part of the book deals with those cognitive and language problems that are closely related in many TBI survivors. Chapter 4 outlines the conceptual issues in the various cognitive rehabilitation approaches employed with TBI survivors. Chapter 5 reviews the neuropsychological assessment procedures that are usually administered to individuals with TBI. Chapter 6 reviews the memory deficits commonly found in individuals with TBI and outline intervention strategies and tools to retrain and augment memory capabilities. Chapter 7 discusses the cognitive and language bases of spoken communication disorders in individuals with TBI and describe an extensive intervention program. Chapter 8 outlines the current scope of practice regarding the literary skills of individuals with TBI. In this chapter the authors report the results of their national survey describing literacy assessment and intervention strategies in numerous, major TBI treatment centers.

In the third part of the book, three chapters focus on the motor control problems associated with communication and swallowing disorders of individuals with TBI. In Chapter 9 the authors detail the assessment and intervention programs of the motor speech disorders that commonly accompany TBI. Chapter 10 provides an excellent description of the augmentative and alternative communication strategies that are used with TBI survivors at various cognitive levels. Chapter 11 outlines a comprehensive approach to the swallowing problems of individuals with TBI, and the author reviews the results of a recent research project focusing on the swallowing problems of individuals with TBI that the author and colleagues completed at Northwestern University.

Communication Disorders Following Traumatic Brain Injury: Management of Cognitive, Language, and Motor Impairments has been written at differing levels of detail to accommodate the backgrounds and needs of personnel serving the communication and swallowing disorders of persons with TBI. This book reflects the contributions of many persons. As the editors, we wish to thank the authors who wrote chapters, willingly revised their manuscripts, and smiled most of the time. We have appreciated the support of Nancy Brown and Becky Jones for their assistance with the manuscripts. We acknowledge the support of the Barkley Memorial Trust and Grant #H133B80081 from the National Institute of Disability and Rehabilitation Research, Department of Education, Washington, D.C.

K.M.Y.
D.R.B.

I.

Service Delivery Issues

CHAPTER 1

Traumatic Brain Injury Changes the Way We Live

DAVID R. BEUKELMAN
KATHRYN M. YORKSTON

Severe traumatic brain injury (TBI) changes the way all of us live—the survivors of the injury, their families, the professionals who serve them, and the society in which we live. For the severely traumatically brain-injured individual, the change is sudden and profound. Immediately following the trauma, once healthy, active children and young adults find themselves fighting for their lives and, if they live, experiencing years of medical care, rehabilitation, and an atypical lifestyle. For the mildly injured, the initial impact of TBI may be deceiving. At times, an injury considered mild from a medical viewpoint may have long-term vocational and educational consequences.

The impact of TBI goes beyond the survivor. Parents who expect to enjoy a more independent lifestyle following the emancipation of their young adult children may face years of unanticipated financial and personal responsibility as they share in the care of a child with TBI. If the survivor has a nuclear family of his or her own, parents often see their grandparenting roles extended to a second generation of parenting. According to Jacobs most survivors of severe TBI

lived with their families, did not work or attend school, and were dependent upon others for skills, finances, and services outside the home. Due to a lack of available programs, families most frequently assumed the major responsibility for the survivor's long-term care despite no training in the area (Jacobs, 1988, p. 425).

In his survey, Jacobs (1988) questioned families about the financial impact of severe TBI. A summary of these results is presented in Table 1-1. Note that over 25 percent of the families indicated that most or all of their family resources had been used because of the TBI. Approximately 33 percent reported a mild or moderate financial drain. Another 33 percent reported no change in financial status. A small proportion indicated that their financial status had improved as the result of receiving additional services or a financial settlement following the injury.

Society at large is also affected by the epidemic of TBI. Society loses the productivity of individuals in whom considerable educational investments have been made. This loss is most obvious when a company or

Table 1-1. Impact of traumatic brain injury on family finances

Financial Impact	Percentage of Families (%)
Most (or all) family resources used	28
Moderate to mild financial drain	34
No change in financial status	34
Financial status improved	3

Source: Jacobs, H. E. (1988). The Los Angeles head injury survey: Procedures and initial findings. _Archives of Physical Medicine and Rehabilitation, 69,_ 425–431.

organization loses a valued employee or a family loses a parent and spouse. The loss is less apparent, but no less significant, when young people are injured during the school years and much of their potential is yet to be realized. Society also absorbs long-term financial commitments for rehabilitation and long-term care of those who survive. Kalsbeek and colleagues (1981) estimated both direct and indirect annual costs of head injury in the United States during 1974 to be $2.43 billion. By the time the Kalsbeek study was published in 1980, the authors estimated that inflation had already increased the figure to $3.9 billion. Their study did not include mild head trauma. As the number of traumatically brain-injured individuals continues to increase, their presence in schools, jobs, recreational facilities, and care centers will become more apparent.

When one considers the profound impact of TBI on survivors, families, and society, it is somewhat surprising that it is considered a "silent" epidemic (National Head Injury Foundation, 1983). Nonetheless, several factors may justify the use of this term. Perhaps the number of individuals experiencing TBI has not changed dramatically through the years, but certainly the number of survivors has. With advances in emergency medicine techniques, trauma units, neurosurgery, and drugs, individuals who would have died in the past are now surviving. These "heroic" efforts are documented and celebrated in the media. However, once the drama of the rescue effort is over and the accident victim has survived, the attention of society and the community turns to other news. The survivors, their families, and their closest friends begin the silent phase of TBI, the journey of recovery.

The nature and demographics of TBI make this journey of recovery long and difficult, requiring family members and professionals to assume roles that are unfamiliar to them. The mosaic of cognitive, physical, communicative, and social disabilities that can occur following TBI interact such that the single-disability intervention model is inappropriate. For example, physical rehabilitation procedures must accommodate the communication, memory, and cognitive deficits that often accompany TBI. Likewise, an augmentative communication team cannot ignore memory and cognitive deficits as they select augmentative and alternative communication options. Because TBI changes survivors as well as those who serve them, this book is prepared as a guide to clinicians in the transdisciplinary rehabilitation of individuals with TBI who have communication and swallowing disorders.

DEMOGRAPHICS OF TBI

Injuries to the head resulting in either temporary or permanent brain damage are common. However, the actual number of persons with TBI is difficult to estimate for at least two reasons. First, such injuries frequently go unreported. If individuals do not lose consciousness or if the loss is brief, they often are not admitted to the hospital or even to the emergency room. Frequently, a visit to a family physician is the extent of the medical care received. This may be followed by a few days rest and a successful or unsuccessful return to the preinjury schedule. Second, no consistent definition of injuries to the head has been used across studies. Given this definitional limitation, reviews of emergency room records reveal that the incidence of TBI is approximately 200 per 100,000 population. Of the 500,000 individuals who sustain TBI each year, approximately 100,000 die, 50,000 to 100,000 survive with severe impairments that prevent independent living, and more than 200,000 suffer continuing sequelae that interfere with daily living skills (Gualtieri, 1988; Jennett and colleagues, 1981; Kalsbeek and colleagues, 1981; Kraus, 1978; Olsen and Henig, 1983). Trauma in the United States is the third leading cause of death, behind cardiovascular disease and cancer (Turnkey, 1983). It is the leading cause of death for those under 35 years of age (Kraus and colleagues, 1984; National Head Injury Foundation, 1983).

Individuals with TBI do not represent a random sample of the total population. More than twice as many males as females are injured. The risk of TBI is also greater among children from 4 to 5 years of age, males from 15 to 24 years of age, the elderly (especially those over 75 years), and individuals who have had previous TBI.

The exact extent of disability from TBI is unknown. The National Head Injury Foundation (1983) estimates that nationwide there are 30,000 to 50,000 individuals severely disabled each year by TBI. In a recent study Jacobs (1988) surveyed the families of 142 survivors of severe TBI. During an extensive interview, these family members reported whether their survivor was independent in many different behavioral skills. A review of Table 1-2 reveals that TBI profoundly affects the survivor's ability to complete daily living tasks independently. A further review of this list reveals the extent of the daily behavioral skills that involve written or spoken communication. Reintegration of individuals with TBI into an independent lifestyle requires intervention in many areas including extensive communication instruction.

Disability following injury is not limited to those with severe TBI. The term *minor head injury* is usually defined as a loss of consciousness for less than 20 minutes, a Glasgow Coma Scale score from 13 to 15 (see Chapter 2), and no abnormality on computed tomographic scan or skull radiographs. More than two thirds of TBI cases are classified as minor. Posttraumatic symptoms occur with great variability. They may include headache, neckache, backache, dizziness, blurred or double vision, sleep disturbance, fatigue, or increased sensitivity to noise or medications. In the cognitive domain, slowing of performance, decreased motivation,

Table 1-2. Independence in discrete behavioral skills as a function of skill complexity

Reading

DISCRETE BEHAVIOR	PERCENTAGE INDEPENDENT (%)
Reads or recognizes directional signs	87.3
Reads or recognizes safety words or symbols	84.4
Reads basic instructions	66.0
Reads package directions	66.0
Reads newspaper	51.8
Reads magazines	50.4
Reads books	45.4

Writing

DISCRETE BEHAVIOR	PERCENTAGE INDEPENDENT (%)
Writes own name	85.2
Writes numerals and letters	81.0
Writes own address	76.8
Writes messages	66.9
Fills out forms	50.0
Writes checks	42.6
Writes letters	46.8
Writes paper or reports	34.5

Telling time

DISCRETE BEHAVIOR	PERCENTAGE INDEPENDENT (%)
Tells relative time	91.5
Knows difference between A.M. and P.M.	90.8
Knows that ¼ and ½ hour are 15 and 30 minutes, respectively	90.0
Tells time on the clock to the minute	88.75
Understands sequencing of events in time	76.1
Estimates the passage of time	65.2
Knows how much time to allocate for specific purposes	65.0

Concentration

DISCRETE BEHAVIOR	PERCENTAGE INDEPENDENT
Stays on task for short periods of time	83.8
Stays on task for a few minutes when not interrupted	77.5
Completes task when working in a quiet setting	66.2
Completes task when working in a noisy or "busy" environment without being distracted	42.6
Concentrates in nondistracting settings	64.3
Concentrates in noisy or distractible settings	37.9

Remembering and being oriented

DISCRETE BEHAVIOR	PERCENTAGE INDEPENDENT
Knows own name	97.9
Knows own address	85.2

Table 1-2. (continued)

Remembering and being oriented (continued)	
DISCRETE BEHAVIOR	PERCENTAGE INDEPENDENT
Knows own phone number	80.6
Knows own age	82.9
Knows day of week	72.7
Knows date (day, month, and year)	66.2
Remembers names of people frequently encountered	62.7
Remembers telephone numbers	57.5
Remembers recent events	37.9
Remembers events of past years	63.4
Knows layout of own residence	92.1
Knows neighborhood layout: locations of stores, houses, etc.	77.5
Knows directions: north, east, west, south	67.4
Can get around city without getting lost	57.0

Source: Jacobs, H. E. (1988). The Los Angeles head injury survey: Procedures and initial findings. *Archives of Physical Medicine and Rehabilitation, 69,* 425–431.

and word-finding difficulties may be present. Anxiety, depression, irritability, and mood swings are some of the most common affective complaints. There has been considerable controversy surrounding the contributions of organic and nonorganic factors in minor head injury; however, there is little doubt that these injuries can have a profound impact. Rimel, and colleagues (1981) reported that of the mildly injured individuals who are described on discharge from the hospital as being "completely normal," 59 percent continued to have memory problems. Thirty-four percent of these mildly impaired individuals who had been employed before the injury had not returned to work 3 months after the trauma.

No comparable study had been reported for children. Various authors have noted that children who sustain even mild head injuries exhibit personality changes, irritability, school learning problems, headaches, and memory and attention deficits (Boll, 1983). Problems resulting from TBI in children may become apparent years after injury, since they reflect the new demands placed on the children that require integration of the damaged systems (Rourke, 1983). Klonoff and colleagues (1977) reported that 26 percent of children with TBI who were less than 9 years of age had failed a grade or been placed in a resource class. Symptoms that commonly interfere with classroom performance include deficits in sustained attention, selective attention to a specific task, alternating attention between more than one activity, memory deficits, and executive functions such as reduced judgment and lack of insight. The incidence of children sustaining TBI is similar to that of adults, with a morbidity of

10 per 100,000 per year (Shapiro, 1983). As with adults, the lives of children are also being saved at a rate that was uncommon just a few years ago. Therefore, the school districts of America are faced with a rapidly increasing number of students with TBI.

CAUSES OF TBI

The causes of TBI are reported for several research studies in different geographic areas of the United States (Table 1-3). As is apparent from this table, motor vehicle accidents are the most common cause, with falls of various types being the second most common cause of TBI. Among school-aged students, recreational and sports injuries such as bicycling, skating, and horseback riding are common causes of TBI. Among adolescents and young adults, assaults, especially in lower socioeconomic groups, are common. A dramatic increase in TBI in the young adult age group also occurs as a result of motor vehicle accidents with the adolescent as driver or passenger. Alcohol or drugs are often involved.

The fact that a large proportion of traumatic brain injuries result from motor vehicle accidents, assaults, and sports injuries has an impact on the role of professionals who serve individuals with TBI. Frequently, individuals with TBI or their families are involved in legal activity intended to recover costs and damages resulting from the alleged negligence, willful disregard, or intent of another. At times, litigation is directed toward insurance companies, employers, individuals, public

Table 1-3 Percentage distribution of brain
injury by external cause in selected U.S. studies

Study location	External Cause (%)					
	Transport	Falls	Assaults	Sports	Firearms	Others
Olmstead County, MN	46	29	4	9	3	9
U.S. population	49	29	NR	NR	NR	22
North Central VA	55	20	9	7	2	7
San Diego County	53	27	9	—	—	11
Chicago	34[b]	24[n]	25[a,b]	9[b]	—	7[b]
Bronx, NY	31	29	33[a]	NR	—	7
San Diego County	48	21	12	10	6	4

[a]Includes firearms.
[b]Unweighted average of three communities.
NR = number of rates not reported.

funding agencies, or government agencies. In any case, professionals are often required to participate in the legal process in the form of reports, depositions, or testimony in court.

LONG-TERM IMPLICATIONS FOR SOCIETY

The decades of life expectancy predicted for children and young adults who survive the initial hours and days following TBI has both societal and personal implications. From a societal perspective, the prevalence of individuals with disability due to TBI will continue to increase for many years as the advanced medical and emergency procedures implemented in the 1970s and 1980s continue to save the lives of individuals who will be severely disabled. As time passes, individuals with TBI will become increasingly prevalent in all age groups in society. Thus, professionals who serve children, teenagers, adults, and geriatric clients will also serve individuals with TBI. As survivors of TBI age and experience other health impairments, the multiple etiologies of TBI plus heart disease, stroke, multiple sclerosis, and cancer will face the individual and the health care system.

Consider the demands placed on the service delivery system by the typical age profile of TBI survivors. Many of the young survivors of TBI have not yet established themselves as independent adults. Therefore, they are required to attempt many of life's major transitions after their injury. Depending on the extent of their disability, they will attempt to finish school, establish family relationships, live independently, and seek employment. Some will be successful, and some will not. In either case, support systems and personnel to manage these programs will be required in increasing numbers during the next decades unless societal or medical influences change the incidence of TBI.

LONG-TERM IMPLICATIONS FOR FAMILIES

ACCEPTANCE OF CHANGING EXPECTATIONS

The survivors of brain injury and their families face a series of challenges. Not the least of these challenges is changing one's expectations about the future. The unexpectedness of TBI occurring at a young age often has a profound impact on one's expectations. Almost without exception, before these injuries these individuals had expected to live a typical lifestyle. Following their injury, many survivors and their families struggle with those unfulfilled expectations. Many of these individuals must gradually reshape their expectations, and some must do so in the presence of the memory, communication, physical, and cognitive problems that result from TBI.

ACQUIRING INFORMATION

A second fundamental challenge to the families of survivors of TBI involves a process of self-instruction and information gathering. Depending on the particular medical service delivery system, the educational process can be a slow and frustrating one. Beth O'Brian describes her need for information as she sought to survive the consequences of an event that threw her life into chaos, the severe traumatic injury of her 14-year-old son.

My usual strategy for dealing with big problems is to fill my head with information. . . . The first hospital had taught me nothing about brain damage; and the books that I found in the local library were of little help. During those long months of acute care, when I wondered if John would ever wake up, I wanted to learn about head injury: What happened to my son's brain? What would he be like? What happens to families in this situation? How do they cope? (O'Brian, 1987, p. 423).

The process of family education can either be helped or hindered by the professional team. There are many ways for the professional team to fail in its educational task. Family reports are filled with examples of such failures. Perhaps the most obvious educational failure is to give no information. O'Brian describes the initial phase of her education

And the neurosurgeon made no attempt to begin my education. Six months later, another hospital physician told us, "What you see is what you get. When are you taking John home?" (O'Brian, 1987, p. 423).

Another common failure in family education is lack of appreciation of the level of knowledge that the family possesses. At times our presentation to a family assumes a level of sophistication that is simply not yet present. In short, we give the family too much information. O'Brian described her initial meeting with the rehabilitation team in the following excerpt

It was very hard for me to admit that I did not understand what I was being told. The first formal meeting with the staff of the center was a nightmare. It was brutally demoralizing to face a set of professionals who had very important information and not be able even to understand their titles, much less their jargon. "Physical therapy" and "speech therapy" made some sense to me, but what did "occupational therapy" mean? Wasn't it a bit early to be thinking about occupations? And what was "cognitive rehabilitation therapy"? And aphasia?

Apraxia? Agnosia? When they first mentioned John's "premorbid" characteristics I thought maybe they were predicting his death?" (O'Brian, 1987, p. 424).

She goes on to suggest that simple written information is mandatory. This information can be

digested piecemeal, shared with friends, and returned to when a new stage of acceptance makes possible a deeper processing of the information (O'Brian, 1987, p. 424).

Another educational dilemma faced by the medical team may be viewed as a lack of sufficient information regarding the natural course of recovery following TBI. We simply are unable to answer with any degree of certainty some of the families' most pressing questions regarding what the future will bring. Because we do not know, most medical professionals tend to be conservative. Family after family has recounted for us the stories of medical personnel who strongly suggest shortly after the injury that the person with TBI would not survive, but he or she did. Families are often told that their survivors will not regain consciousness, but they do. Families are told that they should expect little recovery, and then the family observes change that occurs slowly but steadily over the years. It is little wonder that the families become skeptical about the knowledge and commitment of professionals who serve their family members. We are learning that recovery from TBI is very different than recovery from stroke. We are learning that recovery from TBI for a young person is different than recovery in an older adult. We are observing long-term recovery patterns in a wide variety of areas. For example, we will report in this book that some TBI survivors begin to speak functionally 3 or 9 or 13 years following their injuries. Clearly, the expectations of the survivors of TBI must be changed in response to the severity of their disability. However, the expectations of personnel who serve them through the years must also change, if the survivors of TBI are to be served effectively, as they slowly continue to improve through the years.

MAINTAINING HOPE

The final long-term challenge described by families of individuals with TBI is one of maintaining hope. The following is a comment made by a mother six years after her son's TBI. At the time these comments were written her son was just beginning to establish an independent lifestyle with the help of a transitional living facility. Again, families who have experienced recovery following TBI say it best

Perhaps they didn't consider John a candidate for rehabilitation: he could not walk, talk, dress, or eat with any semblance of independence. But we had hope. Thank God we had hope! Suppose we had given up? (O'Brian, 1987, p. 422).

The task of the rehabilitation team when attempting to educate families is not an easy one. Families need information that is clear, accurate, and consistent with their current level of understanding and acceptance. They need information presented in such a way that it does not decrease their ability to deal with the realities of today or reduce their ability to plan optimistically for the future.

DEALING WITH SOCIAL ISOLATION

Psychological problems are often cited as one of the most disabling aspects of TBI. Thomsen (1974) reported perhaps the longest group outcome data on TBI survivors with severe disabilities. Forty patients were studied 2.5 years post-trauma and again 10 to 15 years post-trauma. Her findings are informative on a number of issues. First, physical impairment, dysarthria, and persistent memory problems were not the most substantial deterrents to reentering a normal lifestyle. Although these problems were certainly important and deserved continued rehabilitative attention, the problems that seem to be most devastating to the individual's ultimate psychosocial adjustment centered around personality disturbances. Again, not unexpectedly, Thomsen reported that from the patients' point of view, the single biggest problem 10 to 15 years following TBI is that of social isolation.

Reports of social isolation are also common in family reports:

The most difficult part of John's injury for both of us has been his terrible loneliness. He yearns for the companionship of other young people, for the activities that are important for anyone his age. If you have any doubts that your work to promote active community re-entry for head injured young people is of value, put them to rest. You help to give meaning to their lives. (O'Brian, 1987, p. 425).

IMPLICATIONS FOR PROFESSIONALS

The communication problems of individuals with TBI have caused clinicians specializing in communication and swallowing disorders to change the scope, pattern, and focus of service delivery. Although the number of individuals with communication and swallowing disorders following TBI have not yet been documented from a demographic perspective, the evidence is clear that among individuals with moderate and severe TBI, these disabilities are common and, in some individuals, persist for many years following the injury. The remediation of the communication problems associated with traumatically brain-injured individuals began in earnest in the United States following World War II. The efforts in military and veterans' hospitals were initially focused on soldiers with head trauma due to penetrating injuries and later on elderly individuals following stroke or neurologic disease. The intervention strategies that were developed during these years tended to focus on the specific modality of communication disorder. Consequently, intervention approaches in aphasia, apraxia of speech, and dysarthria were developed.

The diffuse neurologic deficits associated with the closed head injury are quite different than those observed with the more focal lesions associated with penetrating wounds or cardiovascular or neurologic disease. Usually, the communication disorders of individuals with TBI occur concomitant with cognitive deficits including attention, memory, judgment, and emotional control. These cognitive impairments tend to exaggerate the specific communication problems, at least in part, because they rob the individual of the ability to compensate for decreased communicative abilities. Thus the pervasive cognitive deficits affect nearly every area of rehabilitation. At times, the specific communication problems demonstrated by a TBI survivor are rather mild, yet the pragmatic problems in communication use that result from the cognitive deficits consitute a major communication disability that interferes with successful educational and social performance.

The growing TBI population has changed the nature and scope of the services delivered by speech and language pathologists. Augmentative and alternative communication options are provided in intensive care units and on a long-term basis if severe communication problems persist. The restoration of appropriate communicative interaction, natural speech, and literacy requires extensive rehabilitation attention for some TBI survivors. As the TBI survivors leave the acute rehabilitation phase of recovery and enter the community reintegration phase, their communication demands can change dramatically as they interact with the uninformed and at times unsympathetic public or as they engage in independent living, education, vocational training, or employment. The breadth of communication-related intervention services is extensive, and the commitment to the TBI survivor is long term.

REFERENCES

Boll, T. (1983). Minor head injury in children—out of sight but not out of mind. *Journal of Clinical Child Psychology, 12,* 74–80.

Gualtieri, C. (1988). Pharmacotherapy and the neurobehavioral sequelae of traumatic brain injury. *Brain Injury, 2,* 101–129.

Jacobs, H. E. (1988). The Los Angeles head injury survey: Procedures and initial findings. *Archives of Physical Medicine and Rehabilitation, 69,* 425–431.

Jennett, B., Snoek, J., Bond, M., and Brooks, N. (1981). Disability after severe head injury: Observations on use of Glasgow Outcome Scale. *Journal of Neurology, Neurosurgery, and Psychiatry, 44,* 285–293.

Kalsbeek, W., McLauren, R., Harris, B., and Miller, J. (1981). The national head and spinal cord injury survey: Major findings. *Journal of Neurosurgery, 53,* S19–S31.

Klonoff, H., Low, M., and Clark, C. (1977). Head injuries in children: A prospective five year follow-up. *Journal of Neurology, Neurosurgery, and Psychiatry, 40,* 1211–1219.

Kraus, J. (1978). Epidemiologic features of head and spinal cord injury. *Advances in Neurology, 19,* 261–279.

Kraus, J., Black, M., Hessol, N., Ley, P., Rokaw, W., Sullivan, C., Bowers, S., Knowlton, S., and Marshall, L. (1984). Incidence of acute brain injury and serious impairment in defined populations. *American Journal of Epidemiology, 119,* 185–201.

National Head Injury Foundation. (1983). *The silent epidemic.* Farmingham, MA.

O'Brian, B. (1987). A letter to professionals who work with head injured people. In M. Ylvisaker and E. M. Gobble (Eds.), *Community re-entry for head injured adults* (pp. 421–430). Boston: College-Hill Press.

Olsen, D., and Henig, E. (1983). *A manual of behavioral management strategies for traumatically brain injured adults.* Chicago: Rehabilitation Institute of Chicago.

Rimel, R., Giodordani, M, Barth, J, Boll, T. and Jane, J. (1981). Disability caused by head injury. *Neurosurgery, 9,* 221–228.

Rourke, B. (1983). Reading spelling disabilities. A developmental neuropsychological perspective. In U. Kirk (Ed.), *Neuropsychology of language, reading and spelling.* New York: Academic Press.

Shapiro, K. (1983). *Pediatric head trauma.* Mount Kisco, NY: Futura Publishing Co.

Thomsen, I. (1974). Patient with severe head injury and his family: Follow-up study of 50 patients. *Scandinavian Journal of Rehabilitation, 6,* 180–183.

Turnkey, D. (1983). Trauma. *Scientific American, 249,* 28–35.

CHAPTER 2

REHABILITATION OF PERSONS WITH TRAUMATIC BRAIN INJURY: A CONTINUUM OF CARE

MARVIN BROOKE
JAY M. UOMOTO
ALVIN MCLEAN, Jr.
ROBERT T. FRASER

By almost any standards traumatic brain injury (TBI) can be considered an epidemic. The National Head Injury Foundation refers to it as the "silent epidemic." So it must seem to families of traumatically brain-injured patients who suddenly may be faced with life-altering decisions related to the best course of action for their loved one. Until recently their voices were not heard. The term *preventable epidemic* can also be applied to the problem. Epidemiologists who study causes and control of the problem suggest that many of the causes of TBI are preventable—motor vehicle accidents, drunk-driving accident, assaults, and gunshot wounds. Unfortunately, one can only speculate how much anguish could have been prevented by such solutions as strictly enforced drunk-driving laws; regulation of the use of seat belts, air bags, and motorcycle helmets; and gun control. Webster's *New World Dictionary* has another definition of epidemic, "the rapid, widespread occurrence of a fad or fashion." In this sense TBI can also be considered an epidemic. Only time will tell whether the explosion of new therapies, organization of services, and consumer awareness will be considered a beneficial aspect of this epidemic. In short, the problems we face offer the medical service delivery community a unique series of challenges. Not the least of these challenges is to organize and understand the explosions of information related to the management of the traumatically brain-injured patient. The goal of this chapter is to provide an organizational framework for understanding the medical and service delivery aspects of TBI.

MEDICAL ASPECTS OF TBI

TERMINOLOGY

Consistent and precise use of terminology is critical in communication among the many health care professionals who help to manage the medical, communication, and psychosocial needs of patients following TBI. The following section provides definitions and critical distinctions among the many terms associated with TBI.

Brain Damage

Perhaps the most general term to describe any brain injury is *brain damage*. Brain damage refers to any type of damage to the brain from an cause and at any age. It is often used to describe conditions as different as cerebral palsy, Alzheimer's disease, cerebral vascular accidents, encephalitis, or toxic injuries to the brain such as those caused by alcohol.

Because the term is such a general one, it carries little information related to such important factors as localization of the lesion, age of onset, natural course, and general prognosis.

Traumatic Brain Injury

Throughout this text, the term *traumatic brain injury* will be used to describe the injury to the brain caused primarily by physical trauma. The term *traumatic head injury* has also been used to describe this population, but this term is a broad one that also includes soft tissue injuries and lacerations, which may not be accompanied by brain damage.

Closed Head Injury

The term *closed head injury* refers to one of the most common types of TBI. The term implies that the trauma did not cause an opening in the skull. Injuries associated with closed head injuries are most commonly caused when the head suffers a sudden acceleration or deceleration, such as against the dashboard of a car. Therefore, they are at times referred to as acceleration-deceleration injuries. They may also be called diffuse axonal injuries because they result in diffuse shearing of axons with their myelin sheaths in the brain. Axonal shearing is felt to be a major cause of unconsciousness in these patients.

Open Head or Penetrating Injuries

When the trauma results in a penetration, as in a gunshot wound or a fracturing of the skull, injuries are referred to as open head or penetrating injures. Such injuries may produce focal lesions rather than the diffuse damage associated with closed head injury. Systematic studies of the consequences of such injuries in the wartime population have been reported (Luria, 1964).

Coma

Coma is not a disease but the product of damage to or depression of the function of the central nervous system (CNS). In TBI, coma may be due to neuronal or axonal injury, hypoxemia, or ischemia. A fully conscious patient is awake and normally aware of both internal and external stimuli. Precise definition of coma is difficult. Typically, the depth of coma is assessed using the Glasgow Coma Scale (Teasdale and Jennett, 1974) (see Table 2-1). A review of the table suggests that scores can range from 3 (with the patients receiving a score of 1 on "eyes open," "best motor response," and "verbal response.") to 15. When the score rises to 9 or more, the person is considered to be out of coma.

Posttraumatic Amnesia

Posttraumatic amnesia is defined as the period following injury when the patient does not have continuous memory of daily events (Russell, 1932; Jennett and Teasdale, 1981). The duration of posttraumatic amnesia is estimated by asking the patient about his or her first and subsequent memories after the injury. It has been suggested that posttraumatic amnesia is a better predictor of outcome than measures such as the duration of coma (Klove and Cleeland, 1972; Russell, 1971).

EARLY MEDICAL INTERVENTION

Emergency Medical Service

The ideal emergency system would provide a prompt and sophisticated level of care at the scene of the injury. This is extremely important because studies show an inverse relationship between resuscitation latency and level of brain dysfunction. Trauma centers have emerged as an important component of medical service delivery to individuals with TBI (Miller and Jones, 1985). The most specialized of these trauma centers have the following components: trauma service, cardiopulmonary surgery, general surgery, neurologic surgery, ophthalmic surgery, orthopedic surgery, ortorhinolaryngologic surgery, pediatric surgery, plastic and maxillofacial surgery, and urologic surgery. Twenty-four-hour-a-day availability is required for both general and neurologic surgery. From the trauma center, patients may be placed in special intensive care units for neurosurgical patients or in the neurosurgery ward where the rehabilitation services will follow the patient from the acute emergent situation until he or she is discharged to either the acute rehabilitation unit or, where appropriate, to the outpatient rehabilitation program. Patients who stay in coma will be referred to a coma center.

Goals of Early Medical Intervention

Stabilization of Medical Condition. The first goal of early medical management is to stabilize the patient. This effort should begin immediately in the field. The patient is first given an adequate airway and ventilation with supplementary oxygen, since many patients are hypoxic when they get to the emergency room. Adequate oxygenation will prevent hypoxic brain damage, and ventilating off the carbon dioxide will prevent its retention, which leads to higher intercranial pressure. The patient's blood pressure is maintained by controlling bleeding and administering fluids as needed. Since TBI injured patients often have cervical spine injuries, they are treated as such with the spine immobilized on a board. The

Table 2-1. Glasgow coma scale

Response	Examiner's test	Patient response	Score
Eye opening	Spontaneous	Opens eyes on own	4
	Speech	Opens eyes when asked in a loud voice	3
	Pain	Opens eyes when pinched	2
	Pain	Does not open eyes	1
Best motor response	Commands	Follow simple commands	6
	Pain	Pulls examiner's hands away when pinched	5
	Pain	Pulls a part of the body away when pinched	4
	Pain	Flexes body inappropriately when pinched (decorticate posturing)	3
	Pain	Body becomes rigid in an extended position when pinched (decerebrate posturing)	2
	Pain	Has no motor response to pinch	1
Verbal response	Speech	Carries on a conversation correctly and tells examiner where he or she is, who he or she is, month and year	5
	Speech	Seems confused or disoriented	4
	Speech	Talks so examiner can understand but makes no sense	3
	Speech	Makes sounds that examiner cannot understand	2
	Speech	Makes no noise	1

Source: Teasdale, G., and Jennett, B. (1974). Assessment of coma and impaired consciousness. *Lancet, 2,* 81.

patient is evaluated with the Glasgow Coma Scale for level of consciousness and an examination for localizing neurologic findings.

Identification of Treatable Conditions. Once the patient is stabilized, aggressive evaluation and treatment of neurosurgical and other problems is begun immediately. Examination and computed tomography (CT) scan are used to find hematomas that may need to be evacuated, bone or other fragments that may need to be removed from the brain, and hydrocephalus or severe edema that may need to be treated surgically. Patients' ventilatory, fluid, and medication interventions are adjusted to decrease intercranial pressure, which is monitored with a Richmond bolt and repeated examinations. Patients are usually begun on prophylactic phenytoin (Dilantin) to prevent seizures. Seizures are more common in patients with depressed fractures, penetration of the dural membrane, and hemorrhage or other irritations inside the brain itself. There is no test to predict who will develop seizures. If a patient's mental status decreases, localizing neurologic signs appear, or a patient's recovery plateaus unexpectedly, the patient is reevaluated for complications such as hematoma, hydrocephalus, or seizures.

Prevention of Secondary Complications. Another important goal of early medical management is to prevent further complicating conditions. These complications will consume time and money and decrease the functional outcome if not prevented. Often the rehabilitation team has the most experience in using medications for spasticity, heterotopic ossification, and agitation as well as in providing behavioral and other approaches to these problems. The importance of minimizing the sedative effects of medication and the destructive effects of behavioral problems is obvious. We have already discussed the importance of maintaining adequate ventilation and blood pressure to prevent additional secondary brain damage caused by their failure.

Ischemic damage can be caused not only by low arterial blood pressure due to blood loss or volume depletion but also by increased intracranial pressure. If the intracranial pressure is too high, the arterial blood pressure will not be able to overcome it and perfuse areas of the brain. There also is a risk after TBI of arterial vasospasm, which causes local ischemia when the local arteriole goes into spasm. Brain injury can interrupt the sophisticated autoregulation of local blood flow that normally directs the proper amount of blood to different areas of the brain. This can cause additional problems with perfusion. If the intracranial pressure becomes too high, this will cause additional brain damage by decreasing perfusion to areas of the brain or by direct compression of brain tissues. This can be treated by hyperventilation, fluid restriction, osmotic agents that increase the bloodstream's osmotic pressure and pull off fluid from the brain, and medications that decrease the brain's inflammation and metabolic activity. If the problem is severe enough, surgery is indicated to remove a bone flap and allow more room for the brain to expand.

Several different types of hematomas may need to be removed to decrease the diffuse intracranial pressure and the local compression they are causing. If an open head injury has occurred with penetrating bone fragments or other tissues, this will no doubt need to be removed and bleeding controlled. An epidural hematoma with high pressure arterial-blood forming above the dural membrane can lead to very rapid expansion and death. This emergency is treated by craniotomy with control of the bleeding and the removal of any large clots. Subdural hematomas with lower pressure blood underneath the dural membrane may be slower but are also life threatening and are removed unless they are very small and chronic. Intracranial hemorrhage into the substance of the brain as well as severe contusions or bruising vary depending on their size, location, and changes. They should be treated surgically if severe or progressive. Patients are monitored for changes, since these hematomas may occur after weeks or months even if not present on admission.

Occasionally, patients develop acute hydrocephalus. This increase in pressure in the ventricles, due to obstruction of the flow of cerebral spinal fluid, may be caused by blood obstructing this flow. Patients occasionally require the placement of an emergency shunt if this is causing their decline in function. Patients also may have seizures that must be controlled to prevent secondary damage from increased metabolic activity of the brain or physical exertion. Most patients are given prophylactic medication to decrease the chance of seizures; if this is not successful, the dosage may need to be increased. Finally, patients are given appropriate nutritional and nursing care to prevent the secondary complications of malnutrition including skin breakdown and contractures. The rehabilitation team can be of great assistance by monitoring for some of these problems and advocating for their control so that complications do not slow recovery later. Prevention of other secondary complications will be described later.

Pathophysiology

There has been a rapid advance in knowledge, not only about early medical intervention but also about the pathophysiology of TBI. We will first look at primary mechanisms of injury. These are mechanisms by which trauma directly causes damage to the brain. We will later look at secondary mechanisms of injury. These are mechanisms such as pressure exerted by a blood clot that are secondary to something such as a blood clot caused by the trauma. These different mechanisms not only have a different prognosis and treatment, but they also give different general patterns of abnormality after the injury.

Primary Mechanisms of Injury. Primary mechanisms of injury are listed below.

1. *Diffuse axonal shearing.* A closed head injury caused by sudden acceleration or deceleration results in diffuse shearing of axons within their myelin sheath in the brain. The axon is the long, vulnerable, thin extension of the nerve cell that goes through the brain and communicates with other nerve cells. The axon is therefore essential to transmitting information and maintaining the level of consciousness. Diffuse axonal injury causes the patient to be unconscious. If the brain is examined microscopically, small lesions are

seen with retraction bulb formation of axons, which have been damaged by shearing forces and retracted back into a bulb shape where the end was broken. Also, microglial clusters are seen where the surrounding tissues of the brain are abnormally clustered together. These are seen in the cortex or surface of the brain first, the diencephalon, where much sensory input is communicated up into the brain, and in the brainstem, where structures maintain alertness and control vital functions such as respiration. In addition to the loss of consciousness, it is easy to see how this type of injury will cause diffuse impairment of cognitive function.

2. *Focal contusions.* Focal contusions are localized areas of bruising with an increase in blood and fluid similar to a bruise on one's arm or leg. There is a continuum of this type of damage due to direct force on the cerebral matter and vascular injury to the smallest blood vessels. The mildest injury would cause edema, or fluid without blood, to collect. Next would be a contusion or bruise, with blood, fluid, and the accompanying swelling. If there is almost pure blood in the damaged area, this would be called a hemorrhage or hematoma, meaning bleed or blood clot with the more severe local damage one would expect. The focal contusions most commonly occur in those exposed lobes of the brain that bounce against the bones surrounding the anterior and middle cranial fossae, and therefore they are most commonly seen in the inferior frontal and temporal cortex bilaterally in an asymmetric pattern. The corpus callosum, which connects the left and right cerebral cortex; the cerebral peduncles, which connect the cerebral cortex with lower structures; and the cerebellar peduncles, which connect the balance and coordination controlling cerebellum with lower structures are all areas of concentrated axons lying next to strong tentorial membranes of the brain. They therefore have an increased frequency of damage when these concentrated axon structures bounce against fixed membranes. The cranial nerves VI, II, VIII, and I are also often damaged because of their exposed positions. The previous habit of ascribing bilateral deficits to "coup" and "contracoup" lesions was felt to explain bilateral deficits on the basis of the brain's bouncing against the skull at the site of a blow, "coup," and the opposite side of the brain, "contracoup," when it bounces back against the skull. Bilateral damage is now known to be due mainly to diffuse axonal shearing and multiple cerebral contusions (Jennett, 1986). The focal contusions will cause more specific localized deficits if they involve one of the structures of the brain that carries out a specific function. They are managed by the same interventions to control intracranial pressure and edema with a more careful observation for progression into frank hemorrhage or hematoma.

Secondary Mechanisms of Injury. Secondary mechanisms of injury are listed below.

1. *Edema.* As indicated above, edema means swelling or increased extracellular fluid in the brain tissues. The danger is that it not only will disrupt local brain activity, but more important, it has no place to expand within the enclosed cranial vault and therefore causes an increase in intracranial pressure. This increased edema and pressure can gradually worsen over hours and days after an injury and lead to a very dangerous decline in consciousness and vital functions. Edema causes local damage to brain tissue and, more important, causes diffuse pressure and disruption of normal physiologic functions throughout the brain. It is treated by a series of interventions that decrease cerebral pressure, such as (a) hyperventilation of the patient to blow off carbon dioxide and cause the cerebral blood vessels to contract slightly, (b) fluid restriction or increase in osmotic pressure to draw fluid off the brain, (c) decreasing the metabolic activity of the brain by controlling seizures and adding sedatives, and (d) if necessary, surgical removal of part of the skull and, if severe enough, the brain tissue itself to allow room for expansion.

2. *Hypoxia.* Hypoxia occurs when an abnormally low amount of oxygen is supplied to the brain tissues. This, as indicated earlier, can occur not only because of decreased respiration in the field immediately after an emergency, but also due to later problems with inadequate ventilation, loss of blood or blood pressure, and disruption of the blood supply to the brain by increased intracranial pressure or disregulation of local blood flow. Anoxic damage occurs most commonly in the hippocampus, which is essential for memory; the basal ganglia, which may result in movement disorders; and in the watershed areas of the cerebral cortex and the cerebellum. The watershed areas are areas at the extreme end of arterial blood supply areas and therefore are the first to suffer damage when oxygen supplies are inadequate. This type of injury occurs not only after cardiac arrest but also after an initial primary closed head injury where shock or airway obstruction interferes with oxygenation. A deceleration injury itself may cause bradycardia and hypotension immediately due to brain injury, and brain injury commonly leads to hypoventilation because the brain is not adequately controlling respiration. Hypoxia and ischemia (inadequate perfusion of an area) are two common problems that are correctable in the early emergency service. It is not uncommon for these secondary problems to be overlooked in medical summaries. It is important to look for documentation, such as low blood pressure or low oxygen level,

in the emergency room. The prognosis is worse after a brain injury with less improvement and often severe memory deficits.

3. *Disruption of cerebral blood flow regulation.* The brain has a very delicate and complicated mechanism to provide adequate blood pressure perfusion and oxygen supply to different areas as their metabolic activity changes and the level of pressure and oxygen in the blood itself changes due to factors outside the brain. This mechanism can be disrupted by TBI. Not only can damage to the brain and blood vessels directly interrupt their ability to regulate themselves, but increased intracranial pressure can also overwhelm this regulatory mechanism. Finally, blood vessels may go into vasospasm or dilate inappropriately due to local damage and other mechanisms that we do not fully understand. This may result in a worsened condition and may also cause more local damage to one lobe of the brain supplied by a malfunctioning blood vessel. In addition to the mechanisms to decrease damage to the brain mentioned above, disruption of cerebral blood flow regulation can be treated by certain medications and by allowing the brain to rest before putting metabolic or surgical stress on it.

Assessment Procedures and Techniques

Speech and language pathologists who provide services to the acutely brain-injured patient may see references in the medical charts to a number of procedures and techniques. The following is a brief description of some procedures common in early medical management of TBI.

Richmond Bolt. A Richmond bolt is a devise placed through a hole in the skull allowing a pressure transducer to measure intracranial pressure. It is used early in management of a comatose patient to guide medical and surgical therapy aimed at keeping the intracranial pressure in the normal range. Pressures that are high and remain elevated for a long time are not only a poor prognostic sign but also tell the neurosurgeon that more aggressive intervention is needed.

Computed Tomography Scan. A CT scan is a computed tomography x-ray image of the body constructed by a computer from multiple x-ray readings to produce tomograms that appear like slices through the brain. This allows the neurosurgeon to detect hemotomas, hemorrhages, edema, bone fragments, and abnormal shifts of the brain tissue itself. It is most commonly used on admission to look for correctable causes of coma or localized neurologic deficits. If there are not localized abnormalities after TBI, it is likely the loss of consciousness is due to the diffuse axonal injury resulting from acceleration and deceleration forces sustained at injury. It is often helpful to correlate the location of abnormalities, when present, with observed or expected functional abnormalities, such as language deficits correlated with left temporoparietal hemotomas. A CT scan may be obtained later to look for hydrocephalus because increased pressure within the ventricles may enlarge them. Localized atrophy may appear on later scans as the damaged brain tissue shrinks.

Nuclear Magnetic Resonance. Nuclear magnetic resonance (NMR) images are a different type of scan produced by a computer reconstructing images from the magnetic properties of tissues after a strong magnetic field is applied. This procedure is not as useful as others in the emergency room because metal and life-support equipment cannot be near the magnetic field. The procedure is not as readily available as CT scans. However, NMR images provide a finer resolution image than CT scan and may, for example, show smaller lesions in the brainstem that would not be visible on CT scan. They may also be useful later to show small areas of bleeding and correlate image abnormalities with functional deficits.

Positron Emission Tomography. A positron emission tomography (PET) scan allows us to see metabolic activity of the brain after appropriately labeled substances such as glucose are injected. Positrons are given off in metabolically active areas, and a scan is reconstructed from this source. Currently, PET scans are the best way to look at metabolic activity that may be decreased in an area after brain injury but is not visible as a structural lesion on a CT or NMR scan. At this time, PET scans are difficult to do and expensive, and they are thus most commonly used as a research tool.

Cranial Nerve Examination. In the cranial nerve examination, a physician assesses the function of the various cranial nerves. The most useful ones in examination of a traumatically brain-injured patient include the optic nerve (cranial nerve II), the three brainstem cranial nerves that control eye movements (III, IV, and VI), facial motor (VII), tongue and pharynx (IX, X and XII), and auditory and vestibular (VIII). These are tested to see if the brain damage involves the vital brainstem functions and if edema or trauma interferes with these functionally important nerves.

Cortical Evoked Potentials. Cortical evoked potentials are measured in several ways (Rappaport and colleagues, 1977). Somatosensory evoked potentials are obtained by stimulated peripheral nerves in the arms and legs while recording electrical brainwave responses over the scalp. Visual evoked potentials are obtained by stimulating the eyes with a changing visual pattern, and auditory evoked potentials are obtained by stimulating the ears with auditory signals. The waveforms that are recorded are compared with normal values and give some information about the location and extent of neurologic damage. If a certain part of the waveform is missing, for example, this may indicate an abnormality in the brainstem as opposed to higher or lower neurologic structures. The values of these potentials in making prognostic statements regarding traumatically brain-injured patients remains an area of controversy. They are most useful for group research studies and for confirming localized neurologic damage to one of the structures being stimulated or its pathway up to the brain.

Neural Transmitter Levels in the Cerebrospinal Fluid. Obtaining neural transmitter levels in the cerebrospinal fluid and use of substrates are new ways of assessing the type and extent of neurologic damage. Cerebrospinal fluid may be evaluated by seeing if the level of epinephrin is abnormally high. At this time these studies are not used clinically but may become more useful for prognosis or localization of the structures damaged.

The Galveston Orientation and Amnesia Test. The Galveston Orientation and Amnesia Test (GOAT) is a standardized test of the patient's orientation and memory function (Levin and colleagues, 1979). The patient is asked questions about orientation such as the date, and about memory, with a score derived from the number of correct responses. This is used to measure the patient's progress and, in particular, the time it takes the patient to regain memory function. The period of posttraumatic amnesia, where the patient does not remember day-to-day events after he or she has come out of coma, is a useful prognostic indicator like the length of coma. It is also useful in planning rehabilitation therapies.

REHABILITATION

PREDICTORS OF OUTCOMES

The Disability Rating Scale

The Disability Rating Scale (Rappaport and colleagues, 1982) is one way of measuring clinical outcome in eight categories of potential disability, each of which is given a numerical value. Under the category of psychosocial adaptability, for example, employable is scored and under cognitive ability for self-care, feeding and toileting are scored. This scale is still being validated in the literature, but it is one useful way to measure level of disability before and after rehabilitation.

The Glasgow Outcome Scale

The Glasgow Outcome Scale (Jennett and Bond, 1975) is a five-point outcome scale. The best outcome is good recovery, meaning the resumption of normal life; the next lower level is moderate disability, meaning the patient is disabled but independent; the next is severe disability, meaning the patient is conscious but disabled and dependent; the next is a persistent vegetative state, meaning the patient is unresponsive and speechless but has some wakefulness or eye opening. The lowest outcome on this scale is death. The scale has obvious discrete points but is limited by the lack of sensitivity to minor changes and rehabilitation effects.

Sickness Impact Profile

The Sickness Impact Profile (*Bergner, and colleagues, 1981*) is a sensitive measure of the impact of any illness on daily activities. The frequency of going shopping, for example, may be decreased in very high level patients. This scale is useful in measuring the functional impact in the real world and in measuring small changes likely to be of value to a patient's function. It is comprehensive and frequently used for research but not for planning rehabilitation care.

The Katz Adjustment Scale

The Katz Adjustment Scale (*Katz and Lyerly, 1963*) measures 205 items of patient behavior and adjustment, each on a four-point scale period. It gives an observer assessment of social, expected performance, and symptom changes produced by illness. It is sometimes supplemented by the Social Adjustment Scale to measure the patient's perception of family and economic relationship. This is one way to measure the impact on the family of a severe illness or the effect of rehabilitation.

PREVENTING SECONDARY COMPLICATIONS

As in the acute medical phase of management of the traumatically brain-injured patient, a number of secondary complications can occur late in the course of the disorder. The following is a brief review of some these secondary complications and their medical management.

1. *Contractures* are decreases in joint range of motion produced by shortening and other changes in muscles, tendons, and ligaments.
2. *Skin breakdowns* are caused by prolonged pressure unrelieved by turning the patient off bony prominences.

3. *Environmentally induced psychosis* is a psychiatric abnormality caused by abnormal environmental stimuli and made worse by cognitive impairment, medication, sleep deprivation, and painful or absent sensory stimulation. It is sometimes called intensive care unit psychosis and may be prevented by avoiding abnormal or decreased sensory stimulation, excessive medication, and sleep deprivation and by attempting to give the patient as much normal orientation and sensory stimulation as possible. Medications may be needed for the symptoms of hallucinations and delusions.

4. *Seizures* are abnormal, repetitive discharges of cortical brain cells causing the familiar tonic-clonic jerking extremity movements, loss of consciousness, and incontinenace brought on by many types of brain damage.

5. *Malnutrition* is often seen after TBI and is due not only to decreased food intake but also to an increased metabolic activity from the brain injury itself.

6. *Agitation* is a frequent complication of TBI and may be very distressing to patient, family, and staff. Many patients become agitated briefly as they come out of their coma and are confused and irritated. For some, agitation persists and interferes with the rehabilitation process.

7. *Heterotopic bone formation* or ossification is the abnormal formation of bone in soft tissues. This is not completely understood but does occur after TBI and is probably caused by the immobilization and small amounts of trauma around joints.

8. *Medication-induced decreases in cognitive function* are common. Patients with brain injuries are more sensitive to medication-induced problems and often are being treated with seizure medications or tranquilizers.

9. *Complications of prolonged intubation* include damage to the vocal cords or nerves controlling phonation from prolonged pressure of an endotracheal tube. This can be prevented by taking the tube out of the inside of the trachea and performing a tracheostomy so that the tube enters the trachea from the front of the neck, avoiding damage to the vocal cords and nerves that supply them. An otolaryngologist can assist by visualizing the vocal cords and adjusting tube type, location, and pressure. An injection to the vocal cords or another surgical procedure may be considered if symptoms do not resolve spontaneously.

VISUOSPATIAL PERCEPTION IMPAIRMENT

Visuospatial disorders are less commonly reported in TBI than other neurobehavioral disorders (Whyte and Rosenthal, 1988). There may be several reasons for this pattern. First, Whyte and Rosenthal suggest that the posterior areas of the brain are less often damaged in TBI than are the frontal or temporal areas. Second, Brain (1941) reports that persons with visual deficits often demonstrate a limited awareness of their disorder. Finally, because of the interaction between visually mediated activities and deficits in attention, problem solving, and poor manual dexterity, the presence of problems in visuospatial perception may be masked by other cognitive deficits.

The frequency and nature of visual problems associated with TBI have not been systematically studied and reported. However, there are patient reports of double vision, blurry vision, hypersensitivity to light, and difficulty judging distance. Formal testing often suggests visuo-spatial confusion, slow visual-motor integration, or unilateral neglect (Sohlberg and Mateer, 1989). Anecdotally, a number of cases of cortical blindness have been observed following TBI. Over the course of acute recovery many patients experience some resolution of their visuospatial problems.

MANAGEMENT OF PHYSICAL IMPAIRMENT

Physical impairments are very frequent after TBI. Patients not only have motor problems from their brain injury but also from associated periph-eral trauma. It is very important to address these problems, since they may significantly complicate rehabilitation of other disabilities, such as communication, and often compound the amount of disability. Despite the fact that physical impairments are not as disabling in terms of out-come measured by employability or independent living, they are a sig-nificant factor in planning rehabilitation. It is encouraging to realize that physical impairments can be addressed with multiple different types of therapy and may respond better to therapy than cognitive deficits.

Type of Motor Impairment

Bradykinesia. Some types of motor impairment are more common after TBI than others. Perhaps the most common, although subtle, defi-cit is impairment in speed of movement. Severe decreases in the speed are termed bradykinesia, but many patients have subtle abnormalities that are not immediately obvious. These abnormalities will slow down all mobility and self-care activities and be especially obvious when pa-tients try to perform a timed task. Subtle abnormalities are often found when a standardized test such as finger tapping is carried out. Many patients will have an easily detectable abnormality when doing rapid alternating movements. Patients will usually have a related abnormality of fine motor control. They may have difficulty manipulating small objects successfully or just be slower and less skillful when carefully observed. These abnormalities are common sequelae of even mild damage to the cerebral motor cortex and pathways.

Spasticity. Spasticity is a rate-sensitive resistance to passive or active movement associated with increased deep tendon reflexes. This is caused by damage to the upper motor neuron pathways and, if severe, will result in clonus, which is a sustained repetitive involuntary movement caused by spasticity. More attention is being paid to the problem of cocontraction. When a patient tries to carry out a movement the agonist muscles, which normally cause that movement, are opposed by involuntary spasticity in antagonist muscles. This makes the movement more difficult, slower, less accurate, and more expensive in energy expenditure. Patients often become fatigued not only due to the primary effect of the head injury but also due to the increased energy expenditure throughout the day while they are doing their self-care activities. The spasticity will also interfere with speech if it affects the muscles of articulation.

Whyte and Rosenthal (1988, p. 597) list the following indications for treatment of increased muscle tone after TBI:

Interference with active movement
Contracture formation or progression in posturing limb
Interference with appropriate positioning or hygiene
Self-inflicted trauma during muscle spasms
Excessive pain on range of motion or during muscle spasms
Excessive therapy time devoted to contracture prevention rather than
    functional activities

Spasticity can be treated in a number of effective ways. Primary therapies include range of motion to decrease the muscle contracture, resting length, and therefore spasticity. Positioning or application of appropriate splints or casts may decrease spasticity by breaking up a synergistic pattern. The most common synergistic pattern is an extensor spasticity pattern in the lower extremity and a flexor pattern in the upper extremity, although patients with deceberate posturing may have extension of all four extremities. Occasionally a patient will have an asymmetric tonic neck reflex, where one upper extremity is flexed and the other upper extremity is extended in the direction the neck is turned. By positioning the patient out of these patterns, one may be able to decrease the spasticity at adjacent joints.

The medical treatment of spasticity is complicated by the side effects of medication and the lack of good research in the TBI population. Diazepam (Valium) is the traditional medication for spasticity but has a side effect of cognitive impairment. Baclofen is a gamma-aminobutyric acid (GABA) inhibitor with less sedation. Although it is officially approved for use in patients with spinal cord injury and multiple sclerosis, it is being more commonly used in head injury in recent years, since it has fewer side effects. Dantrium is a third medication without cognitive side effects but with a primary effect of decreased muscle strength and occasional toxicity, so that frequent liver enzyme assays should be obtained. With all these medications it is important to monitor a functional clinical outcome as a guide to dosage such as improvement in ambulation or dysarthric speech. In addition to watching for side effects, one should be aware that the primary effect, decreased spasticity, may decrease a patient's function if they were using the spasticity.

Other therapies for spasticity include motor point blocks, nerve blocks, and surgery. It is often helpful to do a temporary nerve or motor point block to sort out the amount of spasticity versus fixed contracture and assess the functional result of the planned block. These therapies also have a more limited area of effectiveness, since only a moderate number of muscles or a few nerves can be blocked. If these considerations indicate potential benefit from the block, the muscle motor points or motor nerve is first localized with electrical stimulation and then injected with Phenol or another destructive agent. More invasive procedures that are used in a small number of selected cases include motor nerve or tendon resection. In a very small number of patients, central procedures such as root or lateral spinal cord destruction may provide some improvement in function despite the risks. It is vital that these interventions be combined with an aggressive program of range of motion, positioning, and functional training.

Ataxia. Ataxia is evidenced by decreased balance, broad-based gait, and poor trunk stability. This can be very disabling and is also relatively hard to treat. It is the result of damage to the cerebral peduncles and connecting pathways more commonly than damage to true cerebral lesions. It often improves slightly with time and with careful training. More commonly, broadening the base is attempted by appropriate use of and training with assistive devices, namely, moving up from the cane to the hemiwalker to the walker to weighted devices and finally to the wheelchair if necessary. A few patients are helped with ankle or wrist weights to decrease the incoordination and ataxia by the inertia of the weight. This is often not very effective and obviously has its side effects. Tremors, a later problem that may impair fine motor skills, are occasionally amenable to treatment with medications such as propranolol (Inderal). Sometimes they gradually improve, but occasionally patients will have the late onset or increase in a tremor months after their head injury.

Hemiparesis. Hemiparesis (weakness contralateral to the side of focal brain injury), and hemiplegia, (paralysis) occur less often than problems of spasticity and fine motor control. Usually traced back to a focal brain or brainstem injury, they have important diagnostic considerations. Patients with hemiparesis should be evaluated for other signs of focal brain damage. It is also important to be aware of the small number of patients with primarily brainstem injuries who have more motor than cognitive impairment. The danger in missing this diagnosis is that a patient who perhaps has severe motor and communication impairment due to spasticity and weakness will be overlooked and thought to have poor cognitive skills. It is also crucial to be aware that despite a striking apparent one-sided lesion, patients almost always have at least subtle motor problems on the opposite "normal" side. With TBI it is rare for a focal lesion to produce unilateral deficits without some impairment of the other side. It is apparent that even true unilateral brain injuries produce some mild abnormality in function of the apparently normal ipsilateral extremities.

Rigidity and Dyskinesia. Rare motor impairments of the traumatically brain-injured population include rigidity and dyskinesia. Rigidity is the constant resistance to movement not related to speed and is most commonly seen in Parkinsonian patients. It resembles a lead pipe or cogwheel resistance to passive movement. Even though this is uncommon after brain injury, it is worth considering a trial of medication with Sinemet if it occurs. The dyskinesias include dystonia, chorea, and athetosis. Dystonia is a striking posturing and severe muscle tone abnormality with minimal movement. Chorea produces continuous, fast, involuntary, proximal movements that are either bizarre or made to seem purposeful by the patient. Athetosis is continuous writhing and variable involuntary movements of distal extremities. Perhaps the most common cause of these abnormalities in brain-injured patients are side effects from medications such as the major tranquilizers. Many of these disorders may have a less obvious impairment of swallowing and speech, and one should look at medications not only for treatment but also a possible unintended cause of these problems. It is also important to be aware that everyday problems such as lack of sleep, fatigue, and anxiety may make these motor problems worse.

Sensation and Motor Control

The importance of sensation for motor control is graphically demonstrated in the patient who has an anesthetic limb. Losing sensation is almost completely disabling to the functional use of an extremity despite preserved motor function. Sensation is most important for fine motor activities and coordination, especially if one's vision is impaired. It is important not only to test touch pressure and pain but also joint position sense. Many patients have subtle abnormalities that are not detected by these straightforward tests. Patients may have a relative inattention to sensory stimuli or neglect. Neglect is manifested by complete lack of awareness of one side of the body or perhaps environment and may result in trauma to the extremity or walking into objects. Many patients have subtle inattention to one side or quadrant of body or visual field, and this should be checked with sensitive testing.

Stereognosis is the sensory and proprioceptive recognition of objects held in the hand. It is important to check this without the person using vision. It is also important to check for two-point discrimination, since the patient may be able to recognize touch but not two points close together. Bilateral simultaneous stimulation is the test for awareness of two stimuli on different spots of the body at the same time. This may also reveal a subtle impairment that should be considered in rehabilitation.

If one looks at what is required for control of movement, one can see how much cerebral control and coordination is required. Multiple muscles must contract with the appropriate amplitude, velocity, and trajectory of movement. Peripheral sensory feedback takes longer than most motor movements and so is more useful for guiding slow movements. Vision is particularly important if peripheral sensation is impaired, and most rapid tasks must be learned. Learning is of course impaired in most brain-injured patients. Further factors of importance in motor control are the postural balance and preliminary movements that must be carried out before an extremity movement.

Motor Learning

Sensation and repetition are both very important in learning new motor tasks. The patient must have sensory feedback to get the motor pattern down correctly. Also, contractions can be preprogrammed and carried out successfully. Learning of tasks is sometimes able to be carried out with just verbal instruction. This will probably take much longer in brain-injured patients. The goal is to provide much repetition in the correct pattern and produce a skilled automatic task. Variables that affect this learning of motor patterns are practice, appropriate feedback for each trial during learning, massing of trials together, and variable training procedures so that there are fewer errors on varied tasks being performed. One hopes that the skill will generalize. It is important to try to learn rules and strategies so that brain-injured patients who have difficulty generalizing to new tasks can do this. Some patients benefit from breaking a task down into steps and learning the most difficult part first. Other patients have difficulty with the sequential learning and must learn things as one unit.

Safety

Impaired judgment, rapid change in activities, and learning in new situations necessitate that the patient be trained for safety. Not only should early mobility skills in self-care be learned in a safe pattern, but patients should also learn to seek appropriate assistance and supervision for additional new tasks. The goal is to have a patient progress to the highest level of function safely so that he or she is not suffering secondary injuries and failures. As a patient is trained and checked for safety, he or she can then be advanced successfully.

BRAIN INJURY CARE CONTINUUM

Figure 2-1 provides an overview of the service components in the ideal care continuum for rehabilitation of the traumatic brain-injured patient. Obstacles to patients' optimal involvement in this care continuum and approaches to removing these obstacles are also reviewed.

TRAUMA CENTER AND EMERGENCY ROOM CARE

Depending on the severity of the injury and available services, a survivor may receive initial trauma care in a variety of settings. A specialized brain injury trauma center (where a team of health care professionals may be available to consult on TBI cases or where emergency beds are designated for TBI or other neurologic insults) may be available. More often, patients will go to the local emergency room of a hospital for initial care. From the emergency room, a patient may be transferred to an intensive care unit based on the severity of the injury and need for life-sustaining measures or monitoring technologies. Frequently, in many of the larger centers, patients with TBI are transferred to neurosurgical intensive care units where specialized services are provided.

Many cases of minor TBI also pass through the emergency room. These individuals are assessed by the emergency room physician with ancillary treatment provided for more immediate needs (e.g., fractures, lacerations, bodily contusions), with some cases receiving initial diagnostic imaging as a precautionary measure. Individuals with these injuries are frequently discharged to home, since the severity of the injury in terms of physical and cognitive sequelae may not warrant further hospitalization. Instructions are given to return should problems with headaches, vision, balance, and nausea persist. Although it is beyond the scope of this chapter to delineate the special needs and treatment issues for patients with minor TBI, it should be noted that many of these

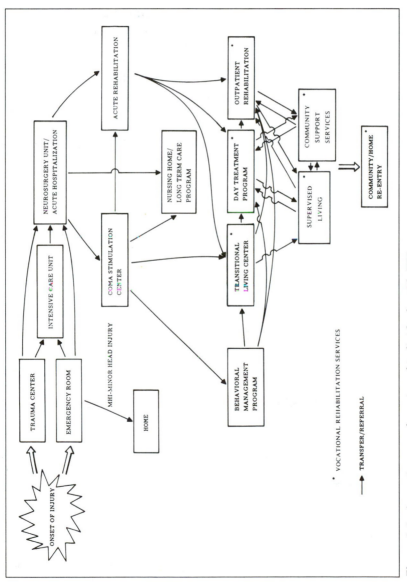

Figure 2-1. A continuum of service of individuals with TBI.

individuals will reappear later in the service delivery system due to continued psychosocial adjustment difficulties.

NEUROSURGERY UNIT AND ACUTE HOSPITALIZATION

From the emergency room or intensive care unit a patient may be transferred to a neurosurgery-neurology medical unit where the goal is medical stabilization, primarily of the patient's neurologic status. Some of these patients may still be in some level of coma or in a posttraumatic amnestic state. Procedures such as craniotomies, shunt placements, monitoring intracranial pressure, and seizure assessments and management take place in this setting. In hospitals without a specialized neurologic service, these procedures may be carried out on a general medicine service. Some patients, on the other hand, sustain severe general trauma such as pneumothorax, a ruptured spleen, or comminuted fractures. With these patients, acute medical care may be provided on a general surgery unit with neurosurgical consultation.

COMA STIMULATION

A proportion of TBI patients remain in a coma at the acute hospitalization phase. It may be decided to attempt bringing the patient out of a coma by a stimulation program. The specific goal of such an approach is to provide a comprehensive sensory stimulation regimen to arouse the patient toward a higher level of awareness. The family, funding sources, and coma treatment facility staff usually negotiate a specified period of time within which to work toward arousing the coma patient. Throughout this phase of treatment, the patient's health and comfort are managed by nursing and medical staff.

NURSING HOME AND LONG-TERM CARE PROGRAMS

Traumatically brain-injured patients may be referred to nursing homes when there appear to be few active or high-level rehabilitation goals to be reached. In other cases, the referral may be made because the TBI survivor requires more labor-intensive nursing care that cannot be handled by family members or home nursing assistants. These individuals may be severely impaired in physical and cognitive realms such that they are unable to benefit from rehabilitation treatment at other facilities.

Unfortunately, there are some TBI individuals currently residing in nursing homes or long-term care facilities who could benefit significantly from transitional or community reentry rehabilitation services. In some cases, this situation is the result of a routine transfer to a nursing home setting due to lack of alternatives. However, this trend is changing with the development and availability of additional treatment options, such as coma stimulation, neurobehavioral, and long-term care programs.

Long-term care facilities have the basic goal of providing interdisciplinary rehabilitation, usually in an inpatient or residential setting. Such facilities serve those clients who may in the past have been placed in a nursing home, those who are in a persistent vegetative state, or those who maintain severe physical and cognitive impairments as a result of TBI. "Long-term" is often defined as months or years of rehabilitation and, in some cases, may be a more permanent living situation. One advantage that such facilities have over nursing home placement can be long-term cost saving as well as specialized management and treatment by professionals trained in brain injury. Ironically, one of the primary reasons for nursing home placement rather than transfer to a more cost-effective, treatment-oriented facility is that the only funding available is for skilled nursing or medically oriented therapies.

NEUROBEHAVIORAL PROGRAMS

Many TBI survivors exhibit behavioral disturbances that are difficult for both family members and health care professional staff to manage. In cases in which maladaptive behaviors interfere with rehabilitation efforts, these individuals can benefit from a structured neurobehavioral program. The goal of such programs is to contain and decrease behavioral disturbances, increase appropriate social behaviors, and prepare the individual for entry into rehabilitation programs such as those described below.

ACUTE REHABILITATION

Once the patient's emergent medical concerns are addressed and there is the capacity to profit from rehabilitation intervention, a transfer to a rehabilitation unit is often initiated. This may be the first step in active TBI intervention carried out by rehabilitation medicine staff. This treatment typically includes the psychiatrist, neuropsychologist, clinical psychologist, speech and language pathologist, occupational therapist, physical therapist, therapeutic recreational specialist, vocational rehabilitation counselor, prosthetic and orthotic specialist, rehabilitation engineer, rehabilitation nurse, social worker, and often a case manager.

Neuropsychological evaluation is performed at this stage of rehabilitation to establish baseline cognitive status and to assist with defining realistic assessment and treatment goals. These goals may include (1) pinpoint basic strategies to compensate for impaired cognitive skills, (2) relearn ways to carry out activities of daily living, (3) improve communication interaction, (4) engage in active physical medicine rehabilitation, (5) initiate training in physical restoration, and (6) begin vocational, educational, and avocational planning. In addition, intervention with the family is often critical at this point. Both counseling and educational services may be necessary to enable family members to have clear expectations of the patient and begin preparing for the task of caregiving (Lezak, 1988).

TRANSITIONAL LIVING CENTER

Transitional living centers are community-based residential programs. TBI residents live within these programs and receive daily therapies provided by an interdisciplinary or transdisciplinary rehabilitation team. The focus of a community reentry program is to provide the individual with TBI with the necessary skills to live as independently and productively as possible within the home community.

There are both financial and clinical benefits to the use of this type of treatment model. It is far less costly to provide services in a community-based, rather than a hospital-based, facility, even when the treatment program is intensive. Clinically, living in such a setting brings the client one step closer to preinjury lifestyle. In addition, the practical skill acquisition on which community reentry programming centers occurs far better in a community than a hospital setting. The reason for this benefit is at least twofold: (1) community resources (local grocery store, on-the-job training site, etc.) needed to relearn skills are more readily available and (2) generalization of skills learned, a notoriously difficult area for the head injured, is greatly enhanced by the similarity between this type of treatment setting and the individual's home community.

DAY TREATMENT AND OUTPATIENT REHABILITATION

Clients who no longer require the intensity and structure of a residential program may continue to receive rehabilitation training in a day treatment or outpatient setting, since recovery from brain injury may allow them to be challenged in terms of cognitive abilities. Clients usually attend such programs five days per week for approximately four to eight hours per day.

In outpatient rehabilitation, a patient's schedule is largely determined by the individual needs of the client and family (e.g., a focus on particular community or vocational goals). Although the setting includes an interdisciplinary treatment team, not all disciplines work with a given client at this level. The group milieu is often an important treatment component of this type of program. Psychotherapuetic services, including group sessions involving both staff members and patients, are frequently a part of the program. Vocational assessment to include job samples and work experience (job station or on-the-job training) activities can be a therapy component of both day treatment and outpatient rehabilitation programs.

SUPERVISED INDEPENDENT LIVING CENTER AND SUPPORT SERVICES

Supervised independent living centers are facilities that emphasize the final reintegration of a TBI patient back into the community. Group homes and apartment units (either purchased or rented by a head injury facility) may be used by head injury programs to provide an independent living experience for the resident. Staff support is provided to create a safety net for those remaining problems that can surface in such an environment. In vivo practice of daily living skills and use of compensatory strategies can be safely tested in a supervised living program.

Community support services provided to TBI survivors in their own homes are another option for those who continue to need some level of assistance. These services include case management, community mobility training, assistance with leisure planning, or a variety of other services that enable the individual to live as independently as possible. Family support and assistance may be equally valuable services. Individuals who are living in a supervised living program or are receiving community support services may also be involved in a day treatment or outpatient rehabilitation program. With this arrangement, generalization of treatment can be addressed by a cooperative staffing effort between treatment facility and the patient's independent living setting.

VOCATIONAL REHABILITATION SERVICES

Represented across several of the previously discussed treatment settings is the integration of vocational services for the TBI patient. These services are essential in order that realistic return to work goals can be established before the patient exist the care system. Having an employment goal can structure the type of treatment the patient receives. Each treatment facility may have its own vocational counselors. In other cases, state or private vocational counselors are enlisted to assist the patient toward returning to some form of employment.

There are a number of issues in the provision of vocational rehabilitation services. Because of the complexity of the injury and a lack of understanding of the injury's implications, it is difficult for the state vocational rehabilitation counselor to make eligibility decisions, to request appropriate evaluations, and to become aggressively involved in vocational planning. Counselors are more specifically confused about their involvement due to the natural recovery time associated with the injury and the unevenness in client patterns of asset and deficit that they encounter. It is most helpful for state agency counselors to confer with an experienced rehabilitation counselor when providing services in this area and to have the input of a qualified neuropsychologist. Evaluations should standardly include neuropsychological assessment to help frame the vocational planning effort. In some cases of mild TBI, identification of an individual's pattern of assets can help direct the establishment of job goals. Areas of deficit can often be avoided or compensatory approaches developed relative to job demands. In cases of a more severe injury, neuropsychological evaluation can still identify areas of asset and diverse areas of deficit that will require some compensatory interventions. Vocational evaluations should standardly include job-relevant work samples and community-based work experiences for those with severe injury. It often occurs that even with some severe areas of brain impairment, an individual remains able to perform a job due to its structure and his or her number of years of experience within the position. Different methods of supported employment can also be used, such as on-the-job training funds to defray the costs of a supervisor's or company owner's time in training, use of a job coach to train the client on the work site, and job sharing or use of another coworker as a training consultant. Residential programs have developed affirmative industries so that they are able to evaluate individuals within the facility and pay them minimum wage or greater for the work that they are performing during the evaluation. Evaluation data from affirmative industries work activity can then be used to assist in targeting a selective placement for supported employment positions within the community.

In TBI vocational rehabilitation, it is still vital that a goal be set early in the rehabilitation process even if it must be reformulated several times. Vocational rehabilitation service dollars are best spent if the vocational evaluation is relevant to job market access points for the individual. For clients with prior work background, much of the evaluation will be spent in job sampling to identify residual generalizable skills and segments of prior work activity that can still be performed by the TBI survivor. For individuals with no job experience, it can be most helpful to use a series of job samples that relate to high-frequency entry level jobs within the employment market. It is important to remember that everything done within the vocational rehabilitation process must relate to generalization of vocational skills that can be applied in the client's home community or discharge site.

After the vocational evaluation has been completed and recommendations have been obtained from the neuropsychologist, the vocational rehabilitation counselor decides whether he or she can handle the case personally or vocational services must be purchased. In considering purchase of services, it is important to purchase services from counselors who are experienced in TBI or at least in working with severe disabilities. It can be helpful to screen for competency by asking counselors to review vocational plans that they have arranged for prior TBI individuals, particularly those with severe injuries. Counselors should have an appreciation for the steps or bridges in the return to work (e.g., nonprofit job stations, on-the-job training, different models of supported employment) and appreciate the need for generalization of learned vocational skills to the client's home community or discharge site. Services purchased from a residential program should also have some linkage to the client's home community to ensure the vocational program's stabilization. There should also be awareness on the part of the vocational counselor that postemployment services can require and include case management, monitoring of the vocational program by a community vocational counselor, a job coach, psychotherapy or substance abuse counselling, or other services that abet position stabilization.

SERVICES FROM CONSUMER GROUP ORGANIZATIONS

In a recent report by the National Head Injury Foundation (1988) concerned with issues in developing and administering community-based programs, a range of services were described that need further clarification and expansion to serve the needs of individuals with TBI. The most frequently cited needs included the need for day programs, respite care, community-based recreation programs, summer camps, and case management. Support for these programs may be established through a mix of public and private funding. A description of these and other programs that can be spearheaded through a local consumer group are described below (day programs have been described earlier in the chapter).

Case Management–Service Coordination Program

A case management–service coordination program is a system that provides the training of family members and significant others, uses professionals willing to do case management, and trains individuals as appropriate to manage their own service needs. This is one of the most critical needs and an underpinning to appropriate service provision in TBI rehabilitation.

Recreational Service

The recreational service provides social and leisure opportunities for TBI individuals. The program can offer activities on weekends or several nights a week. This can be an invaluable program because of the isolation of many traumatic brain-injured individuals and can be coordinated by either a stable volunteer or through a paid professional. Staffing can be augmented by use of other volunteers.

Respite Service

The respite service is designed to give significant others and family members of traumatic brain-injured individuals a break from caring for the TBI individuals. In some cases these services are provided through a residential program, and in others they are provided by private individuals within the home. To improve and support the psychosocial functioning of families and significant others of traumatic brain-injured individuals, the availability of respite services had been identified as an invaluable asset.

Family-to-Family Programs

In family-to-family programs, family members are trained as volunteers to support and assist other families in dealing with the occurrence of TBI within their family. This type of family-to-family program is often used during crisis periods to support, educate, and sensitize the significant others of a TBI individual and offer potential courses of action. This type of support can provide some sense of order in a situation that can quickly become out of control for the family trying to absorb the injury's impact and take practical steps to assist a loved one.

In-Home Services

The purpose of in-home services is to bring care and rehabilitation services to TBI individuals within the home. These types of programs can include a range of services such as personal care, domestic assistance, financial advisement, and assistance in structuring the TBI survivor's day.

Self-Help Group Services

A number of consumer organizations around the country have developed self-help group networks. These types of groups are helpful for both the TBI survivors and their significant others. In some instances, groups are set up specifically for parents and spouses of the TBI survivor. Groups are also established for TBI survivors at different age levels and for those at different career levels. Some very strong bonds can be built through these groups that not only support the rehabilitation momentum but also assist in recreational and other social outlets. The self-help groups also serve as educational networks for TBI survivors and their families.

ANCILLARY SERVICES

Other ancillary services in the community exist from which TBI patients may receive assistance. Several universities and community colleges have disabled student services available to assist students in reintegrating into the academic setting after acquiring a disability. Although the majority of these programs are not specialized in TBI, many of those working within such services have experience and knowledge of the problems associated with brain injury (e.g., various cognitive, behavioral, and physical sequelae) and the obstacles these pose in college settings. Similarly, school psychologists and special education specialists within school systems can help children and adolescents with TBI. Specialists within state departments of vocational rehabilitation or workers' compensation departments may have expertise in head injury and other physical disabilities. Often rehabilitation nurses will fill such positions. Home health care professionals (e.g., registered nurses and licensed practical nurses) can provide respite for family caregivers of TBI patients when activities of daily living, health education, or temporary supervision needs are present.

OBSTACLES TO TBI CARE CONTINUITY

Burke sees the need for integration and coordination of TBI services so that the various components of the system "provide a continuum of care for individual patients within a flexible system, so that the patient may move smoothly from one facet to another according to need" (Burke, 1987, pp. 195–196). This certainly is a worthy goal; however, it has been our experience that there are some significant obstacles for moving patients through the current system. These obstacles include some of the following issues.

1. *Funding.* TBI rehabilitation is labor intensive and requires an extended rehabilitation period. Consequently, it is a costly endeavor. Inpatient acute costs can generally be covered, but as the patient must move on through the care continuum, services coverage can rapidly decline.

2. *Weak knowledge base.* Although the National Head Injury Foundation and other groups are increasing information dissemination efforts, often families, insurance carriers, and health care and legal professionals do not understand fully the consequences of TBI. This lack of knowledge contributes to the confusion of not understanding what the most appropriate services are for an individual and how to access them.
3. *Nature of the injury.* Brain injury can result not only in physical consequences but also in cognitive, behavioral, interpersonal, emotional, and vocational problems. For the survivor, family members, and helping professionals, severe injuries present a particular challenge because of the multiple needs and required services involved.
4. *Accessibility.* Many of the described service components within the care continuum are not well coordinated even when they exist in urban areas. In rural areas, rehabilitation treatment for TBI victims is almost nonexistent. Service accessibility can be a major issue even when funding exists.

Acknowledgment. This chapter was supported in part by Grant #H133B80081 from the National Institute of Disability and Rehabilitation Research, Department of Education, Washington, DC.

REFERENCES

Bergner, M., Bobbitt, K.A., Carter, W.B., and Gibson, B.S. (1981). The Sickness Impact Profile: Development and final revision of a health status measure. *Medical Care 19,* 787–805.

Brain, W. (1941). Visual disorientation with special reference to lesions of the right cerebral hemisphere. *Brain, 64,* 244–272.

Burke, D. C. (1987). Planning a System of Care for Head Injuries. Brain Injury 1, 189–198.

Jennett, B. (1986). Head trauma. In A.K. Asbury, G.M. McKann, and W.I. McDonald (Eds.), *Diseases of the nervous system* (pp. 1282–1991). Philadelphia: Saunders.

Jennett, B., and Bond, M.R. (1975). Assessment of outcome after severe brain damage: A practical scale. *Lancet, 1,* 480–484.

Jennett, B., and Teasdale, G. (1981). *Management of head injuries* (pp. 317–332). Philadelphia: Davis.

Katz, M.M., and Lyerly, S.B. (1963). Methods of measuring adjustment and social behavior in the community. I. Rationale, description, discriminative validity and scale development. *Psychological Reports, 13,* 503.

Klove, H., and Cleeland, C.S. (1972). The relationships of neuro-psychological impairment to other indices of severity of head injury. *Scandinavian Journal of Rehabilitation Medicine 4,* 55.

Levin, H.S., O'Donnell, V.M., and Grossman, R.G. (1979). The Galveston Orientation and Amnesia Test: A practical scale to assess cognition after head injury. *Journal of Nervous and Mental Disorders, 167,* 675–684.

Lezak, M.D. (1988). Brain damage is a family affair. *Journal of Clinical and Experimental Neuropsychology, 10,* 111–123.

Luria, A.R. (1964). *Higher cortical functions in man.* New York: Basic Books.

Miller, J.D. and Jones, P.A. (1985). The work of a regional head injury service. *Lancet,* 1:1141–1144.

National Head Injury Foundation. (1988). *The role of the National Head Injury Foundation and state associations in developing and administering community-based programs.* Southborough, MA.: unpublished manuscript.

Rappaport, M. et al. (1977). Evoked brain potentials and disability in brain damaged patients. *Archives of Physical Medicine and Rehabilitation, 58,* 333.

Rappaport, M., Hall, K.M., Hopkins, H.K., and Belleza, T. (1982.) Disability rating scale for severe head trauma: Coma to community. *Archives of Physical Medicine and Rehabilitation, 63,* 118–123.

Russell, W.R. (1932). Cerebral involvement in head injury. *Brain, 35,* 549–603.

Russell, W.R. (1971). *The traumatic amnesias.* London: Oxford University Press.

Sohlberg, M., and Mateer, C. (1989). *Introduction to cognitive rehabilitation: Theory and practice.* New York: The Guilford Press.

Teasdale, G., and Jennett, B. (1974). Assessment of coma and impaired consciousness. *Lancet, 2,* 81.

Whyte, J., and Rosenthal, M. (1988). Rehabilitation of the patient with head injury. In J. Delisa (Ed.), *Rehabilitation medicine: Principles and practices* (pp. 585–611). Philadelphia: Lippincott.

CHAPTER 3

PSYCHOSOCIAL DISTURBANCES AFTER HEAD INJURY

JO ANN BROCKWAY

Most if not all clinicians who work with individuals with traumatic brain injury (TBI) could attest to the numerous problems, generally categorized as psychosocial, experienced by these individuals after their head injury. These so-called psychosocial sequelae of head injury include such difficulties as social isolation, relationship problems, sexual dysfunction, inappropriate sexual behavior, difficulties with family role, legal problems, and vocational difficulties. Recovery from head injury does occur, but over time. It may take hours, weeks, months, or even years. Although few individuals with severe traumatic head injury are likely to recover completely with no psychosocial sequela, most will recover some degree of psychosocial function (Grant and Alves, 1987). Bond (1984), for example, found some recovery of psychosocial function in most patients but stated that it was difficult to predict psychosocial recovery from early postinjury status. There is, in fact, a lack of consensus among clinicians and investigators on the type and extent of impairment likely to occur following a head injury of a given type and severity. This lack of consensus results in part from differences in characteristics of individuals with TBI at different treatment facilities. Moreover, significant issues related to research methods contribute to the inconsistencies in findings.

This chapter aims to provide the reader with an overview of psychosocial disturbances after head injury. It will include a brief review of some of the relevant literature on psychosocial disturbances after head injury and will address intervention strategies used for psychosocial rehabilitation. This chapter is not intended to be an exhaustive review of the literature but is meant to acquaint the reader with clinical aspects of psychosocial sequelae to TBI.

FACTORS CONTRIBUTING TO PSYCHOSOCIAL DISTURBANCES AFTER TBI

PREMORBID FACTORS

There has been little research done to date on the impact of premorbid factors on psychosocial sequelae of head injury. Clinically, it often appears that some of the individual's less pleasing premorbid personality or behavioral characteristics are exacerbated after TBI. A number of authors have hypothesized that certain premorbid personality styles may predispose individuals to emotional and psychological difficulties after head injury (Bond, 1975; McMillan and Glucksman, 1987; Fordyce and colleagues, 1983). It is certainly clear that head injury is not a random event. The highest incidence of head injury is among young males. Low socioeconomic status, prior head injuries, and prior neuropsychiatric difficulties, chemical dependence, and substance abuse are overrepresented in the population of individuals with head injury (Brooks, 1984; Rimel and colleagues, 1981; Levin and colleagues, 1982; Annegers and colleagues, 1980). These preexisting conditions may affect postinjury psychosocial functioning in two ways. First, individuals with such preexisting conditions may already have impaired cognitive, psychologic, and psychosocial functioning even before their injuries. Second, it is not unreasonable to hypothesize that these conditions may well interact with the effects of the head injury. This is not to say, however, that all individuals with TBI had poor premorbid coping skills, preexisting psychiatric difficulties, or histories of substance abuse. It is important to note that a large number of individuals with TBI may have had no significant preexisting problems and may have functioned quite well before injury. The point is, there are individual differences in the preinjury characteristics of individuals with TBI that interact with other factors to influence psychosocial functioning after TBI.

COGNITIVE-INTELLECTUAL AND EMOTIONAL-BEHAVIORAL SEQUELAE

The negative consequences of head injury may be broadly divided into three categories: neurologic-physical, cognitive-intellectual, and emotional-behavioral. Neurologic-physical deficits include motor impairments such as posttraumatic epilepsy, impaired coordination, motor weakness, vision deficits, gait disturbances, and sensory deficits. Cognitive-intellectual impairments include short-term memory deficits, decreased attention, word-finding problems, and impaired judgment. Emotional-behavioral sequelae include personality changes, lack of self-awareness, episodic dyscontrol, and disinhibition.

Clinical experience suggests that cognitive-intellectual deficits and emotional-behavioral difficulties are both more persistent and more contributory to psychosocial disability following head injury than are physical impairments. Bond (1975), for example, reported that psychosocial difficulties after head injury were due primarily to impaired cognitive functions and changes in personality rather than to physical difficulty and that families were more concerned with the cognitive and personality changes than they were with physical disability. Other investigators have reported similar findings (e.g., Oddy, 1984; Brooks and colleagues, 1987).

Cognitive-intellectual and behavior changes occur with considerable frequency after head injury. There is general agreement that approximately two thirds of individuals with head injury manifest significant changes in behavior (Grant and Alves, 1987). Reports in the literature indicate that cognitive and emotional difficulties can occur with relatively high frequency even when there are no documented physical or neurologic difficulties (Dikmen and Reitan, 1976; Gronwall and Wrightson, 1974). In a study of more severely injured individuals, Brooks and McKinlay (1983) found that 49 percent of the relatives interviewed reported undesirable personality changes in their family members with brain injury. At a five-year followup, Jennett and colleagues (1981) found personality changes in two thirds of their subjects with head injury.

Emotional-behavioral disorders following TBI include unrealistic self-appraisal and decreased social awareness, socially inappropriate behavior, depression, aggressive disorders, paranoia, and anxiety. A number of personality changes appear to be a direct result of the organic effects of brain injury and often contribute to psychosocial difficulties after TBI. The lack of self-awareness leads to poor-quality control and a lack of appreciation of one's own skills and deficits. A lack of social awareness may result in the individual's not appreciating social signs and signals from those around him or her, and therefore the person may engage in socially inappropriate or socially inept behavior.

Many authors have indicated that "depression" is a frequent sequel to head injury. McKinlay and colleagues (1981), for example, indicated that slightly over half their subject group complained of depressed moods at 3, 6, and 12 months after injury. It is not always clear to what extent depression is an organic effect of brain injury, is a reaction to brain injury, or is a premorbid characteristic. Depressed mood may well be a reaction to the changes in abilities or losses of reinforcing activities that may follow the onset of the head injury. Feelings of depression are common after head injury and appear to be related to the injured individual's increasing awareness of the physical, cognitive, and social consequences of the injury (Bond, 1984). Onset of depression may be seen as a positive sign of decrease in denial and increase in awareness and understanding of one's limitations (Rosenthal, 1983). Clinicians working with individuals with TBI often note that early on the individual with TBI may have severe cognitive deficits and be quite unaware of them, but that as the individual "gets better" (i.e., becomes more aware of deficits and difficulties), he or she may "get worse" (i.e., becomes more emotionally distressed). Individuals who experience depression after TBI may report feelings of worthlessness, helplessness and hopelessness, guilt, decreased initiation of activities, social withdrawal, decreased libido, suicidal ideation, and even a suicide attempt. Depression after head injury is common but does not appear to be related to severity of injury (Lishman, 1978, Levin and Grossman, 1978) or level of neurologic impairment (Prigatano, 1985). Such depression may interfere with the individual's ability to participate in the rehabilitation program, may interfere with his or her adequate functioning in the family, and may lead the individual with head injury to avoid the very support and reinforcing activities that could help decrease the depression.

Aggressive behavior is another fairly frequently reported and problematic symptom following head injury and is among the sequelae most disturbing to others. Irritability is common in the early stages of recovery preceding full consciousness; in some cases that includes combative behavior (Wood, 1984). Aggressive behavior may continue until the later stages of recovery, generally lessening somewhat as the ability to control emotions increases. Nonetheless, in some patients episodic aggressive behavior disorders have been described in relationship to head injury. One, episodic dyscontrol, is impulsive, unprovoked behavior that is thought to be related to abnormal electrical activity in the brain (Lishman, 1978). Aggressive behavior of this kind is thought to begin abruptly and to have an explosive quality. A second appears to be more related to poor emotional control, i.e., the inability to maintain emotional equilibrium or to control emotional expression and to involve a lowered threshold for aggressive behavior (Lishman, 1978). Both may be exacerbated and maintained by environmental responses. Such aggressive behavior may impair relationships with family and friends, rehabilitation efforts, and ability to return to work. Approaches to treatment of aggressive disorders following head injury have included pharmacologic management (e.g., Yudofsky and colleagues, 1987) and behavioral interventions (e.g., Francen and Lovel, 1987), but little has been done to study systematically the efficacy of various treatment strategies.

Paranoid symptoms can also emerge in patients with TBI. Often individuals who show paranoid symptoms manifest language and memory difficulties that may affect their ability to communicate and to perceive realistically what goes on around them. They may misinterpret others' intentions or actions and may become suspicious and uncooperative. Often there is significant cognitive dysfunction, typical in temporal lobe damage (Prigatano, 1987).

Anxiety symptoms may also occur following head injury. Some patients report a period of "feeling as if I were going crazy" occurring after they became aware of their functional difficulties in certain situations but before they were aware enough to understand why they were having difficulties. One individual described this as feeling "thick-headed." He found that he often felt "thick-headed" when he was attempting a new activity or something that he had experienced difficulty on previously (although after his injury). He found, however, that once he realized that he was able to perform the task adequately, the "thick-headed" feeling disappeared.

A variety of factors have been hypothesized to contribute to the incidence of cognitive-intellectual and emotional-psychological sequela of

TBI. A number of studies have looked at severity of injury as a possible factor. Levin and colleagues, (1987), for example, looked at a group of individuals with TBI of differing severities. They found that severity of injury was related to cognitive impairment, impairments in language functioning, poor planning, and decreased awareness of self. Injury severity has generally not been found to be related to emotional distress. (Bond, 1975; Levin and colleagues, 1987, Levin and Grossman, 1978, Keshavan and colleagues, 1981).

Litigation has also been investigated as a factor in the incidence of cognitive-intellectual and emotional-psychological sequel to head injury. Although there have been some reports that persistent postconcussive symptoms are related to litigation or industrial compensation (e.g., Miller, 1961), other investigators have found that similar symptomatology occurs in patients not involved in litigation (e.g., McMillan and Glucksman, 1987; Kelly, 1975).

RESPONSE OF THE ENVIRONMENT

Another factor in psychosocial disabilities may be the response of the environment to the individual with TBI. There has been considerable attention paid in recent years to the impact of TBI on the family (e.g., Lezak, 1988; Romano, 1976), but little attention has been paid to the impact of the response of the environment on the psychosocial rehabilitation of the individual with TBI. Kozloff (1987) indicated that environmental support facilitates good long-term recovery from head injury. Families and friends may respond with what appears to the individual with head injury to be a lack of understanding of his or her difficulties. As one individual with TBI said, "I walk, I talk, I look like I'm okay. They can't see how difficult it is for me to do things now. They think I'm just pretending." Some family members respond with overprotectiveness, while others seem to minimize or even not to recognize the individual's deficits following head injury. At one extreme, the family may reinforce inappropriate behavior and increase dependency; at the other extreme, the family may inappropriately expect the individual to resume preinjury roles and responsibilities fully.

Clinically, many individuals find that after TBI their social network has shrunk. Their world becomes narrowed and more focused on a few other individuals, most often family. Some individuals, after head injury, become involved with new or old "friends" who take advantage of them. One trusting and lonely young man received a settlement that allowed him a $1,500 per month income. He often had difficulty paying his rent, however, because he did such things as loan $200 to his "friend" to post bail and allowed another "friend" to make $400 in long-distance telephone calls for which he was never repaid. After each time he would verbalize that he had used poor judgment and vow not to let it happen again.

The response of the work environment may also play a significant role in the economic sequela of head injury. The employer who allows return to work on a gradual basis, in a changed capacity, or with environmental or job description modifications may assist with the long-term psychosocial recovery of the individual with TBI.

PSYCHOSOCIAL REHABILITATION

The process of psychosocial rehabilitation after TBI may necessitate the individual's reassessment of self, including abilities, areas of difficulties, and goals in a variety of life's areas (e.g., work, relationships, recreation). This reevaluation may lead to a redefinition of self and a modification of goals and expectations. It is part of the work of the TBI rehabilitation team to facilitate and assist with this process.

The first step in the rehabilitation process is the establishment of a productive relationship between the individual, the family, and the rehabilitation team. A number of general principles are both simple and obvious but are often forgotten. The first and perhaps the most important is that of establishing a therapeutic relationship in which the client is treated with respect. This includes respecting the client's privacy and listening to the concerns of the individual and the family. Feedback should be given to the individual and family in a straightforward but supportive manner. Feedback should be nonjudgmental and presented in language the individual or family can understand. It is important to provide information regarding the individual's difficulties, but it is equally important to provide feedback regarding the individual's abilities, successes, and gains. It may be necessary to repeat information and feedback numerous times to make certain that it is understood and remembered.

The second step of rehabilitation involves a thorough evaluation of the individual, including an assessment of the individual's current abilities, disabilities, and goals and the environment to which the individual will return. Evaluation should include information regarding prior neurologic-physical, cognitive-intellectual, and emotional-behavioral abilities and disabilities and prior psychosocial status. This will allow the development of treatment goals and strategies appropriate to the individual in the context of the individual's environment.

A well-coordinated rehabilitation team is integral to the psychosocial rehabilitation of the individual after TBI. This team provides a therapeutic milieu in which the individual may practice psychosocial skills, i.e., an environment in which the individual may exhibit behaviors and receive therapeutic feedback in a variety of situations and with a variety of individuals to facilitate learning of psychosocial skills. The psychosocial rehabilitation process may include intervention through behavioral modification techniques, individual, couple, or family counseling, group counseling, or psychopharmacologic therapies integrated into the total treatment program.

It is imperative that the team clearly define goals and strategies for achieving those goals and that each member of the team work with the individual toward those goals, using the strategies decided on by the team. Specific and concrete goals, a consistent approach by a well-organized and well-integrated team, and frequent and appropriate feedback are highly important in working with individuals after TBI, perhaps more important than for individuals with other disabilities, because of the difficulties individuals with TBI often have in learning, in coping with the unexpected, and in dealing with ambiguity.

Another essential aspect of psychosocial rehabilitation is that of generalization and reintegration into the community. Individuals with TBI often have difficulty generalizing skills to different environments, and it is often necessary to provide opportunity to practice what has been learned in the rehabilitation program in a variety of community settings with gradually decreasing supervision. It may be necessary to provide followup assistance for some months after formal discharge from the rehabilitation program.

REFERENCES

Annegers, J.F., Grabow, J.D., Kurland, L.T., and Laws, E.R. (1980). The incidence, causes, and secular trends of head trauma in Olmstead County, Minnesota. *Neurology, 30,* 912–919.

Bond, M.R. (1975). Assessment of psychosocial outcome after severe head injury. In *Outcome of Severe Damage to the CNS.* CIBA Foundations Symposium, Amsterdam: Elsevier-Excerpta Medica, 34, 141.

Bond, M. (1984). The psychiatry of closed head injury. In N. B. Brooks (Ed.), *Closed head injury: Psychological, social and family consequences.* New York: Oxford University Press.

Brooks, N. (1984). Head injury and the family. In N.B. Brooks (Ed.), *Closed head injury: Psychological, social and family consequences.* New York: Oxford University Press.

Brooks, N., et al (1987). The effects of severe head injury on patient and relative within seven years of injury. *Journal of Head Trauma Rehabilitation, 2,* 1–13.

Brooks, N., and McKinaly, W. (1983). Personality and behavior change after severe blunt head injury—a relative's view. *Journal of Neurology, Neurosurgery and Psychiatry, 46,* 336–344.

Dikmen, S., and Reitan, R.M. (1976). Psychological deficits and recovery of functions after head injury. *Trans-American Neurological Association, 101,* 72–77.

Dikmen, S., and Temkin, N. (1987). Determination of the effects of head injury and recovery in behavioral research. In: H.S. Levin, H.M. Eisenberg, and J. Grafman (Eds.), *Neurobehavioral recovery from head injury.* New York: Oxford University Press.

Fordyce, D., Rouche, J., and Prigatano, G. (1983). Enhanced emotional reaction in chronic head trauma patients. *Journal of Neurology, Neurosurgery and Psychiatry, 46,* 620–624.

Francen, M.D., and Lovel, M.R. (1987). Behavioral treatment of aggressive sequela of brain injury. *Psychiatric Annals, 17,* 389–396.

Grant, I., and Alves, W. (1987). Psychiatric and psychological disturbances in head injury. In H.S. Levin, J. Grafman, and H.M. Eisenberg (Eds.), *Neurobehavioral recovery from head injury,* New York: Oxford University Press.

Gronwall, D., and Wrightson, P. (1974). Delayed recovery of intellectual function after minor head injury. *Lancet, 2,* 605–609.

Kelly, R. (1975). The post-traumatic syndrome: An iatrogenic disease. *Forensic Science, 6,* 17–24.

Keshavan, M., Channabasavann, S., and Reddy, G. (1981). Post-traumatic psychiatric disturbances: Patterns and predictors of outcome. *British Journal of Psychiatry, 138,* 157–160.

Kozloff, R. (1987). Networks of social support and the outcome from severe head injury. *Journal of Head Trauma Rehabilitation, 2,* 14–23.

Levin H.S., Benton, A.L., and Grossman, R.G. (1982). *Neurobehavioral consequences of closed head injury.* New York: Oxford University Press.

Levin, H., Grossman, R., Rose, J., and Teasdale, G. (1979). Long-term neuropsychological outcome of closed head injury. *Journal of Neurosurgery, 50,* 412–422.

Lishman, W.A. (1978). *Organic Psychiatry.* Oxford: Blackwell.

McKinlay, W.W., Brooks, D.N., Bond, M.R., Martinase, D.P., and Marshall, M.M. (1981). The short-term outcome of severe blunt head injury as reported by relatives of the injured persons. *Journal of Neurology, Neurosurgery and Psychiatry, 44,* 527–533.

McMillan, T., and Glucksman, E. (1987). The neuropsychology of moderate head injury. *Journal of Neurology, Neurosurgery and Psychiatry, 50,* 393–397.

Miller, H. (1961). Accident neurosis: Lecture C. *British Medical Journal,* April 1, 919–925. Accident neurosis: Lecture D. *British Medical Journal,* April 8, 992–998.

Oddy, M. (1984). Head injury and social adjustment. In N. Brooks (Ed.) *Closed head injury.* New York: Oxford University Press.

Prigatano, G. (1985). Personality and psychosocial consequences of head injury. In G. Prigatano (Ed.), *Neuropsychological rehabilitation after brain injury.* Baltimore: Johns Hopkins University Press.

Prigatano, G. (1987). Psychiatric aspects of head injury: Problem areas and suggested guidelines for research. In H. S. Levin, J. Grafmann, and H. M. Eisenberg, (Eds.), *Neurobehavioral recovery from head injury,* New York: Oxford University Press.

Rimel, R., Giordani, M., Barth, J., Boll, T., and Jane, J. (1981). Disability caused by minor head injury. *Neurosurgery, 9,* 221–228.

Rosenthal, M. (1983). Behavioral sequela. In M. Rosenthal, E. Griffith, M. Bond, and J. Miller (Eds.), *Rehabilitation of the head injured adult.* Philadelphia: Davis.

Wood, R.L. (1984). Behavior disorders following brain injury: Their prevalence and psychologic management. In Brooks MD (Ed.), *Closed head injury psychological, social and family consequences.* New York: Oxford University Press.

Yudofsky, S.C., Silver, J.M., and Schneider, S.E., (1987). Pharmacologic treatment of the aggression. *Psychiatric Annals, 17:*397–405.

PART   II

Cognitive/Language Issues

CHAPTER 4

Conceptual Issues in Cognitive Rehabilitation

DAVID J. FORDYCE

Interest in head trauma rehabilitation has grown at an astonishing rate in the 1980s. There has been an explosion in the number of treatment programs and the size of the professional literature. This growth has been fueled by the increased appreciation of the long-term consequences of head trauma (Levin and colleagues, 1982), the evolution of the discipline of neuropsychology, the research on environmentally induced changes in the brain structure of lower organisms after injury (Rosenzweig, 1966, 1984), the formation and growth of the National Head Injury Foundation, and the perceived profitability of brain injury rehabilitation activites. As Leonard Diller (1988) has recently noted, it is no longer possible for a single individual to be generally familiar with the relevant research or the currently existing treatment programs. This was not the case a few years ago.

Cognitive rehabilitation has played a central role in the current head injury rehabilitation movement. It refers to a set of developing strategies of varied nature and scope, which have as their goal the improvement of cognitive impairments following brain injury or the minimization of their impact on daily functioning. These concepts are not new. Zangwill (1947) suggested that some psychological skills could be "retrained" through direct stimulation and that this would augment the more natural "compensation and substitution" reflective of natural recovery. A few studies appeared in the 1950s and 1960s exemplifying early cognitive rehabilitation attempts (Birch and colleagues 1961; Birch and Bortner, 1967; Shapiro, 1953).

Cognitive rehabilitation is a subject that generates both controversy and passionate discussion among neuroscientists and rehabilitation professionals. General reviews of head trauma rehabilitation practices, including cognitive rehabilitation, are beginning to accumulate (Caplan, 1987; Christensen and Uzzell, 1988; Meier and colleagues, 1987; Prigatano and colleagues, 1986; Rosenthal and colleagues, 1983; Uzzell and Gross, 1986). Cognitive rehabilitation, broadly defined, clearly plays an important role in comprehensive head trauma rehabilitation (Prigatano and colleagues, 1986; Prigatano, 1987). There is concern, however, that the current enthusiasm may promote naive practices based on a theoretical and empirical foundation more apparent than real. This chapter will attempt to outline theoretical and practical issues suggesting the need for a critical approach to cognitive rehabilitation. Such a critical perspective ensures that these strategies will continue to make an important and appropriate contribution to the general spectrum of head trauma rehabilitation practices and lends a note of caution to the untempered marketing and implementation of techniques of questionable validity.

COGNITIVE REHABILITATION: CONCEPTUAL ISSUES

There are essentially two related controversies concerning the current practice of cognitive rehabilitation. The first, and most primary, is whether cognitive rehabilitation activities affect meaningful life behaviors in any significant way. This is a question of the *criterion validity* (Cronbach and Meehl, 1955) of such procedures with the additional emphasis of meaningfulness, a concept captured by the term *ecologic validity* (Hart and Hayden, 1986). The second issue is whether changes in performance during cognitive rehabilitation reflect improvements in core cognitive skills (the amelioration of deficits) versus more basic changes in performance of a particular behavioral skill. Stated differently, do cognitive rehabilitation activities have *construct validity?* Note that affirmation of one of these need not require affirmation of the other. That is, changes in underlying cognitive processes could occur but remain insignificant with respect to daily life, and reliable transfer of training to a functional skill could occur without implying a general change in cognitive processes. Despite growth of cognitive rehabilitation activities for the brain injured, there are few data that adequately address either one of these two central questions. Before these points are discussed further, a few critical issues are reviewed.

METHODOLOGICAL ISSUES OF IMPORTANCE

History and Focal Brain Injury

The history of cognitive rehabilitation evolves from the study of individuals suffering from focal brain injuries (cerebral vascular accident, gunshot wound, tumor). For example, the treatment of language deficits following brain injury exemplifies a robust and relatively mature, although controversial, cognitive rehabilitation literature based primarily on the study of left hemisphere cerebral vascular accidents. With respect to "nonlanguage" cognitive functions, the body of knowledge is considerably smaller. Luria's (1963) classic discussion of the rehabilitation of complex cognitive skills was set within the framework of his theory of functional systems of human cognition and cerebral localization. This theoretical framework was derived primarily from his study of individuals with focal brain injuries (Luria, 1966). Much of the current practice of cognitive rehabilitation for victims of traumatic brain injury (TBI) rests on the pioneering work of rehabilitation psychologist from New York University Medical Center (Ben-Yishay and colleagues, 1970; Ben-Yishay and colleagues, 1974; Diller and Weinberg, 1977; Weinberg and colleagues, 1977, 1979). These authors published sophisticated accounts of the evaluation and remediation of visuoperceptual deficits among those suffering from stroke (primarily right hemisphere).

Although there is some commonality in the cognitive deficits shown by individuals with focal nontraumatic brain injuries and those suffering from TBI, the constellation of cognitive and behavioral deficits following head trauma appears in many ways qualitatively unique. Empirically, it remains to be demonstrated whether models and practices derived from the study of individuals with focal brain injury apply to the head trauma population (Gordon, 1987). Philosophically, core impairments in information-processing speed, inattention, learning and memory, abstraction, emotional and behavioral control, judgment, and personal awareness accompanying head trauma suggest the need for a unique set of cognitive rehabilitation strategies. Differences in age, premorbid characteristics, and existing psychosocial environments between TBI patients and those suffering cerebral vascular accidents (CVA) also lead to differing rehabilitation strategies and goals. Models of cognitive deficit, and accompanying methods of cognitive rehabilitation, specific to the brain-injured population have been developed in the 1980s (Ben-Yishay and Diller, 1983a, 1983b; Hagen and colleagues, 1979). Preliminary outcome data are accumulating, but further research is needed to determine whether these techniques are effective. It is clear, however, that the study of focal brain injury provides a rich heritage in the speech and language therapy literature, the work of Luria, and the excellent controlled studies of the New York University group.

Other Subject Variables

Studies attempting to demonstrate the efficacy of cognitive rehabilitation techniques need to employ appropriately controlled experimental designs. The heterogeneity of behavior and multiple complex determinants of dysfunction following head trauma suggests that both group and single case studies are needed (Gordon, 1987; Wilson, 1987). Rehabilitation efficacy must be demonstrated within an experimental setting that accounts for processes of natural recovery, natural variability, and alternative explanations for changes in function after treatment. Untreated or alternatively treated matched controls must be employed in group studies, while stability of dependent measures before, after, or during treatment must be demonstrated in single case design experiments. Controlled outcome studies are difficult, but not impossible, to implement in clinical settings (Prigatano and colleagues, 1984; Sohlberg and Mateer, 1987). Unfortunately, very few such studies are currently available.

Measurement Issues

Cognitive impairments are typically identified and assessed through neuropsychological tests. This "psychometric" tradition in neuropsychology was founded in efforts to diagnose brain lesions (Diller, 1987; Hart and Hayden, 1986). Most neuropsychological test batteries are composed of instruments that have demonstrated some validity for this enterprise. The relationship between these same tests and the daily problems in functioning experienced by those surviving severe TBI remains unclear. This issue will be discussed in more detail in a later section.

A problem impeding the development of ecologically valid cognitive assessment and retraining instruments is the relative absence of reliable and valid methods of measuring or quantifying the behavioral disturbance or psychosocial difficulties of the TBI patient (Hart and Hayden, 1986). Behavioral observation methods applied to the brain-injured individual's natural environments would be most helpful but are time-consuming and expensive to develop, validate, and use. Rating scales based on behavior observed in clinical settings (Levin and colleagues, 1987) may assist in expanding on strictly psychometric measures of impairment. Such instruments, however, also must be validated against overt behavior in appropriate natural environments. Rating scales of behavioral and emotional dysfunction completed by cohabitating relatives are available (Brooks and McKinlay, 1983; Prigatano and colleagues, 1984; Thomsen, 1974; Weddell and colleagues, 1980) but are biased by the attitudes and perceptions of the particular relative. Until reliable measures of behavioral dysfunction in the natural environment of the individual with TBI are established, demonstrations of meaningful changes in function as a result of cognitive rehabilitation will prove problematic.

Levels of Analysis and Intervention

Clinicians attempting to assist individuals in overcoming the consequences of TBI delimit a set of rehabilitation targets. This process presupposes a decision about apparent levels of intervention of great conceptual importance. The distinction between impairments and disabilities is helpful in understanding these conceptual issues as they relate to the practice of cognitive rehabilitation. As elaborated by Diller (Ben-Yishay and Diller, 1983a; Diller, 1987, 1988), impairments are losses of cognitive "structures or functions," while disabilities refer to difficulties in performing functional daily activities. Disabilities are more overt behavioral expressions of impairments, but there is no one-to-one correspondence between the magnitude of "tested" impairment and the degree of disability. This is demonstrated at the level of both group (Bond, 1975; Hart and

Hayden, 1986; Heaton and colleagues, 1978) and individual (Diller, 1987; Hart and Hayden, 1986) case analyses by the often modest relationships between neuropsychological test performance and apparent psychosocial competency. Disabilities become "handicaps" when they affect the person's capacity to perform in various specific natural settings or statuses (Diller, 1987). Thus, a memory impairment, contributing to a disability in meeting scheduled appointments, could lead to a handicap in a work environment (status) demanding such behavior. If the handicap is sufficiently severe, a major change in status (unemployment) could occur, a result all too common to the survivors of severe TBI.

A question of great importance, given the current knowledge base, concerns the level at which scarce rehabilitation efforts and resources should be allocated. For cognitive rehabilitation, this translates into a question of what should be emphasized: impairment remediation or the development of skills or systems that might act to minimize the impact of such impairments (see several discussions in Meier and colleagues, 1987). Since it is now clear that even the most severely amnestic individuals can learn and develop some new skills if provided with the appropriate learning opportunities (Squire and Butters, 1984, Schachter and Glisky, 1986), intervention at the level of disability has some empirical foundation. Further support for the practice of skill development in rehabilitation derives from the traditional rehabilitation literature. It would clearly be desirable to facilitate recovery of central cognitive impairments. This could lead to a general reduction in disability or handicap without the need for multiple skill training enterprises specific to each of the major roles or statuses confronted by the brain-injured individual (Bracy, 1984). Unfortunately, very few data suggest that the chronic cognitive impairments resulting from TBI can be improved through systematic rehabilitation efforts. At this time the available literature is most suggestive of a modest increase in the individual's capacity to employ existing cognitive functions (Ben-Yishay and colleagues, 1985; Prigatano, 1987). As will be seen, even this augmented efficiency must be viewed with caution.

CONSTRUCT VALIDITY, ECOLOGICAL VALIDITY, AND GENERALIZABILITY

Cognitive rehabilitation typically employs computer programs, paper and pencil materials, or other procedures that appear to require or elicit responses phenomenologically related to the targeted cognitive process. That is, cognitive rehabilitation procedures possess a reasonable degree of face validity (Cronbach and Meehl, 1955). For example, Weinberg and colleagues (1977) attempted to reduce disability associated with left visual neglect by training 25 individuals suffering right hemisphere CVA on a set of cued reading and visual scanning materials that maximized the probability the individual would look to the left. They also employed a visual scanning machine, a clearly nonpsychometric method. Sohlberg and Mateer (1987) trained four brain-injured individuals (two with head trauma, one with a ruptured aneurysm, one with a gunshot wound) on a series of increasingly more difficult tasks requiring focused, sustained, selective, alternating, and divided attention to paper and pencil auditory and visual information. They employed a single-case, multiple-baseline study. Although the training data for these two studies were not provided, it appears the subjects improved their performance with guided practice on these face-valid tasks. It is not clear, however, that core attentional impairments were "remediated" in either case. Rather, these results may indicate that a particular psychomotor skill, performance on tasks similar to those used in training, has been learned or made more efficient.

In the neuropsychology and cognitive rehabilitation literatures, tests are typically seen as markers for an underlying cognitive function (or deficit). Thus, "attention," "memory," and "executive function" are not directly determinable but aspire to be theoretical constructs in the traditional psychological sense (Cronbach and Meehl, 1955; Hogan and Nicholson, 1988). Improved performance on training or testing indicators does not imply that the underlying psychological construct (cognitive process) has *probably* been improved. Such affirmation is possible only if validated through systematic research strategies based on, and defining, a system of laws and supporting empirical relationships. Although a conceptual framework for establishing the validity of the construct of *remediable cognitive processes* has been reasonably well outlined (see, for example, Gordon, 1987; Seron, 1987), there are only limited supporting data. As cognitive rehabilitation techniques continue to proliferate, this state of affairs would seem to dictate a certain degree of professional discomfort.

It certainly is possible to perform a weak test of the hypothesis, either in research or clinical settings, that cognitive processes can be retrained following TBI. The central requirement of such a test is that there be reliable accompanying changes in behaviors dissimilar, but conceptually related, to the operationally defined processes being trained and that there be no change in responses conceptually unrelated to training procedures (e.g., Campbell and Fiske, 1959). Thus, the cognitive rehabilitation construct validation process requires the demonstration of the generalization of gains to related untrained behavioral indicators. Note that in the clinical setting there is an added burden of demonstrating that functional behaviors of importance to the brain-injured individual are affected.

Most cognitive rehabilitation outcome studies test efficacy on instruments similar to those used for training. Rarely are functional measures obtained to determine whether interventions reduced some important aspect of disability. These demonstrations become crucial given the standard practice of rehabilitating cognitive processes in settings removed from the complexities of the everyday world. Such methods follow from the reasonable need to simplify and control the stimuli impinging on, and range of response alternatives available to, the brain-injured individual (Ben-Yishay and Diller, 1983b). Even demonstrations of transfer of training to related psychometric instruments are subject to interpretations other than those implying that a cognitive function has been remediated.

Weinberg and colleagues (1977) appear to have demonstrated some degree of treatment generalization for individuals suffering from CVA on three sets of test and rating scale measures varying in their similarity to the training materials. The more similar the neuropsychological test measures were to the training tasks, the more robust the apparent effects of treatment. Sohlberg and Mateer (1987) assessed efficacy on a test of auditory attention (Paced Auditory Serial Addition Test) not grossly dissimilar to some of the materials used in their attention training program. In this multiple baseline study, control tests of visuoperceptual processing did not improve during attention training (even though attention might be thought to play a role in such a process). Analyses of parallel change in functional disability levels were not undertaken in either the Weinberg and colleagues (1977) or the Sohlberg and Mateer (1987) studies.

Rattok and colleagues (1982) and Ben-Yishay and colleagues (1987) analyzed the impact of an auditory and visual attention training program on 40 survivors of severe head trauma well beyond the early stages of recovery. Note that training occurred within the framework of an intensive day treatment program in which other therapeutic activities also were present. Training data are provided, and the mean scores of the head trauma group improved to average levels and even exceeded those obtained by normal controls. The dependent psychometric measures, including ratings of social and behavioral competency, showed modest and variable gains after treatment, with the most improvement seemingly again on tests similar to the training tasks.

The Ben-Yishay and colleagues (1987), Rattok and colleagues (1982), Sohlberg and Mateer (1987), and Weinberg and colleagues (1977) studies suggest a gradient of psychometric generalizability, whereby the relative absence of transfer of training implies a greater degree of functional independence between the processes being trained and the test measures (Seron, 1987). Again, the obtained psychometric generalization does not necessarily imply that the core cognitive deficit presumably tapped by such instruments has been improved. The more parsimonious explanation is that the cognitive rehabilitation activities led to the learning of a specific behavioral skill, which is emitted more effectively in circumstances most like those present during initial training. Given the modest evidence for transfer of training to psychometric instruments, it becomes more difficult to accept, without validation, that such transfer would occur to complex behaviors needed to function in daily living situations. The fact that the correlation between psychometrically measured impairment and psychosocial dysfunction is often small also dictates caution in expecting that practice on such instruments would affect functional disabilities.

A few examples of the demonstrated transfer of gains realized in the cognitive rehabilitation of visuoperceptual skills are available. Ben-Yishay and colleagues (1987) present a case study of head trauma suggesting carryover of attentional training to more functional daily behaviors. This is a narrative report, however, without empirical analysis. The authors further note that among the larger group studied there was great variability among subjects in both the degree of improvement resulting from training and the degree of transfer to more functional behaviors. Diller and colleagues (Diller and colleagues, 1974; Diller and Weinberg, 1977) present data suggesting transfer of visuoperceptual training effects to some behaviors of daily living (eating) among victims of CVA. One study has been found that compared ratings of disability among brain-injured individuals (primarily TBI) receiving 30 sessions of outpatient cognitive rehabilitation to those obtained by similar untreated patients (Fryer and Haffey, 1987). The authors maintain that treatment effects were still apparent at 1 year followup. Replication of these results with alternatively treated controls, behavioral measures of disability, and blind ratings of outcome are needed before assuming that cognitive rehabilitation alone was responsible for the effects. The specific methods of retraining are not described but were reported to be directed toward a range of cognitive processes.

The rehabilitation of nonlinguistic cognitive processes other than attention are less frequently described. A review of the memory retraining literature is presented elsewhere in this text. This literature suggests little evidence for systematic changes in memory processes or for the demonstration of meaningful generalization for any changes obtained (O'Connor and Cermak, 1987; Schachter and Glisky, 1986).

In summary, the construct of cognitive rehabilitation for the TBI patient has yet to be validated. This is especially true with respect to the requirement of generalization to real-life behaviors of functional significance likely dependent on the trained responses. This does not mean that core cognitive impairments cannot be improved, although that is certainly a possibility. If changes are occurring, it is not yet clear whether they yield any meaningful improvement in the brain-injured individual's overall level of psychosocial functioning. The author does not feel that cognitive rehabilitation strategies should be abandoned. In fact, they play a crucial role in comprehensive head trauma rehabilitation activities. The next section will describe ways in which cognitive rehabilitation work can promote more positive psychosocial outcome.

COMPONENTS OF COMPREHENSIVE REHABILITATION

HOLISTIC REHABILITATION AND LEVELS OF INTERVENTION

Comprehensive holistic rehabilitation strategies for the multitude of disabilities and handicaps accompanying TBI have been described (Ben-Yishay and colleagues, 1985; Prigatano and colleagues, 1986). These programs intervene at multiple levels for various problem domains, all occurring within a social rehabilitation environment. Thus a specific cognitive deficit is addressed at the level of impairment through cognitive rehabilitation strategies; at the level of specific disabilities through appropriate skill building, compensation development, and role playing; and at the level of handicaps and statuses through guidance and practice in managing everyday environments and recommendations on specific environmental modifications. Individual and group rehabilitation interventions are constructed so that the relevant cognitive, physical, emotional, and social impairments are addressed at these different levels in an integrated fashion.

There are multiple reasons why this approach makes sense. First, we have seen that there is little evidence that cognitive rehabilitation alone will have a significant general impact on important disabilities. The behavioral manifestations of disability after head injury must be addressed directly. Second, the most disabling aspects of the cognitive sequelae accompanying head trauma are those affecting social functioning in the family, leisure, and vocational environments. That is, a memory impairment is significant to the extent that it creates social disability. Because any improvements derived from cognitive rehabilitation appear not to transfer to the level of social disability, rehabilitation must take place in environments that foster such generalization. Isolated individual cognitive rehabilitation would not seem to be a particularly meaningful enterprise. Individuals suffering brain injury need active guidance and instruction in generalizing learned strategies to meaningful life settings (Ben-Yishay and Diller, 1983b). Finally, in the author's experience, it is rare that cognitive dysfunction (narrowly defined) serves as the major hurdle preventing adequate psychosocial adjustment. The distinction between cognitive deficits and emotional dysfunction is arbitrary (Hart and Hayden, 1986). Yet it appears that it is the brain-injured individual's capacity to understand, accept, and adjust to the residual losses that appears to determine the ultimate degree of psychosocial success (Prigatano and colleagues, 1986). Often this adjustment process depends as much on the individual's personality, social, intellectual, and emotional characteristics before the injury than on the degree of post traumatic cognitive impairment. Isolated cognitive rehabilitation without a parallel emphasis on emotional and social dysfunction makes little sense for most individuals with TBI.

THE ROLE OF COGNITIVE REHABILITATION

Cognitive rehabilitation, in the form of the systematically organized practice of cognitive skills, does play an important role in the general framework of holistic rehabilitation of brain-injured individuals. The purposes of such techniques include the following:

Potentially Improved Cognitive Efficiency

Despite the generally cautionary note emphasized by the author, it is important that cognitive rehabilitation research continue. Clinical practice should be undertaken in a fashion that maximizes the chances that meaningful program evaluation data are obtained. That is, those practicing cognitive rehabilitation from the narrow perspective of "retraining" impaired skills have an obligation to attempt to demonstrate treatment efficacy. Single-case-design methodologies may be particularly helpful in that process (Wilson, 1987). At this point there is a suggestion that multiple hours of cognitive rehabilitation practice *may* increase general skills on tests of attention and speed of information processing (Ben-Yishay and colleagues 1985; Prigatano, 1987), although it is not clear there is functional generalization. It would be reasonable to retain cognitive rehabilitation within holistic rehabilitation practices if these general improvements are a desired outcome. The relatively small average changes in test scores, given the amount of treatment provided (Schachter and Glisky, 1986) is sobering, however.

Specific Skill Development

As noted, even the most severely amnestic individuals can acquire new complex psychomotor and cognitive skills through systematic and repetitive practice. As conceptualized by Cohen (1984), individuals with brain injury are often better at learning procedures (how to do things) then they are at learning new content or information. Guided practice in cognitive rehabilitation materials may be the only effective way to learn some new skills that are of importance to the individual's overall adjustment. Schacter and Glisky (1986), for example, demonstrate a program whereby individuals with memory impairments were taught the procedures of microcomputer operation as a preliminary step to helping them use the computer to manage other aspects of their lives more effectively. There may be a multitude of skills related to home or work environments that could be learned and developed within the confines of typical cognitive rehabilitation settings. Note that there still must be some active attempt to assist with generalization to environments in which such skills will be used.

Enhanced Awareness of Impairments and Skills

It is now widely recognized that many individuals surviving severe head trauma may have limited awareness, and acceptance, of the nature or magnitude of residual deficits in thinking and psychosocial functioning (Prigatano and colleagues, 1986; Fordyce and Roueche, 1986). Limitations in awareness or acceptance appear to have significant negative implications for adequate psychosocial adjustment. Individual cognitive rehabilitation practices are powerful tools in simplifying and clarifying the nature of residual impairments in thinking so that the brain-injured individual may better understand them. Group cognitive rehabilitation sessions have the added benefit of allowing the participant to view the thinking and behavioral deficits of others, providing an additional perspective for understanding his or her own cognitive inefficiencies. When these cognitive rehabilitation sessions are actively linked by the therapist to the behavioral and social impairments evidenced in other aspects of the holistic rehabilitation program, the opportunity for the patient to gain some degree of personal insight is maximized.

Whether the information obtained during rehabilitation activities is accepted by the individual is, of course, another matter. The interweaving of cognitive rehabilitation with more general rehabilitation activities in a social environment would seem to have the best chance of promoting such acceptance, however. In fact, a nonconfrontive hypothesis testing approach to self-awareness during cognitive rehabilitation may be most effective in overcoming denial (Prigatano, 1987). Finally, while many brain-injured individuals have trouble with awareness or acceptance of deficits, a significant number are emotionally devastated and are unable to acknowledge their cognitive skills (Fordyce and Roueche, 1986). Cognitive rehabilitation work can apprise participants of their thinking talents as well as their difficulties. Such activities may serve as a tool in helping individuals deal with depression.

*Provide a Forum for Exploring
Appropriate Compensations in Light
of Residual Cognitive Deficits*

In addition to fostering skill development and enhancing awareness, cognitive rehabilitation settings offer an opportunity for the therapist and brain-injured individual to explore compensations and adaptations that may prove effective in minimizing the psychosocial impact of residual cognitive impairments. An opportunity to practice these "new" ways of doing old things in the relatively safe and restricted environment of the cognitive rehabilitation setting provides a type of "ground school" on which later direct practical applications can be based. Memory books for forgetfulness, or verbal compensations for communication deficits, are examples of strategies most effectively learned first in individual cognitive rehabilitation sessions.

CONCLUSIONS

This chapter has attempted to outline a conservative appreciation of the practice of cognitive rehabilitation. There is considerable work that remains to be accomplished in understanding how best to facilitate recovery from severe TBI. In general, it appears that significant cognitive impairments are relatively resistant to rehabilitative efforts given our current state of knowledge. It is suggested, however, that formal cognitive rehabilitation work is an important component of more general intervention strategies. It must be viewed at this time, however, as something more than a set of techniques to improve central cognitive impairments. The cost effectiveness of intensive postacute holistic rehabilitation for the TBI patient is not yet known. It now appears that approximately 50 percent of head trauma survivors have some major improvement in psychosocial status as a result of comprehensive rehabilitation (Prigatano, 1987). With time and additional research it may be possible to improve these figures. For now, we are left with admittedly expensive programs that are supported by some initial outcome data, are based on reasonable clinical practices, and appear to offer the best chance for overcoming the tragedy of TBI.

REFERENCES

Ben-Yishay, Y., and Diller, L. (1983a). Cognitive Deficits. In M. Rosenthal, E.R. Griffith, M.R. Bond, and J.D. Miller (Eds.), *Rehabilitation of the head injured adult* (pp. 167–184). Philadelphia: Davis.

Ben-Yishay, Y., and Diller, L. (1983b). Cognitive Remediation. In M. Rosenthal, E.R. Griffith, M.R. Bond, and J.D. Miller (Eds.), *Rehabilitation of the head injured adult* (pp. 367–380). Philadelphia: Davis.

Ben-Yishay, Y., Diller, L., Gerstman, L.J., and Gordon, W.A. (1970). Relationships between initial competence and ability to profit from cues in brain damaged individuals. *Journal of Abnormal Psychology, 75*, 248–259.

Ben-Yishay, Y., Diller, L., Mandelberg, I., Gordon, W.A., and Gerstman, L.J. (1974). Differences in matching persistence behavior during block design performance between older normal and brain damaged persons: A process analysis. *Cortex, 10*, 121–347.

Ben-Yishay, Y., Piasetsky, E.B., and Rattok, J. (1987). A systematic method for ameliorating disorders of basic attention. In M. Meier, A. Benton, and L. Diller (Eds.), *Neuropsychological rehabilitation* (pp. 165–181). New York: The Guilford Press.

Ben-Yishay, Y., Rattok, J., Lakin, P., Piasetsky, E.B., Ross, B., Silver, S., Zide, E., and Ezrachi, O. (1985). Neuropsychologic rehabilitation. *Seminars in Neurology, 5*, 252–258.

Birch, H.G., Belmont, I., Reilly, T., and Belmont, L. (1961). Visual verticality in hemiplegia. *Archives of Neurology, 5*, 444–453.

Birch, H.G., and Bortner, M. (1967). Stimulus competition and concept utilization in brain damaged children. *Developmental Medicine and Child Neurology, 9*, 402–410.

Bond, M. (1975). Assesment of psychosocial outcome after severe head injury. *CIBA Foundation Symposium, 34*, 141–153.

Bracy, O. (1984). Editor's note. *Cognitive Rehabilitation, 2*, 2.

Brooks, M., and McKinlay, W. (1983). Personality and behavior change after blunt head injury: A relative's view. *Journal of Neurology, Neurosurgery, and Psychiatry, 46*, 336–344.

Campbell, D.P., and Fiske, D.W. (1959). Convergent and discriminant validity in the multitrait-multimethod matrix. *Psycholgocial Bulletin, 56*, 81–105.

Caplan, B. (Ed.) (1987). *Rehabilitation psychology desk reference.* Rockville: Aspen Publishers.

Christensen, A., and Uzzell, B. (Eds.) (1988). *Neuropsychological rehabilitation.* Boston: Kluwer Academic Publishers.

Cohen, N.J. (1984). Preserved learning capacity in amnesia: Evidence for multiple memory systems. In L.R. Squire, and N.R. Butters (Eds.), *Neuropsychology of memory* (pp. 83–103). New York: The Guilford Press.

Cronbach L. J., and Meehl, P.E. (1955). Construct validity in psychological tests. *Psychological Bulletin, 52*, 281–302.

Diller, L. (1987). Neuropsychological rehabilitation. In M. Meier, A. Benton, and L. Diller (Eds.), *Neuropsychological rehabilitation* (pp. 3–17). New York: The Guilford Press.

Diller, L. (1988). Rehabilitation in traumatic brain injury—observations on the current US scene. In A. Christensen and B. Uzzell (Eds.), *Neuropsychological rehabilitation* (pp. 53–68). Boston: Kluwer Academic Publishers.

Diller, L., Ben-Yishay, Y., Gerstman, L.J., Goodkin, R., Gordon, W., and Weinberg, J. (1974). Studies in cognition and rehabilitation in hemiplegia. *Rehabilitation Monograph 50*, New York University Medical Center, New York.

Diller, L., and Weinberg, J.M. (1977). Hemi-inattention in rehabilitation: The evolution of a rationale remediation program. In E.A. Weinstein and R.P. Friedland (Eds.), *Advances in neurology.* New York: Raven Press.

Fordyce, D., and Roueche, J.R. (1986). Changes in perspectives of disability among patients, staff, and relatives during rehabilitation of brain injury. *Rehabilitation Psychology, 31,* 217–229.

Fryer, L., and Haffey, W. (1987). Cognitive rehabilitation and community readaptation: Outcome from two program models. *Journal of Head Trauma Rehabilitation, 2,* 51–63.

Gordon, W.A. (1987). Methodological considerations in cognitive remediation. In M. Meier, A. Benton, and L. Diller (Eds.), *Neuropsychological rehabilitation* (pp. 111–131). New York: The Guilford Press.

Hagen, C., Malkmus, D., and Durham, P. (1979). Levels of cognitive functioning. In *Rehabilitation of the head-injured adult: Comprehensive physical management*. Professional Staff Association of Ranchos Los Amigos Hospital, Downey, CA.

Hart, T., and Hayden, M.E. (1986). The ecological validity of neuropsychological assessment and remediation. In B. Uzzell and Y. Gross (Eds.), *Clinical neuropsychology of intervention* (pp. 21–50). Boston: Martinus Nijhoff Publishing.

Heaton, R., Chelune, G., and Lehman, R. (1978). Using neuropsychologcial and personality tests to assess the likelihood of patient employment. *Journal of Nervous and Mental Disease, 166,* 408–416.

Hogan, R., and Nicholson, R.A. (1988). The meaning of personality test scores. *American Psychologist, 43,* 621–626.

Levin, H.S., Benton, A.L., and Grossman, R.G. (1982). *Neurobehavioral consequences of closed head injury*. New York: Oxford University Press.

Levin, H.S., High, W., Goethe, K., Sisson, R., Overall, J., Rhoades, H., Eisenberg, H., Kalisky, Z., and Gary, H. (1987). The neurobehavioral rating scale: Assessment of the behavioral sequelae of head injury by the clinician. *Journal of Neurology, Neurosurgery, and Psychiatry, 50,* 183–193.

Luria, A.R. (1963). *Restoration of function after brain Injury*. Oxford: Pergamon Press.

Luria, A.R. (1966). *Higher cortical functions in man*. New York: Basic Books.

Meier, M., Benton, A., and Diller L. (Eds.) (1987). *Neuropsychological rehabilitation* New York: The Guilford Press.

O'Connor, M., and Cermak, L. S. (1987). Rehabilitation of organic memory disorders. In M. Meier, A. Benton, and L. Diller (Eds.), *Neuropsychological rehabilitation* (pp. 260–279). New York: The Guilford Press.

Prigatano, G.P. (1987). Recovery and cognitive retraining after craniocerebral trauma. *Journal of Learning Disabilities, 20,* 603–613.

Prigatano, G.P., Fordyce, D.J., Zeiner, H.K., Roueche, J.R., Pepping, M, and Wood, B.C. (1984). Neuropsychological rehabilitation after closed head injury in young adults. *Journal of Neurology, Neurosurgery, and Psychiatry, 47,* 505–513.

Prigatano, G.P., and Others (1986). *Neuropsychological rehabilitation after brain injury*. Baltimore: Johns Hopkins University Press.

Rattok, J., Ben-Yishay, Y., Ross, B., Lakin, P., Silver, S., Thomas, L., and Diller, L. (1982). A diagnostic remedial system for basic attention disorders in head trauma patients undergoing rehabilitation: A preliminary report. In Y. Ben-Yishay (Ed.), *Working approaches to remediation of cognitive deficits in brain damaged persons* (pp. 177–187). *Rehabilitation Monograph 66,* New York University Medical Center, New York.

Rosenthal, M., Griffith, E.R., Bond, M.R., and Miller, J.D. (Eds.) (1983). *Rehabilitation of the head injured adult*. Philadelphia: Davis.

Rosenzweig, M.R. (1966). Environmental complexity, cerebral change, and behavior. *American Psychologist, 21,* 321–332.

Rosenzweig, M.R. (1984). Experience, memory, and the brain. *American Psychologist, 39,* 365–376.

Schachter, D.L., and Glisky, E.L. (1986). Memory remediation: Restoration, alleviation, and the acquisition of domain-specific knowledge. In B. Uzzell and Y. Gross (Eds.), *Clinical neuropsychology of intervention* (pp. 257–282). Boston: Martinus Nijhoff Publishing.

Seron, X. (1987). Operant procedures and neuropsychologcial rehabilitation. In M. Meier, A. Benton, and L. Diller (Eds.), *Neuropsychological rehabilitation* (pp. 132–162). New York: The Guilford Press.

Shapiro, M.B. (1953). Experimental studies of a perceptual anomaly. III. The testing of an explanatory theory. *Journal of Mental Science, 99*, 394–409.

Sohlberg, M., and Mateer, C. (1987). Effectiveness of an attention training program. *Journal of Clinical and Experimental Neuropsychology, 9*, 117–130.

Squire, L.R., and Butters, N. (Eds.) (1984). *Neuropsychology of memory.* New York: The Guilford Press.

Thomsen, I. (1974). The patient with severe head injury and his family. *Scandinavian Journal of Rehabilitation Medicine, 6*, 180–183.

Uzzell, B., and Gross, Y. (Eds.) (1986). *Neuropsychology of intervention.* Boston: Martinus Nijhoff Publishing.

Weddell, R., Oddy, M., and Jenkins, D. (1980). Social adjustment after rehabilitation: A two-year follow-up of patients with severe head injury. *Psychological Medicine, 10*, 257–263.

Weinberg, J., Diller, L., Gordon, W., Gerstman, L., Lieberman, A., Lakin, P., Hodges, G., and Ezrachi, O. (1977). Visual scanning training effect on reading-related tasks in acquired right brain damage. *Archives of Physical Medicine and Rehabilitation, 58*, 479–486.

Weinberg, J., Diller, L., Gordon, W., Gerstman, L., Lieberman, A., Lakin, P., Hodges, G., and Ezrachi, O. (1979). Training sensory awareness and spatial organization in people with right brain damage. *Archives of Physical Medicine and Rehabilitation, 60*, 491–496.

Wilson, B. (1987). Single-case experimental designs in neuropsychological rehabilitation. *Journal of Clinical and Experimental Nueropsychology, 9*, 527–544.

Zangwill, O. (1947). Psychological aspects of rehabilitation in cases of brain injury. *British Journal of Psychology, 37*, 60–69.

BIBLIOGRAPHY

Cronbach L. J., and Meehl, P.E. (1955). Construct validity in psychological tests. *Psychological Bulletin, 52*, 281–302.
This important paper provides a classic discussion of the relationship between tests and the underlying traits they purport to measure. It highlights the experimental and logical steps required to understand what a particular test score signifies.

Meier, M., Benton, A., and Diller L. (Eds.) (1987). *Neuropsychological rehabilitation.* New York: The Guilford Press.
This edited text provides a recent review of the methodologic factors important in understanding and practicing cognitive rehabilitation techniques as well as a critical review of the outcome data currently available.

Prigatano, G.P., and Others (1986). *Neuropsychological rehabilitation after brain injury.* Baltimore: Johns Hopkins University Press.
This book includes a series of papers describing aspects of a comprehensive brain injury rehabilitation approach with a strong emphasis on psychosocial dysfunction. It places

cognitive rehabilitation enterprises within a framework emphasizing the psychological issues of awareness and acceptance of deficits.

Sohlberg, M., and Mateer, C. (1987). Effectiveness of an attention training program. *Journal of Clinical and Experimental Neuropsychology, 9,* 117–130.

This paper provides excellent examples of how it is possible to research the efficacy of cognitive rehabilitation techniques with single-case experimental designs. Although indicating eloquent changes in test scores as a result of systematic cognitive retraining activities, it fails to assess generalization to related functional behaviors.

CHAPTER 5

Evaluation of Neuropsychological Status After Traumatic Brain Injury

JAY M. UOMOTO

A mind of slow comprehension is, accordingly, not necessarily a weak mind, just as one of quick comprehension is not always profound but is often very superficial. . . . Lack of judgment, in the absence of wit, is stupidity (stupiditas). The same lack, wit being present, is absurdity. He who shows judgment in business is clever. If he has wit along with it, he is called smart. . . . Simple-minded is he who cannot take much into his mind; but he is not on that account stupid, unless he misunderstands what he does take in (From Immanuel Kant, *Classification of Mental Disorders*, 1798)

Kant's typology of mental disorders was rather simple, with four major disturbances—senselessness, madness, absurdity, and frenzy. Although these labels are obviously outdated, the method remains essentially the same as in neuropsychology today. Based on systematic observation of the patient, differentiation of what is observed, testing hypotheses about behavior, and classifying the result, the neuropsychologist is able to infer aspects of brain functioning and make predictive statements about an individual's behavior. Hence, neuropsychological assessment is based on a thorough understanding of brain-behavior relationships.

The behavioral output of the patient seen during the course of neuro-psychological evaluation must be understood within the context of a model of cognitive functioning and organization. Reitan and Wolfson (1985) have outlined such a model. Each component of the model presented in Figure 5-1 corresponds to a set of evaluation procedures. A three-part organization of the CNS is hypothesized with verbal and language abilities, visuospatial abilities, and conceptual reasoning skill represented. At the outset, sensory input must be received by the individual. Specifically input is received primarily through visual, auditory, and tactile modalities. Impairment at this level can lead to functional deficits in any of the above areas. Reitan and Wolfson (1985) refer to this stage of processing as the "registration phase" (p. 6).

Attention, concentration, and memory is the next level of processing in the Reitan-Wolfson model. The individual must be able to sustain concentration on the task at hand to the point that a memory trace of the event is encoded and information is stored in short-term memory. Higher-order cognitive skills such as abstract reasoning and concept formation may be intact; however, if basic attentional processes are impaired, then the individual's functional output may be impaired. The next mode of processing occurs with lateralized function performed by the cerebral hemispheres. Verbal reasoning and language abilities are primarily left cerebral hemisphere tasks, whereas visuospatial and perceptual skills involve mainly right cerebral hemisphere functions. At the highest level of analysis, the individual must integrate all that has occurred in other stages of cognitive processing and use this information to reason logically. Abstract reasoning, complex problem solving,

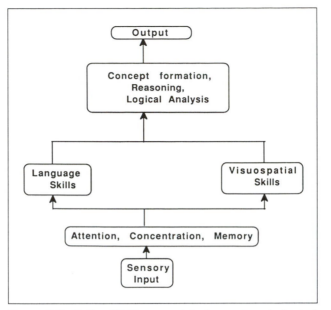

Figure 5-1. Reitan-Wolfson model of neuropsychological functioning.

and logical analysis represent the final function of the brain before the actual behavioral output. Although this model presents a somewhat simplified view of the cognitive processes that occur in any action, it is a rather testable model and has been used as the basis for many neuropsychological measures, particularly the Halstead-Reitan Neuropsychological Battery.

In a comprehensive review of the functions associated with the frontal lobes Stuss-Benson (1986) proposed a model of higher cortical functioning (Figure 5-2). The first level of processing in this hierarchical model includes attention to cognition itself. As one moves up in the hierarchy, functions such as drive, sequencing, and anticipation involve the frontal lobes to an increasingly greater degree. The highest level of processing is that of self-awareness, which includes the ability to self-evaluate and self-consciousness. Impairment in self-awareness in the patient with traumatic brain injury (TBI) can lead to difficulties in community safety due to the patient's having little self-knowledge of cognitive deficits (e.g., marked reduced recent memory ability; limited complex problem-solving skills). A person with TBI may see no reason to avoid driving despite poor quick decision-making ability and dense memory deficits that may lead to an accident or getting lost. Many of the aspects of this model are impaired in persons with TBI.

Conducting neuropsychological evaluations with TBI patients must

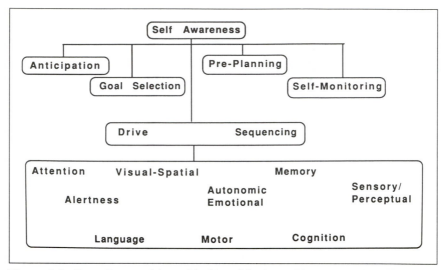

Figure 5-2. Stuss-Benson hierarchical model of cognitive processing. Emphasis is placed on the frontal lobe's role in mediating behavior.

also take into account a host of noncognitive variables that inevitably change the interpretation of test results. Figure 5-3 depicts cognitive functioning within the larger framework of the social, vocational, emotional, and physical variables that affect the daily lives of individuals with TBI. For example, the presence of acute or chronic pain (e.g., intermittent or persistent posttraumatic headaches, low back pain secondary to a motor vehicle accident, acute burn pains) can add attentional deficits due to preoccupation with the pain. An individual who may have been in a manual labor occupation may be less affected on the job by a language problem than a business marketer or salesperson.

Neuropsychological evaluation may yield extensive information about the patient; however, it does not specify the sequences of causality that occur. For example, in Figure 5-4, although decreased attention-concentration ability may be diagnosed by a neuropsychological evaluation, it does not specify whether or to what extent this is the cause or effect of a sequence of events. In this example, emotional dyscontrol (such as anger or depression) may lead to decreased attention. This in turn can affect memory ability, thus leading to impairment in functional daily skills (e.g., remembering important appointments). Furthermore, one's self-coping abilities are taxed, leading to further emotional dyscontrol, and the cycle continues. These sequences underscore the need to interpret beyond the testing data per se and include the environmental context, both internal and external to the patient.

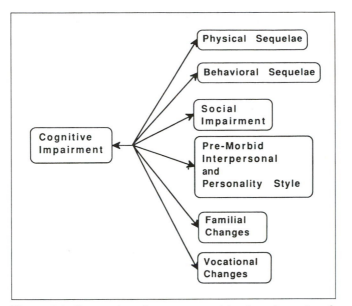

Figure 5-3. Interactions between cognitive impairment and noncognitive variables.

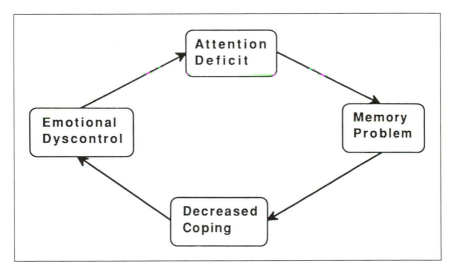

Figure 5-4. Sequences of causality between cognitive variables and emotional-coping responses.

MAJOR PURPOSES OF NEUROPSYCHOLOGICAL EVALUATIONS IN TRAUMATIC BRAIN INJURY

NEUROLOGIC DIAGNOSIS

After a minor head injury, individuals may experience brief loss of consciousness, transient posttraumatic amnesia, and Glasgow Coma Scale scores of between 13 and 15. These individuals may experience a set of neurobehavioral sequelae often referred to as a postconcussion syndrome (Horwitz, 1960). Diffuse axonal stretching and sheering may occur that cannot be identified outside of neuropathologic studies on autopsy. Neuropsychological evaluation may document cognitive impairments that are not found by medical testing and thus lend some explanation for the behavioral sequelae seen in minor head injury.

Another issue in the use of neuropsychological testing is in the differential diagnosis of psychological disorders and brain damage. A common case is that of differentiating between clinical depression and brain dysfunction resulting from trauma. Affective dysfunction is a very common concomitant to brain damage (Ruckdeschel-Hibbard and colleagues, 1986). Depression contributes to additional cognitive deficits in terms of decreased concentration, recent memory deficits, and slowed psychomotor response. Part of the task of neuropsychological assessment is to identify the presence of depression and determine if it contributes to cognitive deficits.

The coexistence of alcohol-drug abuse and brain injury is not uncommon, and such dual diagnoses can pose difficult questions when one is asked to determine prognosis and develop rehabilitation strategies. Neuropsychological assessment may be necessary to differentiate deficits due to chronic alcoholism (e.g., recent memory deficits) and those attributable to TBI. Although some trends in the pattern of test results have been shown among alcoholics (Brandt and Butters, 1986; Ryan and colleagues, 1980) and drug abusers (Carlin, 1986), less is known about the combined effect of brain injury and alcohol-drug abuse.

IDENTIFICATION OF ASSETS AND DEFICITS

Even though a large part of medical practice is focused on deficit remediation and prevention of secondary medical complications, in rehabilitating the brain-injured patient it is equally important to identify and capitalize on the patient's cognitive and behavioral assets to plan appropriate rehabilitation. It can be argued that this is the primary use of neuropsychological evaluation in the TBI population, and this adds unique and important information over and beyond that obtained by medical tests. Testing results can be used to predict which training methods are likely or unlikely to work with a particular patient. For example, if a patient demonstrates greater difficulty in verbal recent memory ability yet maintains good visual retention skills, the training strategy will be to "show" rather than "tell" the patient what to do. This information can also help family members understand why the individual with TBI becomes confused with lengthy discussions or instructions. Assessment of the speed with which a person processes cognitive information may yield information about the rate of learning capacity a patient possesses and thus implicate a "step-at-a-time" approach to training. By maximizing the particular strategies that best enable the patient to perform tasks, it is hoped that over the long term, costs of treatment will be reduced.

Functional diagnosis based on neuropsychological data may involve determining rehabilitation potential. Since comprehensive rehabilitation programs for individuals with TBI are costly, it is important to identify those areas that can be affected the most by treatment and that will be of most lasting benefit to the patient. For example, if a patient's neuropsychological test results show preserved verbal expressive ability and poor complex problem solving, such as patient may present as being of normal functioning to the casual observer. In fact, this patient may not be able to implement tasks or possess the ability to solve problems and mobilize those intact verbal skills in a work or social situation. Rehabilitation should then be focused on a particular vocational or avocational goal that can capitalize on good verbal skills yet minimize the need for complex problem solving. Similarly, neuropsychological assessment can yield information regarding the pattern of cognitive assets that can be mobilized to assist with rebuilding other deficit areas. For example, a patient may exhibit significant attentional deficits yet demonstrate a potential for better recent memory skill. In this case, the cognitive training strategy would be to enhance basic attention and concentration abilities through focused attention training and the minimization of distractability.

Kay and Silver (1988) remark that neuropsychological evaluation is becoming "something of a catchword in the field of vocation rehabilitation of injured persons" (p. 65). They note that it is beneficial for vocational counselors to know information about several areas of the patient's neuropsychological functioning to develop a vocational plan that is both realistic and feasible. The neuropsychological evaluation can provide a component of information needed to identify a fit between patient's assets, deficits, interest, past and present skills, and behavior with prospective job placements—certainly a most difficult task.

Finally, the neuropsychological evaluation may assist in determining case disposition, for example, from an acute hospitalization setting. The level and type of cognitive functioning will determine in part the type of brain injury rehabilitation facility most appropriate for referral. If the patient demonstrates excellent recovery of cognitive functions, that person may be more appropriately discharged to an outpatient or more vocationally oriented treatment setting versus another patient who exhibits significant behavioral or executive function disturbances. In the latter case a more structured day treatment or transitional living setting may make a better disposition plan.

MONITORING PATIENT PROGRESS

Although neuropsychological evaluations can be costly, repeated testing can be useful to measure cognitive change over time. In the case of closed head injury, one expects cognitive function to improve with time. When decline in functioning is seen on repeated testing, a medical examination may be appropriate to identify the reason for the decline. Ideally, repeated testing can identify whether cognitive rehabilitation strategies are effective, although it is difficult to differentiate those effects due to training versus that attributable to recovery. Another application is in examining the impact of medication on cognitive functioning. For example, a patient taking seizure medication may be tapered off the medication, and a partial clearing of cognitive functioning may result. This could be monitored by pretaper versus posttaper assessments. The same method can be employed to examine the effects on cognitive function of depression treatment (e.g., psychopharmacologic or psychological intervention).

LITIGATION

Cases of TBI will frequently go to litigation, perhaps because of the pervasive and long-term ramifications involved with brain damage. Physical, cognitive, interpersonal, social, vocational, and recreational competencies can all be affected by brain injury and result in long-lasting disability. Very few patients return to preinjury level of functioning after moderate and severe brain injury. Documentation of the extent of damage and issues of prognosis are standard questions raised in litigation cases. The neuropsychological evaluation can provide objective data regarding the patient's cognitive status and how it may have been affected by a trauma or acquired condition. There are a number of different issues to address in litigation cases, such as (1) what is a "normal" neuropsychological profile, (2) what is the "expected" recovery curve in TBI, (3) what was the patient's preinjury or premorbid level of functioning, and (4) how much of the cognitive deficits seen on testing can be attributable to brain damage versus psychological overlay problems. As more research is conducted and data gathered, neuropsychological evaluations may be able to answer these questions more specifically.

The extent and speed of recovery of cognitive functions following minor head injury is a topic of considerable debate. Dikmen and colleagues (1986) report that many studies may have overestimated head injury–related deficits in this population because of the lack of control for the effects of preinjury characteristics and of other system injuries such as fractures sustained at injury. In this study, the neuropsychological results were clinically unremarkable one month after injury when preinjury variables were taken into consideration. On the other hand, Rimel and colleagues (1981) have reported significant neuropsychological difficulties three months after minor injury. For the neuropsychologist whose evaluation and subsequent testimony rests on testing data gathered at a single point in time, it may be difficult to differentiate preexisting conditions from injury-related cognitive impairment.

THE NEUROPSYCHOLOGICAL EVALUATION

DIFFERENT APPROACHES
IN CLINICAL NEUROPSYCHOLOGY

Over the course of development in clinical neuropsychology, a number of approaches or "camps" have emerged. Each camp developed out of a specific history or tradition, and each has its proponents. This situation is analogous to American psychology in general where differing views of human nature will lead to diverse conceptualizations and models to explain behavior. Intrapsychic and developmental models of human behavior thus led Sigmund Freud to take what is now known as a psychodynamic view, while stimulus-response theory of human behavior outlined by John B. Watson and B. F. Skinner has lead to modern behavioral models of human health and pathology. So, too, the particular view of how the brain functions lays the foundation for the particular approach used in clinical neuropsychology. Note also that the same models of brain-behavior relationships (e.g., the Reitan-Wolfson model mentioned earlier) can undergird diverse approaches to neuropsychological assessment. As with any discipline in which there is much diversity of method, ongoing debates persist over which are preferred or useful and under which conditions (Filskov and Boll, 1981, 1986; Grant and Adams, 1986; Incagnoli and colleagues, 1986; Lezak, 1983).

A distinction between *fixed* versus *flexible* battery approaches is often made in the neuropsychology literature. Fixed battery approaches are those that employ a standard set of measures or procedures to each patient seen. This allows for comparison of results to normative (without known neurologic impairment) and to reference groups (e.g., TBI; cerebral vascular accident [CVA]; tumor). In the flexible battery, a set of measures are chosen for the individual case. It may include tests that are given across patients as well as other measures that suit the referral question. It is thought that questions about a case may be answered more specifically in this way. Each approach has it own merits and shortcomings. Neither of these approaches is used more than the other, and use tends to be somewhat setting and geographically specific. The approach employed will largely depend on the neuropsychologist's training background and experience.

Fixed-Battery Approaches

Perhaps the most frequently employed fixed-battery approach with TBI patients is the Halstead-Reitan Neuropsychological Test Battery (HRNB) (Reitan and Wolfson, 1985). It consists of seven standardized tests originally developed by Ward Halstead in 1947. The measures that comprise the core of the HRNB are the Category Test, Tactual Performance Test, Seashore Rhythm Test, Speech–Sounds Perception Test, and Finger Oscillation Test. From these is derived the Impairment Index that provides a quantification of the level of overall cognitive impairment. A number of other measures are routinely administered and are often referred to as "allied procedures." These include the Wechsler Adult Intelligence Scale (WAIS), Trailmaking Test, Reitan-Klove Sensory Perceptual Examination, Reitan-Indiana Aphasia Screening Test, and Minnesota Multiphasic Personality Inventory (MMPI). A more detailed explanation of the skills and abilities assessed by test measures will be discussed later.

The Luria-Nebraska Neuropsychological Battery (LNNB) (Golden and colleagues, 1985) was pioneered by Charles Golden in an attempt to objectify and systematize the behavioral neurologic method of A.R. Luria. Much of the now revised LNNB was based on the earlier work of Anne-Lise Christensen, a neuropsychologist who developed a set of stimulus cards and procedures known as Luria's Neuropsychological Investigation. The LNNB consists of 212 items in 14 subscales that are purported to measure the full range of cognitive abilities. Various methods of combining items for scoring the LNNB lead to lateralization and localization diagnoses. The controversies surrounding the LNNB basically involve issues of reliability and discriminant validity to identify localization of brain lesions and ability to differentiate neurologic groups (Adams, 1984; Spiers, 1982; Stambrook, 1983).

Flexible-Battery Approaches

As the phrase implies, this assessment approach employs a variety of measures that vary across different patients. What drives the assessment are the particular issues to be addressed by the neuropsychological evaluation. In the Boston Procas Approach whose main proponent is Edith Kaplan (Milberg and colleagues, 1986), a common set of measures (e.g., Wechsler Adult Intelligence Scale-Revised (WAIS-R); Wechsler Memory Scale) are administered in standardized fashion but are often followed by augmentative procedures. For example, on the WAIS-R, the block design subtest (in which the patient must look at a two-colored pattern and use blocks to construct a pattern identical to the original pattern) is modified by following the process by which the patient solves the problem. Two individuals taking the test may each achieve the same score; however, one could use a systematic yet slow method while the other may work quickly on a trial-and-error basis. This then assists the neuropsychologist in commenting on the method of problem solving as well as looking at the outcome.

In the hypothesis-testing approach (Lezak, 1983) the neuropsychologist generates a *priori* hypotheses about a particular patient's performance. For example, it may be observed that after head injury, family members notice the patient to have great difficulty in recalling events that occur an hour previous to asking the patient about an event. Several hypotheses may explain this behavior. Are there sensory impairments (such as visual or auditory) that preclude the patient from obtaining information initially? Are there basic attentional deficits that do not allow for encoding into recent memory storage? Are recent memory deficits primarily visual, verbal, or both? To what degree does the passage of time and distraction impair memory abilities? Do word-finding difficulties disrupt the patient's ability to output verbally what is stored initially? Measures are then selected to test and confirm or reject these hypotheses.

TESTING SETTING AND PROCEDURES

Neuropsychological tests are commonly administered by both the neuropsychologist or a trained technician. The latter may be nondoctoral personnel (technicians, psychometrists, psychometricians, psychological assistants) who administer and score neuropsychological tests (Division 40 Task Force on Education, Accreditation, and Credentialing, 1989). For reliable and valid results to be obtained in neuropsychological evaluations, tests must be administered in a standardized fashion. Most measures have standardized instructions for administration and are printed verbatim in a manual format (e.g. HRNB, LNNB, WAIS). This helps ensure that results can be compared with reference and normative groups.

The testing setting is usually one in which an examiner faces opposite the patient being tested. A large table is used for the presentation of stimulus materials and provides work space for the patient. The room is ideally large enough to be physically comfortable for two people and is relatively free from outside noises or distraction. This to ensure conditions for maximum performance. In the case of TBI, the patient may perform better in this setting than, for example, in an occupational therapy setting where there may be more opportunity for distraction. Each set of data are equally important.

The test examiner is skilled at obtaining maximum performance from the patient with TBI. An example is where an individual may naturally tend to discontinue a task easily when faced with error. The score may not reflect so much cognitive deficits as much as test-taking style in this case. Others may approach the test with a more impulsive style by answering questions too quickly or execute a perceptual-motor task with precision due to anxiety. The examiner will take note of these behaviors and record them to be included in the interpretation of the test results.

COMPONENTS OF A
NEUROPSYCHOLOGICAL EVALUATION REPORT

Neuropsychological reports differ widely according to the context in which the patient with TBI is being tested (e.g., an update for an impatient team about recovery versus a report to be used in a large litigation suit), style of the neuropsychologist, and the audience to which a report is directed. There is no one common format. Emphasis may be placed on a more general running narrative of the results to a more detailed test-by-test analysis. Test scores may or may not be included. Details regarding summary statements and recommendations will vary greatly. Reports may be in letter format, appear as a progress note in a medical chart, or be in a variety of report forms. The length varies from one to as high as 20 pages. The content can include voluminous historical information, or it may contain just simple identifying information. Given these variations, it is sometimes difficult to compare results between individuals or across retesting. Table 5-1 shows some of the common elements found amongst neuropsychological evaluation reports.

Identifying information is a brief synopsis of the patient. It is usually a one or two sentence section such as "The patient is a 23-year-old single Caucasian male who was involved in a motor vehicle accident on 3/11/90 resulting in a severe closed head injury and multiple fractures." This may be followed by the *referral question* to place the report in context. An example is, "The patient was referred for neuropsychological evaluation by Dr. Justus Lehmann in Rehabilitation Medicine at University of Washington Medical Center to further delineate cognitive assets and deficits that may assist the inpatient team with treatment and discharge planning."

Table 5-1. Common aspects of neuropsychological evaluation report

1. Identifying Information
2. Referral question and context
3. Background information
   a. Onset of brain injury; severity rating
   b. Initial medical findings
   c. Medical history
   d. Initial symptoms after TBI
   e. Current symptoms and behaviors
   f. Psychiatric, drug-alcohol abuse history
   g. Legal history and ongoing litigation
   h. Family constellation and history
   i. Social history and current status
   j. Education history
   k. Vocational history and current status and goals
   l. Financial status
4. Evaluation procedures
5. Behavioral observations during test administration or clinical interview
6. Test results
7. Summary of neuropsychological evaluation
8. Synthesis
9. Recommendations
10. Clinical impressions

The amount of *background information* included in a report will be different depending on the context of the report. This section is often generated as a result of a review of medical records, diagnostic interview with the patient, family member, or significant other (friend, coworker), or discussion with other health care professionals. Details of the onset of TBI can assist with making preliminary determinations of the severity of the head injury. Indexes such as initial Glasgow Coma Scale scores, length of coma, length of posttraumatic amnesia, presence of retrograde amnesia, and time to follow commands can assist in making hypotheses about recovery and prognosis. Initial medical findings such as diagnosis imaging results showing brain damage (hematomas, contusions) can also assist with prognostic hypotheses. There are also a number of areas that can assist the neuropsychologist in drawing conclusions about deficits that are injury related, those that predate the injury, and how the current clinical presentation is influenced by variables and circumstances that occur after the injury. Background information can also put into context any summary statements or recommendations that follow. Again, each neuropsychologist will differ in terms of the weight given to this information.

Evaluation procedures usually list the tests that were administered or procedures that were employed to generate the report. Included may be details of the documents that were reviewed, who was interviewed, any procedures appended to the tests that were given (e.g., Wechsler Memory Scale, Form 1 with delay procedure; Bender Motor Gestalt Test with interference procedure).

As mentioned previously, it is important to know how the patient approaches the testing situation. *Behavioral observations* take note of impulsivity, anxiety, lowered frustration tolerance with irritability and anger, depressed affect, distractability, physical fatigue, pain complaints, request for repeating instructions, or tendency to abort tasks easily. These factors can influence the interpretation of test scores. Ultimately, it is desired that patients put forth their maximum effort without the influence of behavioral impairments so that test results are a valid representation of the patient's current level of functioning.

The *test results* section usually includes a narrative of the outcome of scores. Some simply report the scores without interpretation, while others will make detailed inferences about the scores. This section frequently is broken down by conceptual areas of cognitive functioning as will be discussed later. Finally, the report concludes with global and specific *summary statements* of the results and presents a case conceptualization in a synthesis paragraph, followed by a listing of treatment or triage recommendations. When these reports appear in medical charts or similar documents, these last sections are the most often read. *Clinical impressions* is a one-line statement of diagnostic hypotheses or conclusions such as "moderate closed head injury; right hemisphere focus; clinical depression without suicide ideation or intent; rule out alcohol dependence."

MAJOR AREAS ASSESSED AND CORRESPONDING TESTS

The Reitan-Wolfson model of brain-behavior relationships provides a view of the general components involved in cognition. A comprehensive neuropsychological evaluation will therefore include measures that assess each component. This is especially important in TBI, since the pattern of brain damage is highly variable across patients. This variability is due in part to the mechanism of TBI, which results in both global deficits and specific areas of impairment. Table 5-2 lists commonly administered neuropsychological tests categorized by major cognitive areas. Detailed descriptions of these tests are available (Lezak, 1983). It is important to bear in mind that many neuropsychological measures have no norms for brain-injured patients, and, as such, it can be difficult to determine readily how a test will react in this population. Interpretation of results therefore is left to the description of the neuropsychologist, whose experience with TBI patients becomes the gauge from which to interpret the result of a test.

Table 5-2. Major areas assessed in a neuropsychological evaluation and corresponding tests and procedures

Variables	Test/Procedures
General neuropsychological functioning	Halstead Impairment Index
	Neuropsychological Deficit Scale
	Wechsler Adult Intelligence Scale
	Revised (WAIS/WAIS-R)
	Full Scale IQ
	Verbal IQ
	Performance IQ
	Digit Symbol (WAIS; WAIS-R)
	Symbol Digit Modalities Test
	General Memory Index (Wechsler Memory
	Scale—Revised)
Intellectual functioning	WAIS, WAIS-R
	Stanford-Binet Intelligence Scale
	Peabody Picture Vocabulary Test
	Quick Test of Intelligence
Academic achievement	Wide Range Achievement Test-Revised
	Review of academic records
Attention and concentration	Digit Span (WAIS, WAIS-R)
	Arithmetic (WAIS, WAIS-R)
	Trailmaking Test–Part A
	Speech-Sounds Perception Test
	Seashore Rhythm Test
	Digit Vigilance Test
	Letter Cancellation Test
	Paced Auditory Serial Addition Test (PASAT)
	Stroop Test
Memory functioning	Wechsler Memory Scale–Russell Revision
	Wechsler Memory Scale—Revised
	Selective Reminding Test
	Rey Auditory-Verbal Learning Test
	California Verbal Learning Test
	Fuld Object-Memory Evaluation
	Benton Visual Retention Test
	Sentence Repetition
	Rey-Osterreith Complex Figure Test
	Memory and Location of the Tactile Performance
	Test
	Rivermead Behavioural Memory Test
Speed of cognitive processing	Trailmaking Test—Part B
	PASAT
	Digit Symbol (WAIS, WAIS-R)
	Symbol Digit Modalities Test
Visuospatial and perceptual motor integration	Tactual Performance Test
	Performance subtests of WAIS, WAIS-R
	Rey-Osterreith Complex Figure Test
	Benton Visual Retention Test

Table 5-2. (continued)

Variables	Test/Procedures
Sensory and motor function	Hooper Visual Organization Test
	Reitan-Indiana Aphasia Examination
	Reitan-Klove Sensory Perceptual Exam
	Tactual Form Recognition
	Finger Oscillation Test (Finger Tapping)
	Strength of Grip
	Fingertip Number Writing
	Purdue Pegboard Test
	Trailmaking Test—Part A
Abstraction, problem-solving, new learning, executive functioning	Category Test
	Wisconsin Card Sorting Test
	Trailmaking Test—Part B
	Tactual Performance Test
	Similarities and Comprehension subtests of WAIS, WAIS-R

General Neuropsychological Functioning

In any assessment an estimate of the patient's general cognitive level is desired. Judgments can then be made about the relative position of each individual test compared with the general index of functioning. The Halstead Impairment Index is based on the HRNB, where seven indexed tests are given (among others) and the number of tests scored in the brain-impaired range (based on cutoff score) determines the level of general impairment. The score ranges from 0 (normal range) to 1.0 (severe impairment). A recent expansion of the Impairment Index is the Neuropsychological Deficit Scale developed by Reitan and Wolfson, (1987). This scale combines cutoff scores from several other tests (WAIS; Reitan-Indiana Aphasia Screening Test) and procedures from the battery to yield a total score. This score then translates into one of four severity categories. The Full Scale Intelligence Quotient (IQ) score from the WAIS and the WAIS-R is often used to suggest general level of functioning. Based on age, education, and occupational background, an estimate can be made of preinjury general intellectual functioning using a regression formula and norms (Matarazzo and Herman, 1984; Wilson and colleagues, 1978), which are then used to compare against current level of IQ. Furthermore, the Digit Symbol subtest of the WAIS has typically been seen as an indicator of brain damage irrespective of the laterality of a brain lesion. The General Memory Index (GMI) of the Wechsler Memory Scale-Revised can be a useful gauge of overall memory functioning in the TBI patient and therefore can be considered a general neuropsychological measure. The level of memory functioning on the GMI is often compared with IQ scores and general impairment ratings.

Intellectual and Academic Functioning

The most widely used test batteries of intellectual functions are the WAIS and WAIS-R. Although not developed as a neuropsychological measure, many of the subtests are sensitive to brain damage and result in profiles unique to brain injury. These tests yield both verbal and performance (nonverbal) scores that can provide useful information not only for neuropsychological purposes but also for academic planning and vocational rehabilitation services for TBI patients. Another, less used battery for brain-injured patients is the Stanford-Binet Intelligence Scale, whose norms range from age 2 to young adult and whose tests vary on the number of verbally loaded tests based on patient age. Other ancillary measures that are good at estimating general intelligence are nonverbal response format tests such as the Peabody Picture Vocabulary Test and the Quick Test of Intelligence. These latter tests require the patient only to point as a response, and thus they can be especially useful in testing those with motor or speech problems.

In assessing the TBI patient, it is helpful to know what level of basic academic abilities exist. On the Wide Range Achievement Test, for example, basic spelling, recognition reading, and written arithmetic skills are assessed with scores reflecting grade-level equivalents. Such information is particularly useful to the vocational counselor who may be seeking a job placement for a brain-damaged patient that is commensurate with the academic skills the patient possesses. Since these data are rather global, obtaining academic records, from elementary to college, can be useful collateral information to examine the patient's strengths and weaknesses. In some brain injuries, the patient may seemingly score well on intellectual and academic tests but complain of being less capable or mentally adept. Examination of records may reveal an individual who had a consistently high grade-point average and who now may have significant academic problems, although the actual performance may be in the high average range. Conversely, the TBI patient may have a preinjury history of a learning disability that would affect test interpretation.

Attention and Concentration

The ability to attend to stimuli and sustain attention is an entry-level cognitive skill: attending to small visual details and listening carefully to sounds or speech are examples of skills in this area. In the Reitan-Wolfson model, attention and concentration are at the level of cognitive processing that feeds into language and visuospatial systems. Therefore, the ability to focus attention, sustain concentration, and minimize distraction will affect other cognitive abilities such as verbal or visual recent memory or complex problem-solving skill. Several factors can influence attention and concentration ability that may be functional in nature, such as clinical depression, excessive medication or seizure prophylaxis medication, and anxiety.

Memory Functioning

A host of memory measures with new scales are developed rather regularly. Listed in Table 5-2 are the more common measures used to assess TBI patients. Memory is a complex process that combines attentional, encoding, storage, retrieval, and recognition mechanisms. Because of the complexity of memory, guidelines have been suggested as to criteria by which adequacy of a memory test should be judged. Erickson and colleagues (1980) have recommended that a good memory test should assess orientation, short-term memory, delayed recall of information, and remote–long-term memory. Mateer, and colleagues (1987) have developed a typology of memory problems in brain-injured patients and factor-analytically derived four memory components: attention–prospective memory (immediate, working memory), retrograde memory (recall of information before brain injury), anterograde memory (memory for episodic and semantic memory with hours of recall), and historic-overlearned memory (overlearned cultural and personal information). Several memory scales will include measures of recent verbal memory, recent visual memory, delayed recall of both verbal and visual information, and recognition memory. Furthermore, tests can assess the degree to which a patient benefits from verbal cues and reminders. It is thus important to examine the literature on the test construction of each memory measure to know what construct or aspect of memory functioning is being assessed. Some measures, such as the memory and location component of the Tactual Performance Test of the HRNB, are a combination of many tasks that include incidental memory (being asked to recall information that the person was not initially asked to remember). Other, newer procedures such as the Rivermead Behavioural Memory Battery use a more in vivo approach to assessing memory by having the patient perform certain tasks within the room of the neuropsychological examination.

Speed of Cognitive Processing

TBI patients may not always make errors in cognitive operations or tasks; however, they may at times exhibit difficulty with processing information quickly. Rapid decision making, or listening to a conglomeration of information and attempting to process that information rapidly, may pose problems. Many timed tests assess this cognitive processing component. For rehabilitation purposes, the patient's ability on these measures assists the practitioner in structuring the method of instruction and the context for rehabilitation activities.

Visuospatial and Perceptual-Motor Functioning

These variables relate to the patient's ability to analyze spatial relationships and make sense out of depth and space terms. Perceptual-motor integration skill refers to the ability to perceive stimuli, formulate a representation of that visual stimuli in memory, and translate that stimuli into a motor response (e.g., drawing a picture of an object that is presented visually). Several of these functions have a right hemispheric focus, with special emphasis on the right parietal regions. These functions become relevant in the return-to-work situation where, for example, a brain-injured patient with visuospatial deficits may wish to do manual dexterity or fine motor coordination tasks but finds it difficult to execute these tasks. In this case the interdisciplinary team may opt to remediate or teach compensatory strategies for visuospatial problems, and the vocational counselor's tasks would be to find a job that minimizes the use of such abilities. A problem with measures of visuospatial and perceptual-motor abilities is the requirement of a motor response. Few tests in this area do not involve use of the hands. The patient's peripheral motor integrity may be compromised secondary to fractures and abrasions with sensory loss, and these may confound test results.

Sensory-Perceptual and Motor Functioning

Lateralized sensory and motor deficits can occur that have a CNS basis. This is to be differentiated from peripheral motor and sensory difficulties that may arise out of previous or existing hand and arm injuries. The interpretation of lateralized findings is generated from multiple sources on the neuropsychological examination and not based solely on specific sensory and motor tests (e.g., speed of finger tapping comparing left and right hands; perceiving shapes of objects with both hands). Motor speed and strength can be influenced by clinical depression, and attention deficits affect the patient's ability to carry out these tests. The majority of the tests that are listed in Table 5-2 include procedures for examining right versus left hand differences. Dominant hand performance is compared with nondominant hand output where significant discrepancies between the two hands are interpreted in light of norms.

Problem Solving and Abstract Reasoning

A critical element of any neuropsychological evaluation is the assessment of higher-order cognitive processing, something that Lezak (1983) refers to as "executive functions." In Lezak's scheme, executive functions involve goal formulation, planning, carrying out goal-directed plans, and effective performances. The Stuss-Benson model underscores the predominant thrust of the frontal lobes' significance for higher-order processing, where anticipation, goal selection, preplanning, and monitoring are included in these executive functions. Stuss-Benson notes that the executive function "represents many of the important activities that are almost universally attributed to the frontal lobes which become active in nonroutine, novel situations that require new solutions" (p. 244). At the behavioral level, these higher-order functions have correlates in terms of ability to use novel strategies to solve newly presented problems, ability to use abstract reasoning to inductively or deductively find solutions to problems, the application of a range of solutions to problems, and ability to learn and generalize from previous learning trials and feedback. The ability to handle and cognitively process from multiple inputs (e.g., listening to verbal instructions while executing a task, coordinating eye-hand movements, and blocking out distracting stimuli) may be considered an executive function. The ability to integrate newly learned material and generalize across situations is an important prognosticator of whether treatment will generalize to another context. In those cases where executive functions are significantly compromised, the rehabilitation strategy is to train the brain-injured patient in the setting that person will be working or living and not rely on generalization.

AUGMENTATIVE TESTING PROCEDURES

Personality Tests

Defining the term *personality* is similar to trying to define intelligence. It is multifactorial, involves interpersonal propensities, and is manifested in everyday behavior depending on the context or situation at hand. More simply, personality is what personality tests measure. For a more thorough discussion of personality and its disorders, see Butcher (1972), Cattell and Dreger (1977), and Millon (1969, 1981).

Probably the most widely used personality test instrument in TBI patients is the MMPI. For a brief review of its development, description, and use, see Butcher and Keller (1984). This 566-item self-report inventory consists of four validity scales and ten clinical scales. This instrument allows the clinician to examine test-taking style, exaggeration or minimization of symptoms, psychological distress (depression, anxiety, and anger), interpersonal traits (social conformity, sociability), somatization, sex roles, and psychotic ideation and experiences. Numerous rationally and empirically derived subscales have been developed since the MMPI was originally released in 1940. Studies on patients with brain injuries abound and attest to the clinical observation that head-injured patients vary in their emotional presentation (Dikmen and Reitan, 1977a, 1977b). The MMPI is currently undergoing a major restandardization effort to reflect more current societal and age-relevant norms.

According to a survey by Butcher and Owens (1978), the next two most frequently administered self-report inventories are Cattell's 16 PF (Cattell and colleagues, 1970) and the Millon Clinical Multiaxial Inventory (MCMI) (Millon, 1982). Cattell's work is founded in the factor analytic tradition of identifying the most basic and consistently occurring personality traits. After a series of extensive and rigorous research studies, Cattell, and his colleagues found 16 traits that are identifiable in a wide variety of cultures and are seen across the age span: warmth, intelligence, emotional stability, dominance, impulsivity, conformity, boldness, sensitivity, suspiciousness, imagination, shrewdness, insecurity, radicalism, self-sufficiency, self-discipline, and tension. Although the instrument holds much potential for TBI patients, to date there are no studies on its use in this population. The MCMI consists of eight basic personality scales (schizoid, avoidant, dependent, histrionic, narcissistic, antisocial, compulsive, passive-aggressive) and three pathologic personality disorder scales (schizotypal, borderline, paranoid) that correspond to current psychiatric nosology. It also measures clinical syndromes such as depression, somatization, psychotic thinking, and substance abuse. Its 175-item format makes it more tolerable for those patients who have a poor attention span.

Mood Assessment

To augment the cognitive data, it is also standard practice that the mood state of the TBI patient be assessed. Depression, anxiety, and anger are the most common emotional sequelae after head injury, and all three can further impair cognition. These mood states can also affect the patient's ability to engage in rehabilitation treatment, adjust to the home environment, or be effective at work. Prigatano (1987) observes that depression commonly occurs several weeks to months after TBI, although specific etiology for the time frame of onset is unclear. Several methods exist for depression assessment, and the majority of these measures have excellent reliability and validity. Probably most popular among the clinical self-report measures is the **Beck Depression Inventory.** A newer instrument is the **Center for Epidemiological Studies Depression Scale,** which was developed on a community population with excellent norms. The **Hamilton Depression Rating Scale** is a clinician rater scale that has often been applied to psychiatric patients and has the advantage of avoiding patient minimization (shallow self-awareness) or exaggeration in self-report. (See Lewinsohn and Lee, 1981, for a review of depression measurement.) Anxiety measures abound, and the State-Trait Anxiety Inventory stands out among the more commonly used and widely researched (Speilberger and colleagues, 1983). State anxiety refers to that which fluctuates from situation to situation and reflects tension, apprehension, and worry at a specific moment in time. Trait anxiety refers to a more enduring pattern of anxiety proneness. Spielberger and his associates have also generalized the State-Trait distinction to the area of anger expression (Spielberger, 1988).

Psychosocial Assessment in Traumatic Brain Injury

It is often helpful to ascertain the everyday impairment, adjustment, and impact of TBI on the patient's psychosocial status. Table 5-3 lists three measures that are often used in research and clinical assessment of brain-injured individuals. The **Sickness Impact Profile** (Temkin and colleagues, 1988) is broken down into 12 areas of daily living in which a patient may perceive impairment as a consequence of TBI: (1) sleep and rest, (2) emotional behavior, (3) body care and movement, (4) home management, (5) mobility, (6) social interaction, (7) ambulation, (8) alertness behavior, (9) communication, (10) pastimes and recreation, (11) eating, and (12) work (or school). An important finding in the literature (McLean and colleagues, 1984) is that 1 month after TBI there are significant limitations in major role activities such as work, school, and home management, along with alternations in pastimes and recreation. Specific neuropsychological instruments measure memory capacity for an

Table 5-3. Augmentative testing and procedures

Realm	Test/Procedure
Personality functioning	Minnesota Multiphasic Personality Inventory
	Millon Clinical Multiaxial Inventory
	16PF
Psychosocial assessment	Sickness Impact Profile
	Memory Questionnaire
	Neurobehavioral Rating Scale
Mood Assessment	Beck Depression Inventory
	Center for Epidemiological Studies Depression Scale
	Hamilton Depression Rating Scale
	State-Trait Anxiety Inventory
	State-Trait Anger Expression Inventory

objective-normative standpoint. It is also helpful to compare this with self-report measures of memory deficit and how such deficits manifest themselves in everyday situations. Sunderland and colleagues (1983) developed the **Memory Questionnaire** to assess the patient's perception of memory problems in five realms of daily behavior: (1) speech (e.g., "letting yourself ramble on to speak about unimportant or irrelevant things,"), (2) reading and writing (e.g., "forgetting how to spell words"), (3) faces and places (e.g., "failing to recognize friends or relative by sight"), (4) actions (e.g., "starting to do something, then forgetting what it was you wanted to do"), and (5) learning new things (e.g., "unable to cope with a change in your daily routine").

CASE EXAMPLE

Background

The following is an example of a full neurophyschological evaluation conducted on a TBI patient and underscores the numerous implications involved with such patients. The patient at the time of his intake to an outpatient brain injury program was a 23-year-old man who had been a doctoral student in engineering and sustained a severe closed head injury in a motor vehicle accident 5 months before intake. Seven days of coma resolved with a period of posttraumatic amnesia estimated to be in the range of 2 to 3 weeks. He received trauma care and inpatient acute rehabilitation and was then transferred for outpatient services. Academic records and estimates of premorbid intellectual abilities suggested that the patient likely functioned in the Very Superior Range (Full Scale IQ > 129) of overall intellectual functioning, at greater than the 95th percentile for an age-peer group. He was independent in all activities of daily living before the injury.

Test Results

At four months post-injury brief neuropsychological testing was conducted. The patient was unable to tolerate more extensive cognitive assessment, attesting to the level of cognitive impairment at that time. A more extensive battery was administered 7 months later (11 months postonset). Table 5-4 shows verbal intellectual functions to be initially in the High Average range, whereas nonverbal abilities were markedly impaired (Intellectual Deficient range). Overall intelligence was in the Low Average range, certainly far below premorbid levels. These scores improved slightly by Time 2 with Speed of Processing, as shown by the Trailmaking Test both with simple psychomotor speed (Trail A) and more complex mental flexibility (Trail B). The latter still remained in the impaired range. Immediate recall for oral story passages (Memory Passages Total) improved across the two testing situations; however, after a delay, the patient's memory remained highly impaired. The same pattern was demonstrated for visual retention on immediate and delayed recall trails. On the Category Test, a task requiring abstract reasoning and new learning ability, the patient did well. When a spatial and speeded component was added to a problem-solving task (TPT), he performed poorly. Basic auditory vigilance and attention (Seashore Rhythm and Speech-Sounds Perception) were also impaired.

Table 5-4. Selected neuropsycholgical test results for the case

Test	Normal Range	Time 1	Time 2
HALSTEAD-REITAN NEUROPSYCHOLOGICAL TEST BATTERY			
Category Test	0–50 errors		10 errors
Tactural Performance Test			
Total Time	< 15.6 minutes (10 blocks)		17.0 (4 blocks)
Memory	> 6 blocks		3
Location	> 5 blocks		0
Seashore Rhythm	25–30 correct		14
Speech-Sounds Perception	0–10 errors		13
Finger Tapping	> 50 taps		52
Impairment Index	0.4		0.7
WECHSLER ADULT INTELLIGENCE SCALE— REVISED			
Verbal IQ	90–109	111	118
Performance IQ	90–109	62	74
Full Scale IQ		85	96
TRAILMAKING TEST			
Part A	< 30 s (no errors)	55 s (1)	32 s (0)
Part B	< 60 s (no errors)	105 s (0)	88 s (1)
WECHSLER MEMORY SCALE			
Memory Passages— Total		12th percentile	46th percentile
Memory Passages— Delay		1st percentile	1st percentile
Visual Reproduction Total		22nd percentile	37th percentile
Visual Reproduction Delay		1st percentile	1st percentile
General Memory	100		85

Analysis

These testing results illustrate several typical aspects of neuropsychological status after TBI. This patient shows evidence for diffuse cognitive deficits with some areas of preserved abilities (e.g., new learning potential). Intellectual deficits are far below expectation and likely impair daily functional capabilities (e.g, cooking a meal). Memory deficits, a cardinal feature of TBI, are dense in this case. Improvement is seen across the two assessments in cognitive speed and immediate memory, and this may be secondary to improved attentional abilities and recovery of cognitive functions. This patient appears also to show relative greater impairment in right hemispheric function as evidenced by marked spatial deficits. At approximately 1 year after injury there remain very significant deficits. Although improvements are likely to continue, at this point it is also likely that a large portion of cognitive change has occurred. Patients who sustain such severe injuries generally do not return to premorbid levels. In this case, the probability is low that the patient will be able to return as a PhD candidate in engineering. With continued rehabilitation and training there is a good chance he would be able to hold a job that requires repetition, minimizes a need for quick decision making, and does not involve a high degree of mechanical-spatial skill. Limitations in several cognitive areas are common among TBI patients and therefore present a challenge for rehabilitation professionals to fit the patient's cognitive assets and deficits to a satisfying social, familial, and vocational environment.

Acknowledgement: This chapter was supported in part by Grant # H133B80081 from the National Institute of Disability and Rehabilitation Research, Department of Education, Washington, DC.

REFERENCES

Adams, K.M. (1984). Luria left in the lurch: Unfulfilled promises are not valid tests. *Journal of Clinical Neuropsychology, 6,* 455–458.

Brandt, J., and Butters, N. (1986). The alcoholic Wernicke-Korsakoff snydrome and its relationship to long-term alcohol abuse. In I. Grant & K.M. Adams (Eds.), *Neuropsychological assessment of neuropsychiatric disorders.* New York: Oxford University Press.

Butcher, J.N. (Ed.). (1972). *Objective personality assessment.* New York: Academic Press.

Butcher, J.N., and Owen, P. L. (1978). Objective personality inventories: Recent research and some contemporary issues. In B. Wolman (Ed.), *Handbook of clinical diagnosis of mental disorders.* New York: Plenum Press.

Butcher, J.N., and Keller, L.S. (1984). Objective personality assessment. In G. Goldstein and M. Herson (Eds.), *Handbook of psychological assessment.* New York: Pergamon Press.

Carlin, A.S. (1986). Neuropsychological consequences of drug abuse. In I. Grant and K.M. Adams (Eds.), *Neuropsychological assessment of neuropsychiatric disorders.* New York: Oxford University Press.

Cattell, R.B., and Dreger, R.M. (1977). *Handbook of modern personality theory.* New York: Wiley.

Cattell, R.B., Eber, H.N., & Tatsuoka, M.M. (1970). *Handbook for the Sixteen Personality Factor Questionnaire* **(16 PF).** Champaign, IL: Institute for Personality and Ability Testing.

Dikmen, S., McLean, A. & Temkin, N. (1986). Neuropsychological and psychosocial consequences of minor head injury. *Journal of Neurology, Neurosurgery, and Psychiatry, 49,* 1227–1232.

Dikmen, S., and Reitan, R.M. (1977a). Emotional sequelae of head injury. *Annals of Neurology, 2,* 492–494.

Erickson, R.C., Poon, L.W., Walsh, O., and Sweeney, L. (1980). Clinical memory testing of the elderly. In L.W. Poon, J.L. Fozard, and L.S. Cermak (Eds.), *New direction in memory and aging.* Hillsdale, NJ: Erlbaum.

Filskov, S.B, and Boll, T.J. (Eds.). (1986). *Handbook of clinical neuropsychology* (Vol 2). New York: Wiley.

Fiskov, S.B., and Boll, T.J. (Eds.). (1981). *Handbook of clinical neuropsychology.* New York: Wiley.

Golden, C.J., Purish, A.D., and Hammeke, T.A. (1985). *Luria-Nebraska Neuropsychological Battery: Forms I and II.* Los Angeles: Western Psychological Services.

Grant, I., and Adams, K.M. (Eds.). (1986). *Neuropsychological assessment of neuropsychiatric disorders.* New York: Oxford University Press.

Horwitz, N.H. (1960). Postconcussion syndrome. *Trauma, 2,* 72.

Incagnoli, T., Goldstein, G., and Golden, C.J. (Eds.). (1986). *Clinical applications of neuropsychological test batteries.* New York: Plenum Press.

Kay, T., and Silver, S.M. (1988). The contribution of the neuropsychological evaluation to the vocational rehabilitation of the head-injured adult. *Journal of Head Trauma Rehabilitation, 3,* 65–76.

Lewinsohn, P.M., and Lee, N.M.L. (1981). Assessment of affective disorders. In D.H. Barlow (Ed.), *Behavioral Assessment of Adult Disorders,* New York: Guilford Press.

Lezak, M.D. (1983). *Neuropsychological assessment* (2nd ed). New York: Oxford University Press.

Matarazzo, J.D., and Herman, D.O. (1984). Relationship of education and IQ in the WAIS-R standardization sample. *Journal of Consulting and Clinical Psychology, 52,* 631–634.

Mateer, C.A., Sohlberg, M.M., and Crinean, J. (1987). Focus on clinical research: Perceptions of memory functions in individuals with closed head injury. *Journal of Head Trauma Rehabilitation, 2,* 74–84.

McLean, A., Dikmen, S., Temkin, N., Wyler, A. R., and Gale, J. L. (1984). Psychosocial functioning at 1 month after head injury. *Neurosurgery, 14,* 393–399.

Milberg, W. P., Hebben, N., and Kaplan, E. (1986). The Boston process approach to neuropsychological assessment. In I. Grant and K. M. Adams (Eds.), *Neuropsychological assessment of neuropsychiatric disorders.* New York: Oxford University Press.

Millon, T. (1969). *Modern psychopathology.* Philadelphia: Saunders.

Millon, T. (1981). *Disorder of personality:* DSM-III, Axia II. New York: Wiley.

Prigatano, G.P. (1987). Psychiatric aspects of head injury: Problem areas and suggested guidelines for research. In H.S. Levin, J. Grafman, H.M. Eisenberg (Eds.), *Neurobehavioral recovery from head injury.* New York: Oxford University Press.

Reitan, R.M., and Wolfson, D. (1985). *The Halstead-Reitan Neuropsychological Test Battery: Theory and clinical interpretation.* Tucson, AZ: Neuropsychology Press.

Reitan, R.M., and Wolfson, D. (1987). Development, scoring and validation of the Neuropsychological Deficit Scale. In R.M. Reitan and D. Wolfson (Eds.), *Traumatic brain injury. II. Recovery and rehabilitation.* Tucson, AZ: Neuropsychology Press.

Rimel, R.W., Giordani, B., Barth, J.T., Boll, O., and Jane, O. (1981). Disability caused by minor head injury. *Neurosurgery, 9,* 221–229.

Ruckdeschel-Hibbard, M., Gordon, W.A., and Diller, L. (1986). Affective disturbances associated with brain damage. In S.B. Filskov and T.J. Boll (Eds.), *Handbook of clinical neuropsychology* (Vol 2). New York: Wiley.

Ryan, C., Didario, B., Butters, N., and Adinolfi, A. (1980). The relationship between abstinence and recovery of function in male alcoholics. *Journal of Clinical Neuropsychology, 2,* 125–134.

Speilberger, C.D. (1988). *State-Trait Anger Expression Inventory.* Odessa, FL: Psychological Assessment Resources, Inc.
Speilberger, C.D., Gorsuch, R.L., Lushene, R., Vagg, P.R., and Jacobs, G.A. (1983). *Manual for the State-Trait Anxiety Inventory.* Palo Alto, CA: Consulting Psychologists Press.
Spiers, P.A. (1982). The Luria-Nebraska Battery revisited: A theory in practice or just practicing? *Journal of Consulting and Clinical Psychology, 50,* 301–306.
Stambrook, M. (1983). The Luria-Nebraska Neuropsychological Battery: A promise that may be partly fulfilled. *Journal of Clinical Neuropsychology, 5,* 247–269.
Stuss, D.T., and Benson, D.F. (1986). *The Frontal Lobes.* New York: Raven Press.
Sunderland, P., Harris, J.E., and Baddeley, A.D. (1983). Do laboratory tests predict everyday memory? A neuropsychological study. *Journal of Verbal Learning and Verbal Behavior, 22,* 341–357.
Temkin, N., McLean, A., Dikmen, S., Gale, J., Bergner, M., and Almes, M.J. (1988). Development and evaluation of modifications to the Sickness Impact Profile for head injury. *Journal of Clinical Epidermiology, 41,* 47–57.
Wilson, R.S., Rosenbaum, G., Brown, G., Rourke, D., Whitman, D., and Grisell, J. (1978). An index of premorbid intelligence. *Journal of Consulting and Clinical Psychology, 46,* 1554–1555.

CHAPTER 6

Compensation for Memory and Related Disorders Following Traumatic Brain Injury

Melissa J. Honsinger
Kathryn M. Yorkston

Consider for a moment the kinds of activities you have been involved with so far today. Now consider what you would like to accomplish during the rest of the day. How many of these activities place some demands on your memory? Even if your day is a routine one, it is likely that you would be able to create a long list of such activities. If you are introduced to an individual recently hired at your workplace, you will attempt to remember that person's name. If you are successful, you have stored that information in long-term memory. If you looked up a telephone number and closed the book before dialing, you have used short-term memory to hold that seven digit-number temporarily. If asked to retrieve that number a half hour later, you probably will be unable to do so. If the operations of your word-processing program are so overlearned that command sequences can be done automatically, you are using procedural memory. At times, you may not be able to tell others how to carry out the same command sequence unless you are sitting in front of your computer and consciously recalling each step in a process as you carry them out. Thus, there is a distinction between procedural memory and declarative memory, the memory required for explicit reporting of processes or procedures. When you remember and retrieve a large number of words to convey precise meanings, you are using semantic memory. You may not remember where or when you learned that information, but you have retained it and can retrieve it at will. If you are able to remember exactly what you did the last time you saw an old friend, you are using episodic memory. The recollection of time- and place-specific experiences is different and more subject to disruption than semantic memory. If you remember to go to your annual dental appointment at 3:30 today, you are using prospective memory, that is, you are remembering to carry out a specified activity at a future time. Thus, memory is a cognitive process that consists of many aspects and memory skills that come into play in almost every aspect of our daily lives. Because any discussion of memory requires the use of so many terms to describe various aspects, a glossary is provided at the end of this chapter.

MEMORY AND RELATED DISORDERS

Disorders of attention and memory are widely viewed as the most common and persistent sequelae of diffuse traumatic brain injury (TBI) (Levin and colleagues, 1982; Levin, 1985). The functional consequences of these memory impairments may be tremendous. They may affect the ability to retrieve old information and to recall personal life events, the ability to learn new information, and the ability to carry out a schedule of activities. Because of the presence of memory deficits in all stages of recovery from TBI and because of our limited ability to predict the extent of recovery of memory skills, assessment and management of memory impairment is a critical component of rehabilitation.

SITE OF NEUROLOGIC LESION

Memory deficits occur when specific structures of the brain are damaged or when there is diffuse cerebral damage (Auerbach, 1986). The fornix, the hippocampus, the mamillary bodies of the diencephalon, and the thalamus are most often cited as being involved in the function of memory. Lesions in the frontal limbic system, particularly the diencephalon, can also produce memory disturbances. In a person with a frontal lobe lesion (often associated with attention deficits), impaired memory may be present secondary to a disorder of attention.

RELATIONSHIP AMONG MEMORY, ATTENTION, AND LEARNING

Because it is necessary to attend to an event to remember it, and because memory skills are the basis for new learning, it is often difficult to distinguish memory, attention, and learning deficits in the clinical setting. Whyte and Rosenthal describe the relationship between memory and attention deficits when they write:

Given the prevalence of attentional deficits in head injury, it appears that much "memory impairment" can be attributed to defective processing of information at the time of presentation (Mack, 1986; Nissen, 1986). Similarly, disorders of planning and organization may lead to a disorganized pattern of information storage and a disorganized mental search at the time of retrieval (Nissen, 1986; Whyte and Rosenthal, 1988) p. 600.

Description of the components of attentional processes also suggests a close relationship between attention and memory. Nissen (1986) suggests that attention has three components—alertness, capacity, and selection. **Alertness** refers to the individuals general readiness to act on information. Theorists in the area of attention suggest that some cognitive processes occur automatically while others require attentional or controlled processing. Because attentional **capacity** is limited, investing attention in one task interferes with performing another task that also requires this capacity. The final component of attention is **selection.** Because of the multiple sources of information and the limited ability to allocate attention simultaneously to all sources, selection is a central feature of attentional skills and memory.

Attention, or the person's ability to focus on a specific internal or external stimulus without being distracted by other stimuli, is often disordered as a result of TBI. Olson and Henig (1983) list four types of attentional deficits in TBI. *Impaired selective attention* reduces the patient's ability to organize and pick out the elements critical for mental activity. To focus attention on one element out of a large array, it is necessary for us to inhibit or disregard all or most of the other stimuli impinging on our sense and thoughts. This is often difficult for individuals with TBI. The disruption of the selection process results in (1) inability to pick out the important things to attend to and (2) erratic jumping from thought to thought and topic to topic without purposeful sequence. The term *perseveration,* or mental inertia, is used to describe the patient who "gets stuck" on one thought or activity and cannot switch to another effectively. The perseverative person can repetitively stay on one topic or verbalization for minutes or hours in acute episodes or can just be mentally clumsy or slow in less severe cases. *Impaired vigilance* refers to the person's inability to focus deliberately on a task, thought, or stimulus for a sustained time. *Hemi-inattention or unilateral neglect* is an organically based denial of disability on the affected side. It can be very detrimental to adaptive functioning of the patient with TBI. In summary, memory and attention are highly related cognitive processes. Memory and learning are also highly related and difficult to separate clinically in the TBI population. Memory disorders can interfere with the storage and retrieval of new information and thus are critical to rehabilitation efforts.

RECOVERY

Memory status associated with TBI can best be considered on a time continuum. Figure 6-1 illustrates the status of memory as a function of time. The period of time preceding the injury that the patient is unable to remember is known as retrograde amnesia. Immediately following the onset of severe brain injury, patients may experience a period of coma that is produced by severe depression of the function of the CNS. A comatose patient is unarousable and unaware of internal or external stimuli (see Chapter 2). As a patient emerges from coma and becomes slightly more responsive, a period of disorientation and confusion often occurs. Posttraumatic amnesia (PTA) has been defined as "the time from the moment of injury to the time of resumption of normal continuous memory" (Lishman, 1978, p. 201). It is characterized by three components— disorientation, anterograde amnesia (difficulty acquiring new information), and retrograde amnesia (Sisler and Penner, 1975). The length of coma and PTA depend on the severity of the injury, and both have been correlated with the degree of recovery (Evans, 1981). During PTA there is impairment in the ability to store and retrieve new information.

The length of PTA is considered the best predictor of permanent mem-

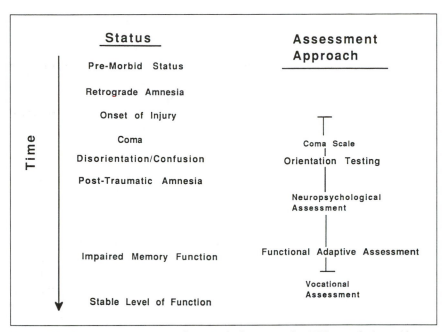

Figure 6-1 Memory status as a function of time in the TBI population. Also illustrated are assessment approaches appropriate during various phases of rehabilitation.

ory impairment (Wilson, 1987). Russell and Smith (1961) reported that 56 percent of individuals with a PTA of more than 7 days developed a long-term memory deficit, while only 8 percent of individuals with PTA of less than an hour did so. A number of studies report the long-term impact of TBI on memory. For example, McKinlay and colleagues (1981) reported that 69 percent of family members indicated that memory problems were still present 12 months after onset. In a 10 year followup study of children with TBI, nearly 25 percent continued to show verbal memory deficits. Thomsen (1984) completed a two-stage followup of patient problems at 2 and 10 to 15 years after onset. Results indicated that 80 percent of relatives of TBI individuals reported poor memory at the first followup; only slightly less, 75 percent, reported memory problems at the second followup. Thus, although many aspects of memory improve following the acute stages of TBI, memory deficits persist in an important proportion of the TBI population.

FUNCTIONAL IMPACT OF MEMORY DEFICITS

The functional impact of persistent memory deficits has been recently investigated using survey and interview techniques. Mateer and colleagues (1987) describe the results of a survey completed by 178 brain-injured and 157 control subjects. Respondents were asked about various types of memory failure or forgetting experiences relating to six memory-related tasks: anterograde episodic and semantic memory, retrograde episodic and semantic memory, working memory, and prospective memory. Subjects with TBI who had experienced a period of coma reported that they most frequently experienced memory failure in attention-prospective memory. This was followed by anterograde memory, retrograde memory, and historical-overlearned memory. A statistical analysis suggested that "the ability to carry out future intended actions depends heavily on attention, perhaps in the form of vigilance relative to time and situational cues" (p. 206).

The initial results of another ambitious survey of discrete functional skills in individuals one to six years after injury were reported by Jacobs (1988). In that survey, 142 families completed a 700-question interview relating to the patient's ability to engage in productive and self-sufficient living skills. Among the 12 general skill areas studied were self care, mobility, communication, and cognition. Each of these general areas was further subdivided. For example, among the seven areas of cognition were reading, writing, concentration, and remembering and being oriented. Table 6-1 contains a listing of specific skills in the area of remembering and being oriented and the percentage of families reporting independence with that skill. The list has been ordered from least independent to

Table 6-1 Behavioral skills as a function of skill complexity in the area of remembering and being oriented. The list has been reordered based on a survey findings.

Discrete behavior	Percentage independent (%)
Remembers recent events	37.9
Can get around city without getting lost	57.0
Remembers telephone numbers	57.5
Remembers names of people frequently encountered	62.7
Remembers events of past years	63.4
Knows date (day, month, and year)	66.2
Knows directions: north, east, west, south	67.4
Knows day of week	72.7
Knows neighborhood layout: locations of stores, houses, etc.	77.5
Knows own telephone number	80.6
Knows own age	82.9
Knows own address	85.2
Knows layout of own residence	92.1
Knows own name	97.9

Source: Jacobs, H.E. (1988). The Los Angeles head injury survey: Procedures and initial findings. *Archives of Physical Medicine and Rehabilitation, 69*, 425–431.

most independent skill. Note, for example, that only 38 percent of families reported independence in "remembering recent events," approximately two thirds reported independence in knowing the date, while nearly all reported independence in the skill "know own name." Thus, lack of independence in memory-related activities is a frequently reported consequence of TBI, and there appears to be a hierarchy of skill complexity in the area of memory and orientation.

ASSESSMENT

A thorough assessment of memory and related functions is necessary for a number of reasons. Because disorders of memory can interfere with an individual's ability to learn new information, a patient's entire rehabilitation program or plan can be affected by memory problems. Therefore, an understanding of the type and severity of memory deficits is necessary for planning intervention. Because the characteristics of memory impairment may vary from patient to patient, assessment must be individualized. Nissan summarizes the need for the comprehensive assessment of memory and related deficits:

Disorders of attention and memory are often selective. Two patients, both with attentional disorders, may present strikingly different patterns of behavior depending upon which aspect of attention is affected in each. Similarly, a patient may be severely impaired in one domain of memory but perform well in another; another patient may show a complementary pattern of deficits (Nissan, 1986, p. 13).

Like many aspects of the rehabilitation of patients with TBI, approaches to the assessment of memory deficits vary as a function of time after onset. Figure 6-1 illustrates the relationships among time, memory status, and general approach to assessment.

ASSESSING THE ACUTELY INJURED PATIENT

For purposes of this discussion the acute management phase will include the period from the onset of the injury through the emergence from PTA. This is often a temporary period of reduced arousal and fluctuating medical and cognitive status. For these reasons, performance may be vastly different from one day to another. Thus, a full neuropsychological evaluation would be inappropriate during PTA. However, Mack (1986) suggests that there are a number of reasons to monitor carefully the cognitive status of patients during PTA. First, sudden declines in cognitive functioning are often the first sign of neurologic complication, such as a delayed hematoma. Thus, cognitive monitoring may help guide medical management. Further, ongoing assessment of the patient's cognitive status provides a means of determining the course of PTA. Finally, determination of the nature and extent of the patient's deficit allows for the early initiation of an individually tailored rehabilitation program. During coma attentional, arousal and responsive to stimuli are usually monitored by the Glasgow Coma Scale (Teasdale and Jennett, 1974) (see Chapter 2).

During PTA, patients are most commonly evaluated by orientation tests. Perhaps the most widely used test of orientation in the acute phase of injury is the Galveston Orientation and Amnesia Test (GOAT) (Levin and colleagues, 1979). This brief, 16-item test asks questions about personal and geographic information (What is your name? Where were you born? Where do you live? Where are you now?), information about the injury (On what date were you admitted to this hospital? How did you get here?), memories before and after the injury (What is the first event you can remember after the injury? Can you describe the last event you recall before the accident?), and information related to current orientation to time (What time is it now? What day of the week is it? What day of the month is it? What is the month? What is the year?). Each incorrect response is given a predetermined number of error points, and these points are subtracted from 100 points. Based on a normative sample of 50 young adults recovering from mild TBI, a score of over 75 falls within the normal range, 66 to 75 falls within the borderline range, and less than or equal to 65 falls within the defective range. It is recommended that the GOAT be administered everyday as a monitor of cognitive status.

ASSESSING THE PATIENT DURING THE CHRONIC PHASE OF REHABILITATION

For purposes of this discussion, the chronic phase of rehabilitation extends from emergence from PTA through community reintegration. At this point, a complete neuropsychological evaluation, including a variety of testing focusing on specific aspects of memory, is appropriate (see Chapter 5).

Evaluation of memory function in the postacute phase of rehabilitation is best carried out in an interdisciplinary setting. In many settings, the neuropsychologist takes the lead in this process by selecting the appropriate tests and interpreting the results. Although such formal testing is invaluable in determining an individualized management plan, other phases of assessment are also necessary. These include a case history and behavioral observation from other members of the team. Observation of functional performance in a variety of settings gives important information about how adequately the patient is functioning, e.g., remembering staff members' names, remembering time and location of therapies, or effectively using memory books. A comprehensive memory assessment would also include evaluation of vision, reading, and writing skills. An understanding of capabilities in these areas is necessary because these skills often form the basis for the development and training of compensatory strategies.

When all the information has been gathered, the many different pieces of a complex puzzle can be assembled to determine the relationships between the formal test results, the patient's everyday memory performance, and other rehabilitation issues. It is only after this has been accomplished that an appropriate management plan can be implemented. Readministration of at least a portion of memory assessment is typically necessary at times when major transitions are being made by the TBI patient. One of the most important and often the most difficult of these transitions is the transition back to work. At this time, a detailed evaluation of the memory demands of potential jobs is conducted.

MANAGEMENT OF MEMORY DEFICITS

The area of management of memory deficits following TBI is not without controversy. Perhaps the debate is fueled by the fact that there are many approaches to the management of memory problems in this population. These approaches, at least on the surface, appear to differ dramatically, with vastly different underlying rationales. However, the goal of any form of intervention in a person with TBI and memory deficits should be to provide the person with the skills needed to perform tasks as independently as possible in as many environments as appropriate. The approach to achieving this goal may vary widely. For purposes of this discussion, approaches will be grouped into four categories—imposition of external structure or cues, process-specific retraining to restore attention and memory, behavioral compensation techniques, and pharmacologic management.

EXTERNAL STRUCTURE AND CUES

During the acute phase of recovery from TBI, attention and concentration deficits may limit the patient's ability to participate in intensive training programs. Therefore, early after-onset it may be most appropriate to modify the environment to provide the patient with appropriate stimulation and activities that can promote a more rapid return of the ability to perform functional tasks. For example, during this time the patient may initially be unresponsive, then only responsive to auditory input early in the morning. An appropriate treatment plan for this patient might be to schedule alternating treatment sessions early in the morning with each discipline involved using auditory stimulation as the primary mode of input (e.g., always pair gestures or actions with a verbal explanation). As spontaneous recovery continues, the same individual may begin to show increasing alertness in the early afternoon and begin to show the ability to tolerate an upright position for a short period. The rehabilitation team may choose to have the person begin to establish some wheelchair tolerance, which can eventually be increased, providing more stimulation to the patient. During this period of spontaneous recovery, it is crucial that the patient not be overstimulated. Overstimulation can cause reduced attention span, increasing confusion and even agitation in a person with TBI.

The Acute Phase of Intervention

During the acute phase of intervention, training of functional activities may initially start with strong cues, which can later be faded. Consider the training program for an acutely injured individual whose attentional and memory deficits interfere with such simple activities of daily living as taking a shower. In this case, the patient may initially need verbal, physical, and written cues to carry out the steps needed for the activity. As the patient gains physical ability, physical cues may be faded, with the patient relying on only the verbal and written cues. As the person becomes better able to learn from written cues, verbal cues may then be faded. The patient then continues to take a shower, relying on written instructions rather than on a combination of verbal, written, and physical cues. With more practice of the steps, it is hoped that the patient can eventually fade the written cues and can independently remember the procedure for taking a shower without external cues. In applying this type of intervention, the clinicians involved must examine and describe all the steps necessary to complete the task, organize the information to present to the patient through the best input method, and carry out the training using the same steps each time the task is performed.

The PostAcute Phase of Intervention

During the postacute phase of rehabilitation, providing external structure and cues may involve providing the patient with calendars, alarm clocks, written schedules, logbooks, or any number of devices to compensate for poor memory. Harris (1978) has proposed that for a cue to be beneficial to patients with memory deficits, it should be (1) given close to the time of the required action, (2) an active rather than a passive cue

Table 6-2 A listing and description of possible memory notebook sections

Orientation: Narrative autobiographical information concerning personal data or information surrounding the brain injury

Memory log: Contains forms for charting hourly information about what patient has done; diary of daily information

Calendar: Calendars with dates and times that would allow a patient to schedule appointments and dates

Things to do: Contains forms for recording errands and intended future actions; includes place to mark due date and completion date

Transportation: Contains maps or bus information to frequented places such as work, schools, store, back, etc.

Feelings log: Contains forms to chart feelings relative to specific incidences or times

Names: Contains forms to record names and identifying information of new people

Today at work: Various forms adapted for specific vocations and settings to allow individuals to record the necessary information to perform their job duties.

Source: Sohlberg, M.M., and Mateer, C. (1989b).

(e.g., an alarm versus a reminder in a book), and (3) specific. Unfortunately, many external memory aids do not possess all these features.

There is growing consensus among rehabilitationists that if external cues and memory aides are to be successful, the aids must be functional and well designed and the individual must be trained to use them effectively. Gradually, descriptions of well-conceived training programs are appearing in the literature. One such program focuses on the memory notebook training program (Sohlberg and Mateer, 1989). Notebooks are individually created depending on the patient's capabilities and needs. Table 6-2 lists and describes possible notebook sections. Sohlberg and Mateer describe a three-stage training program. During the *acquisition* stage, the patient learns the names, purpose, and use of each notebook section through a question-answer format. During the *application* stage, the patient learns appropriate methods of recording in a notebook through role-play situations. Finally, in the *adaptation* stage, the patient is monitored as he or she demonstrates appropriate memory notebook use in naturalistic settings.

At times, use of external memory aids is complicated by severe physical disability. The following case illustrates use of an augmentative communication systems as a memory aid. P.M. is a 34-year-old woman who suffered a TBI as a result of a motor vehicle accident. She was seen for evaluation of her communication and memory skills for 2 years following her injury. At the time of the evaluation, P.M.'s speech was unintelligible to all but her parents and her primary caretaker. In addition to her severe dysarthria, P.M.'s caretakers also reported severe memory deficits that were interfering with her goals of returning to a community college course. After completion of P.M.'s evaluation, an augmentative communication device, SpeechPac (Adaptive Communication Systems), was recommended. This communication system was to serve two purposes. It would enable P.M. to communicate with persons in her environment who were not familiar with her speech and it also served as an external memory aid when combined with a watch timer and a written cueing sheet. P.M. used her SpeechPac communication device as a memory aid by using some of the device's memory and quick access techniques to cue her to perform some daily tasks. P.M.'s caregivers would set the timer on her watch to go off at specific times of the day when she needed to take her medicine, get ready to catch her bus to go to school, eat her lunch, and leave the school library to catch her bus for her ride home at the end of the day. When P.M.'s watch alarm went off at 9:00, she would enter 09 into her communication system. P.M. or her caregivers had then stored under that code 09 the task that she was to perform at that particular time of the day (e.g., take medicine at 9:00). When her alarm went off at 3:00, P.M. would enter the code 15, which was short for 1500 hours, and her communicator would remind her to leave the library to go catch her bus home. Because the communication system produced printed output as well as synthesized speech, P.M. was also able to use a communication system in other ways to increase her independence. At the end of each day, she would type in a list of events or activities that she needed to complete the following day. She would then tape these lists to her wheelchair lap tray to be used as a visual reminder for her.

PROCESS SPECIFIC RETRAINING TO RESTORE MEMORY

Efforts to restore memory function through repetitive drills have been notably unsuccessful. Sohlberg and Mateer (1989b) suggest that such approaches "have repeatedly documented their failures in either enhancing scores on untrained memory tasks or, of greater importance, in impacting functional memory outside the clinic (Godfrey and Knight, 1985; Prigatano and colleagues, 1984; Schacter and colleagues 1985)." (p. 204). Expressing similar arguments, Glisky and Schacter write:

Typical memory-retraining packages require patients to try to remember letters, digits, words, shapes, or location on a computer screen. The materials used often have no real world relevance and learning them typically has no obvious practical value. . . . In view of the fact that careful experimental work has failed to produce any evidence that repetitive practice or drills yield general improvement in memory function, there is no reason to expect that computerized presentation of training materials will produce positive outcomes (Glisky and Schachter, 1986, p. 55).

The area of exercises and drills to improve memory function has not been completely abandoned. Rather than taking the general memory exercise approach, Sohlberg and Mateer (1989a) outline what they call a process-specific approach to attention training. They suggest that because attention or concentration deficits are frequent underlying problems interfering with memory, improving concentration and attention will have a beneficial impact on memory function. Their attention process training (Sohlberg and Mateer, 1986) includes the areas of *focused attention* (the ability to respond discretely to specific visual, auditory, or tactile stimuli), *sustained attention* (the ability to maintain a consistent behavioral response during continuous or repetitive activity), *selective attention* (the ability to maintain a cognitive set that requires activation and inhibition of response depending on discrimination of stimuli), *alternating attention* (the capability for mental flexibility that allows for moving between tasks having different cognitive requirements), and *divided attention* (the ability to simultaneously respond to multiple tasks). A variety of drills are employed, including visual exercises based on a variety of cancellation tasks, in which the patient scans an array of targets and crosses some out. There are also auditory exercises in which the patient responds to audio-taped sequences by pushing a buzzer when the target is heard. Results of a multiple baseline, single-case-design study with four subjects have been reported (Sohlberg and Mateer, 1987). These preliminary results suggest that the patient's attention is improved with training when attention was measured by the Paced Auditory Serial Addition Task (PASAT) (Gronwall, 1977).

BEHAVIORAL COMPENSATION TECHNIQUES

Behavioral compensatory strategies may be viewed as a deliberate, self-initiated application of a procedure or sequence of behaviors to achieve a goal that is difficult to achieve because of impaired functioning (Ylvisaker and colleagues, 1987). Thus, this form of intervention involves teaching the person ways to cope with deficits rather than attempting to restore cognitive function to a more normal level. These techniques are most frequently employed with patients who have progressed through the stage of spontaneous recovery and are still left with memory deficits that interfere with their daily activities.

Mnemonic Techniques

The use of behavioral compensatory strategies can involve the use of mnemonics, visual imagery, or other memory or learning strategies. Some studies have suggested that recall performance in memory-disoriented patients can be improved through training use of such internal mnemonic learning schemes (Gianutsos and Gianutsos, 1979). However, Mateer and Sohlberg (1989) point out that none of these studies has provided support that use of these strategies generalizes to naturalistic settings.

As with many intervention techniques, a word of caution is appropriate before such techniques are applied uncritically to the TBI population. Many of the mnemonic techniques found in the popular literature to help remember lists of items or names of individuals simply do not work well for many individuals following TBI. Glisky and Schacter (1986) present a number of reasons why mnemonic techniques fail to address many of the needs of the brain-injured population. First, many everyday memory problems do not present themselves in the form of paired associates, which are the materials most often used in laboratory training. Other compensatory approaches may be much more appropriate for remembering lists of items. For example, it may be much more efficient to create a written list of grocery items than to try to commit such a list to memory through a mnemonic strategy. Finally, imagery mnemonics are often difficult to learn. Considerable memory ability may be involved in acquiring the mnemonic itself, and the use of that strategy may require considerable effort. There is little evidence that patients use mnemonic strategies spontaneously. Evidence of maintenance and generalization is also weak. Despite these rather pessimistic cautions, mnemonic techniques may be usefully applied for the acquisition of a body of information that is specific and finite, such as medication dosages and schedules.

Orientation, Comprehension, and Memory Techniques

Ylvisaker and colleagues (1987) present a number of behavioral compensatory strategies for TBI individuals with cognitive impairments. To facilitate orientation, patients should be taught to select anchor points or events during the week and then attempt to reconstruct either previous or subsequent points in time (e.g., "My birthday was on Wednesday and that was yesterday, so this must be Thursday"). Other suggestions include requesting time, date, and similar information from others when necessary and learning to scan the environments for landmarks. To facilitate auditory comprehension, patients may be taught to give feedback to speaker (e.g., "Please slow down: Speak up: Break information into smaller "chunks") and to request repetition of information in another form (e.g., "Would you please write that down for me?"). Strategies to facilitate memory include the use of self-questions (e.g., "Do I understand? Do I need to ask a question? How is this meaningful to me? How does this fit with what I know?) to ensure that comprehension of the material has been adequate. Ylvisaker and colleagues (1987) also suggest that patients be taught to build "frames" or background for new information that is of particular significance or interest and to relate the information to personal life experiences and current knowledge. Rehearsal both overt and covert, in a variety of modalities (auditory-vocal or motor) may facilitate remembering. Patients may also be taught to verbalize visuospatial information as a means of remembering.

Study Skills Techniques

Another type of behavioral compensation draws from the field of study skills development. For example, the PQRST technique (Robinson, 1970) is being used extensively in the clinical management of TBI patients. PQRST is an acronym for "Preview, Read, Question, State, and Test." This and a similar technique know as "SQR3" (Survey, Question, Read, Recall, and Review) (Rowntree, 1983) help to facilitate comprehension and storage of written information.

The procedure in PQRST is as follows:

1. Preview: Preview the material to be remembered; i.e., skim through it briefly.
2. Question: Ask important questions about the text; for example, "What is the main point the author is trying to convey? In what country does the action take place? How many people were injured?"
3. Read: Read the material thoroughly to answer the questions.
4. State: State the answers. If the answers to the key questions are not clear, read through again until they are.
5. Test: Test at frequent intervals for retention of the information.

Wilson (1987) reviews a number of studies suggesting that memory-impaired patients can acquire some new information through the PQRST study technique. She indicates that one explanation for the success of PQRST might be that it provides better retrieval cues than does rehearsal alone. Lewinsohn and colleagues (1977) have described a similar procedure for improving recall of stories by teaching patients to break each story down into the main ideas and to remember as many of these as they can. The method involves an additional stage called the "Probe" and is labeled "PQRSTP." The last stage requires probing for information available in the passage but not contained in the answers to the questions.

PHARMACOLOGIC MANAGEMENT

The final approach to the management of memory is pharmacologic intervention. It is known that individuals with TBI are often hypersensitive to drug effects. Many medications used for other purposes have negative effects on arousal, attention, and general cognitive function. Anticonvulsants such as phenytoin and phenobarbital, antihypertensives such as methyldopa and propranolol, and antispasticity drugs such as diazepam, baclofen, and dantrolene may all impair cognitive performance (Thompson and Trimble, 1982; Solomon and colleagues, 1983; Young and Delwaide, 1981a and 1981b). On the positive side, Whyte and Rosenthal (1988) reported that stimulant medications have been used clinically to increase alertness and decrease distractibility. Cope (1986) suggests that to date no drug has been demonstrated to improve memory, attention, or general cognitive function reliably in a clinically useful manner. Recently the effectiveness of combination of cholinergic agonists in producing an additive enhancement on memory has been reported (Flood and colleagues, 1985; Goldberg and colleagues, 1982). Nootropics are a relatively new class of pharmacologic agents felt to result in increased vigilance and memory. Drugs such as physostigmine, scopolamine, and pramiracetam are thought to be selective in activating the higher-level brain functions while leaving brainstem function unaffected. Preliminary clinical studies are encouraging (McLean and colleagues, 1987).

Acknowledgment This chapter was supported in part by Grant #H133B80081 from the National Institute of Disability and Rehabilitation Research, Department of Education, Washington, DC.

GLOSSARY

For a more comprehensive discussion of these terms as they relate to models of memory and its disorders, a number of excellent sources are available, including Brooks, 1983; Lezak, 1979; Sohlberg and Mateer, 1989; and Wilson, 1987.

Amnesia. Memory disorder that exists independent of a confusional state or other cognitive disturbance.

Anterograde amnesia. Cause of the difficulty in acquiring new information and a common sequelae of TBI. Damage to the medial temporal lobes and hippocampus or to portions of the thalamus can lead to profound anterograde amnesia with relative preservation of other cognitive capacities (Auerbach, 1986).

Attention. Generally refers to a person's ability to focus on a specific internal or external stimulus without being distracted by other stimuli.

This process is predicated on the person's ability to be alert enough to respond to the environment in general (Olson and Henig, 1983).

Coma. An abnormal state of depressed responsiveness to internal and external stimuli due to CNS damage.

Declarative memory. Involves conscious awareness and the ability to report something explicity (as opposed to procedural memory).

Episodic memory. Involves the recollection of time- and place-specific experiences.

Longer-term memory. Secondary memory, which allows one to memorize, store, and retain information over longer periods. Long-term memory consists of a number of components including visual and verbal memory as well as semantic and episodic memory.

Posttraumatic amnesia (PTA). Period after TBI when a patient is unable to remember events or information from one day to the next. This period is characterized by disorientation and confusion during the reemergence from coma.

Procedural memory. Ability to learn rule-based or automatic behavioral sequences, such as motor skills, conditioned response, performance on certain kinds of rule-based puzzles, perceptual motor tasks, and the ability to carry out sequences for running or operating things. Procedural learning may occur even though the individual does not remember having done it and cannot talk about it (Sohlberg and Mateer, 1989, p. 148).

Prospective memory. Involves the ability to carry out assigned or required tasks at a specific future time.

Retrograde amnesia. Time interval preceding the injury that the patient is unable to recall. It is typically much briefer than PTA, and in some cases there may be a brief period of retrograde amnesia that is irreversible.

Semantic memory. Knowledge of word meanings, classes of information, and ideas.

Short-term memory. Often referred to as working or primary memory. Short-term memory has a limited capacity, holding only a small amount of information for a limited time.

REFERENCES

Auerbach, S.H. (1986). Neuroanatomical correlates of attention and memory disorders in traumatic brain injury: An application of behavioral subtypes. *Journal of Head Trauma Rehabilitation, 1,* 1–12.

Brooks, N. (1983). Disorders of memory. In M. Rosenthal, E.R. Griffith, M.R. Bond, and J.D. Miller (Eds.), *Rehabilitation of the head injured adult* (pp. 185–196). Philadelphia: Davis.

Cope, N. (1986). The pharmacology of attention and memory. *Journal of Head Trauma Rehabilitation, 1,* 34–42.

Evans, C.D. (Ed.). (1981). *Rehabilitation after severe head injury.* Edinburgh: Churchill Livingston.

Flood, J.F., Smith, G.E., and Cherkin, A. (1985). Memory enhancement: Supraadditive effect of subcutaneous cholinergic drug combinations in mice. *Psycholpharmacology, 86,* 61–67.

Gianutsos, R., and Gianutsos, J. (1979). Rehabilitating the verbal recall of brain-injured patients by mnemonic training: An experimental demonstration using single-case metholology. *Journal of Clinical Neuropsychology, 2,* 117–135.

Glisky, E.L., and Schacter, D.L. (1986). Remediation of organic memory disorders: Current status and future prospects. *Journal of Head Trauma Rehabilitation, 1,* 54–63.

Godfrey, H., and Knight, R. (1985). Cognitive rehabilitation of memory functioning in amnesiac alcoholics. *Journal of Consulting and Clinical Psychology, 43,* 555–557.

Godfrey, H.P.D., and Knight, R.G. (1988). Memory training and behavioral rehabilitation of a severely head-injured adult. *Archives of Physical Medicine & Rehabilitation, 69,* 458–460.

Godfrey, H.P.D., and Knight, R.G. (1987). Interventions for amnesics: Review. *British Journal of Clinical Psychology, 26,* 83–91.

Goldberg, E., Gertsman, L.J., Mattis, S., Hughes, J.E., Bilder, R.M., Jr., and Siro, C.A. (1982). Effects of cholingergic treatment on posttraumatic anterograde amnesia. *Archives of Neurology, 39,* 581.

Gronwall, D. (1977). Paced auditory serial addition task: A measure of recovery from concussion. *Perceptual Motor Skills, 44,* 367–373.

Harris, J.E. (1978). External memory aids. In M. M. Gruneberg, P. Morris, and R. Sykes (Eds.), *Practical aspects of memory.* London: Academic Press.

Jacobs, H. E. (1988). The Los Angeles head injury survey: Procedures and initial findings. *Archives of Physical Medicine and Rehabilitation, 69,* 425–431.

Levin, H.S. (1985). Outcome after head injury: Clinical consideration and neurobehavioral recovery. II. Neurobehavioral recovery. In D. P. Becker & J. T. Povlishock (Eds.), *Central nervous system trauma status report—1985* (pp. 281–302). Washington, DC: National Institutes of Health NINCDS.

Levin, H. S., Benton, A.L., and Grossman, R.G. (1982). *Neurobehavioral consequences of closed head injury.* New York: Oxford University Press.

Lewinsohn, P. M., Danaher, B. G., and Kikel, S. (1977). Visual imagery as a mnemonic aid for brain-injured persons. *Journal of Consulting and Clinical Psychology, 45,* 717–723.

Lezak, M. D. (1979). Recovery of memory and learning functions following traumatic brain injury. *Cortex, 15,* 63–72.

Lishman, W. (1978). *Organic psychiatry.* Oxford: Blackwell Scientific Publications.

Mack, J.L. (1986). Clinical assessment of disorders of attention and memory. *Journal of Head Trauma Rehabilitation, 1,* 22–33.

Mateer, C., Sohlberg, M., and Crineon, J. (1987). Perceptions of memory function in individuals with closed head injury. *Journal of Head Trauma Rehabilitation, 2,* 74–84.

Mateer, C. A., and Sohlberg, M. M. (1988). A paradigm shift in memory rehabilitation. In H. A. Whitaker (Ed.), *Neuropsychological studies of nonfocal brain damage: Dementia and Trauma.* (pp. 202–225). New York: Springer-Verlag.

McKinlay, W.W., Brooks, D.N., Bond, M.R., Martinage, D.P., and Marshall, M.M. (1981). The Short-term outcome of severe blunt head injury as reported by relatives of the injured persons. *Journal of Neurology and Neurosurgery and Psychiatry, 44,* 527.

McLean, A., Stanton, K., Cardenas, D., and Bergerud, D. (1987). Memory training combined with the use of oral physostigmine. *Brain Injury, 1,* 145–159.

Nissen, M. J. (1986). Neuropsychology of attention and memory. *Journal of Head Trauma Rehabilitiation, 1,* 13–26.

Levin, H. S., O'Donnell, V. M., and Grossman, R. G. (1979). The Galveston orientation and amnesia test: A practical scale to assess cognition after head injury. *Journal of Nervous and Mental Disorders 167,* 675–684.

Olson, D., and Henig, E. (1983). *A manual of behavioral management strategies for traumatically brain-injured adults.* Chicago: Rehabilitation Institute of Chicago.

Prigatano, G., Fordyce, D., Zeiner, H., Rouche, J., Pepping, M., and Wood, B. (1984). Neuropsychological rehabilitation after closed head injury in young adults. *Journal of Neurology, Neurosurgery, and Neuropsychiatry, 47,* 505–513.

Robinson, F. B. (1970). *Effective study.* New York: Harper & Row.

Rowntree, D. (1983). *Learn how to study.* New York: Harper & Row.

Russell, W. R., and Smith, A. (1961). Post traumatic amnesia in closed head injures. *Archives of Neurology, 5,* 4–17.

Schacter, D., Rich, S., and Stampp, A. (1985). Remediation of memory disorders: Experimental evaluation of the spaced-retrieval technique. *Journal of Clinical and Experimental Neuropsychology, 7,* 79–96.

Sisler, G., and Penner, H. (1975). Amnesia following severe head injury. *Canadian Psychiatric Association Journal, 20,* 333–336.

Sohlberg, M., and Mateer, C. (1989a). *Attention process training (APT).* Puyallup, WA: Association for Neuropsychological Research and Development.

Sohlberg, M., and Mateer, C. (1989b). *Introduction to cognitive rehabilitation: Theory and practice* New York: The Guilford Press.

Sohlberg, M.M., and Mateer, C. (1987). Effectiveness of an attention training program. *Journal of Clinical and Experimental Neuropsychology, 9,* 117–130.

Solomon, S., Hotchkess, E., Saravay, S.M., Bayer, C. Ramsey, P., and Blum, R.S., (1983). Impairment of memory function by antihypertensive medication. *Archives General Psychiatry, 40,* 1109–1112.

Teasdale, G., and Jennett, B. (1974). Assessment of coma and impaired consciousness. *Lancet, 2,* 81.

Thomsen, I.V. (1984). Late outcome of very severe blunt head trauma: A 10–15 year second follow-up. *Journal of Neurology, Neurosurgery, and Psychiatry, 47,* 260–268.

Thompson, P.J., and Trimble, M. R. (1982). Anticonvulsant drugs and cognitive functions. *Epilepsia, 23,* 531–544.

Whyte, J., and Rosenthal, M. (1988). Rehabilitation of the patient with head injury. In J. Delisa (Ed.), *Rehabilitation medicine: Principles and practice* (pp. 585–611). Philadelphia: Lippincott.

Wilson, B. A. (1987). *Rehabilitation of memory.* New York: The Guilford Press.

Ylvisaker, M., Szekeres, S. F., Henry, K., Sullivan, D. M., and Wheeler, P. (1987). Topics in cognitive rehabilitation therapy. In M. Ylvisaker and E.M. Gobble (Eds.), *Community re-entry for head injured adults.* Boston: College-Hill Press.

Young, R. R., and Delwaide, P. J. (1981a). Drug therapy: Spasticity: I. *New England Journal of Medicine, 304,* 28–33.

Young, R. R., and Delwaide, P. J. (1981b). Drug therapy: Spasticity: II. *New England Journal of Medicine, 304,* 96–99.

CHAPTER 7

Cognitive and Language Bases
for Communication Disorders

MARY R. T. KENNEDY
FRANK DERUYTER

The area of language disorders following traumatic brain injury (TBI) has challenged our thinking perhaps more than any other area of communication disorders. We have been forced to deal with issues of language use or pragmatics to an extent that far exceeds other acquired neurologic communication disorders. At times, the language disorders found among those with TBI are more than simply a reflection of underlying cognitive deficits. At other times, specific language processing deficits occur in conjunction with cognitively related communication disorders.

As neurobehaviorists, we continue to wrestle with terminology to describe adequately the cognitive and language disorder that has come to be associated with TBI. The devastating effect of TBI on cognitive and language processes results in behavioral changes that occur in a distinctly different manner than other causes or etiologies. However, we have tried to place it into our already existing categories for language disorders, thereby labeling it as something it is not. Terminology we are familiar with, such as aphasia, subclinical aphasia, and language of confusion, have been used frequently to identify this neurobehavioral disorder.

The terms *aphasia* and *subclinical aphasia* emphasize the focal language components of the disorder while neglecting its cognitive counterpart and the interplay between cognition and language. "Language of confusion" narrows the category too severely. If a person is not confused after TBI but has difficulty with language "use," yet another descriptive term is required. Language *disorganization* and *cognitive-communication disorder* are new terms that have been created. Others have claimed, however, that impaired cognitive processes can exist in isolation without affecting language or its use. Thus, statements such as the following appear in medical reports: "the individual demonstrates severe cognitive impairment, in the form of inappropriate interaction with the environment, but does not demonstrate a language disorder." *Language disorganization* is one of the many possible results of the underlying disorder, but use of this term does not include the other deficits.

Recently, the term *cognitive communication disorders* has been used to describe the many deficits that affect communication as the result of underlying cognitive disruption. Although this term is more inclusive than the former ones, its exact meaning and implication are in question. Use of *cognitive* appropriately focuses attention on the underlying cause of the impairment. However, by not including *language*, the implication is that language deficits are a result of impaired cognition, when in fact language is both the result of cognitive processing and functions as a copartner in an integral-reciprocal relationship between cognitive and language processes. Second, confusion may be generated by this term, since *communication* could be interpreted to include dyspraxia, dysarthria, voice disorders, impaired hearing, and so on.

The authors recommend the use of the term *cognitive-language disor-*

ders(s) to describe the deficits in processes of cognition and language and the resulting language behaviors following TBI. This is not an entirely new term (Hagen, 1981), but its use emphasizes the integral relationship between cognitive and language processses. Vygotsky (1962), Piaget and Inhelder (1969), Guilford (1967), and others have structurally and philosophically shown that language and thought are entwined, while Luria (1973, 1980) linked both to neuropathology. Cognitive and language processes can only be seen through the window of language behavior (e.g., disorganization, dysnomia, impaired pragmatics) and nonlanguage behavior (e.g., slowing of responses, inattentiveness, perseveration). Even though both language and nonlanguage behavior are products of mental activity, language is a part of the essence of mental activity. Thus, the use of *cognitive-language disorder(s)* to describe the neurobehavioral impairment following TBI includes all aspects of the cause (both cognition and language), allowing the vast variety of resulting behaviors to be described as products of the impairment rather than as the impairment itself.

A CONCEPTUAL FRAMEWORK FOR COGNITIVE LANGUAGE DISORDERS

Establishing a conceptual framework assists our understanding of brain-behavior relationships in the following manner: a discussion of this type reminds us that (1) cognitive-language relationships and their relevance to brain injury is not a new concept; (2) cognitive-language deficits are the result of diffuse or focal damage to the brain and therefore require a team approach to evaluation and remediation; (3) a framework organizes descriptions of deficits that span a broad range and type; (4) a framework allows for establishment of goals by focusing, prioritizing, and selecting a hierarchy of tasks; and (5) a framework generates and directs continued research (Malkmus, 1980; Szekeres and colleagues, 1985).

The interdependent relationship between cognition and language provides us with the basis to understand and identify the disordered communication behavior both verbal and nonverbal, following TBI. Three theoretical models have contributed to our understanding of brain-behavior relationships: information processing theories, cognitive development theories, and neuropathologic theories. It is the combination of all three, that is, how they work together and influence each other, that gives us perspective on the complexity of cognitive language disorders.

INFORMATION PROCESSING THEORIES

Information processing theories provide a broad perspective of cognition. It is viewed as a complex system in which information is processed within mental and environmental structures (Dodd and White, 1980). Three theories comprise the current view of how information is processed. Lurian theory is a blending of neuroanatomical and processing theory and proposes that higher mental functions emerge from several subsystems working together (Luria, 1967 and 1973). Hemispheric processing theory proposes two types of processing mediated in the right and left hemispheres (Nebes, 1974). The left hemisphere is responsible for the analysis and synthesis of serial, sequential, and detailed information, while the right hemisphere provides the "gestalt", serving as an organizer-synthesizer (Kirby, 1980; Kaplan, 1983; Lezak, 1983; Gazzaniga, 1979; Cummings, 1985). For further information, the reader is referred to Galin (1974), Gazzaniga and Hillyard (1971), Gazzaniga (1979), Springer and Deutsch, (1981) and Kirby (1980). Organizational-structural theory of information processing was first proposed by Atkinson and Shiffrin (1968). Information is processed in a sequential organization involving perception and short and long term storage. For detailed discussion of various types of organizational theories the reader is referred to Guilford (1967), Chapey (1986), Broadbent (1958), Neisser (1976), Flavell (1977), Kirby and Biggs (1980), and Parril-Burnstein (1981).

COGNITIVE DEVELOPMENT THEORIES

It is well accepted that development of basic cognitive processes must occur prior to the initial attachment of symbolic codes or language (Piaget, 1969; Bruner, 1964; Piaget and Inhelder, 1969). There is no doubt that cognitive development theory has molded our view of how cognition and language are intertwined. As Vygotsky (1962) stated, "thought is not merely expressed in words; it comes into existence through them." (p.121)

NEUROPATHOLOGICAL THEORIES

Researchers have studied the relationship between types of brain injuries, specific areas of damage, and the clinical symptomatology (Adams and Victor, 1981; Gennarelli and colleagues, 1981, 1982). However, as Alexandar (1987) states, there exists no model for explaining the relationship between neuropathology and neurobehavior after TBI because of a wide combination and diversity of damage, the range of severity of damage, and the broad age range. However, several researchers have investigated types of injuries, types of brain damage, and clinical symptoms and outcome. In 1941, Denny-Brown and Russell looked at the type of injury and loss of consciousness. They found that acceleration-deceleration forces produced immediate loss of consciousness and speculated that movement of the brainstem was in part responsible. A blunt blow to the head could cause brain injury without loss of consciousness. Strich (1961) used the microscope to discover axonal shearing in white brain matter. The Gennarelli and colleagues (1981,1982) studies addressed types of damage (axonal, subdural hematoma, intracerebral hemorrhage) in association with various types of blows to the head (blows and falls versus acceleration-deceleration injuries). The presence of hematoma is apparently not related to any particular clinical syndrome, as several investigators have noted (Bricolo and colleagues, 1980; Rimel and colleagues, 1982). In isolation, age as a predictor of outcome is not significant when the sample groups were divided at 30 years of age (Brooks and colleagues, 1980). However, in general, the older the individual, the lower the eventual outcome (Najenson and colleagues, 1974).

Alexandar (1987) summarized three common neuropathologies with distinct behavioral consequences in TBI patients. Diffuse axonal injury (Adams and colleagues, 1982; Gennarelli and colleagues, 1982) occurs in the parasagittal area, resulting in impaired motor function in the legs, with less impairment in integrative brain functions, such as language and visual processing. Abrupt loss of consciousness and length of coma are indicators of severity of diffuse axonal injury. Focal cortical contusions (Courville, 1937; Clifton and colleagues, 1980) frequently result in damage to the fronto-orbital and anterior-temporal regions, with clinical symptoms in the areas of emotion, social behavior, and pragmatics (limbic functions). The behavioral consequences of hypoxic-ischemic injury include memory loss, dementia, persistent vegetative state (from necrosis), and visual impairment. Diffuse axonal injury and hypoxic-ischemic injury are difficult to diagnose neurologically. In patients with TBI, two or three combinations of tissue damage are usually present. Clinically this makes the identification of patterns difficult. For example, severe damage in the motor regions by diffuse axonal injury may have less implication for eventual outcome than would minor damage to the hypothalmus (Alexandar, 1987). The relationship between cognition and language following TBI requires the integration of normal development, processing theories, and the impact of damage to specific as well as diffuse areas of the brain.

COGNITIVE-LANGUAGE RELATIONSHIP

Bloom and Lahey define language as "a knowledge of a code for representing ideas about the world through a conventional system of arbitrary signals for communication. Language consists of some aspect of content or meaning that is coded or represented by linguistic form for some purpose of use in a particular context" (Bloom and Lahey, 1978, p. 23). Each aspect of language (content, form, and use) involves cognitive processing, and impairment in any process can affect any or all parts of language. Depending on the individual's cognitive development initially, language eventually serves to shape and organize the environment, thereby shaping further cognitive development (Piaget and Inhelder, 1969; Vygotsky, 1962). "The evolution of representational thought, made possible through language, allows the child to break away from the restrictions of . . . time, space and action," as identified by the boundaries of sensorimotor action and perception (Malkmus and Becker, 1983, p. 2). Language becomes a cognitive instrument for categorizing, associating, and synthesizing information. It is the interdependent relationship between cognition and language that allows the individual to generate, assimilate, retain, retrieve, organize, monitor, respond to, and learn from the environment.

The American Speech-Language-Hearing Association's subcommittee on Language and Cognition notes that there is no "accepted theoretical framework or model with which cognitive activity is described" (ASLHA, 1987, p. 53). The report summarizes cognition as:

specific processes which include but are not limited to attention, discrimination, sequencing, memory processes, organizational processes, comprehending, reasoning and problem solving; that use of these processes is based on knowledge (general information, rules, etc.); that use of these processes included the executive functions (execution, monitoring and adjustment of behavior or response) (ASLHA, 1987, p. 53).

It is because of this relationship that cognitive dysfunction produces language and other communicative dysfunction. Cognition allows for goal-directed activity, both mental and behavioral. "It supports, generates and guides man's covert and overt behaviors by serving as the primary means of structuring relations between man and his internal and external environments" (Malkmus and Becker, 1983, p. 3). The ASLHA Subcommittee of Cognition and Language identifies several aspects of cognition that may affect language (ASLHA, 1987):

1. Impaired attention, perception, or memory
2. Inflexibility, impulsivity, or disorganized thinking or acting
3. Inefficient processing of information (rate, amount, and complexity)
4. Difficulty processing abstract information
5. Difficulty learning new information, rules, and procedures
6. Inefficient retrieval of old or stored information
7. Ineffective problem solving and judgment
8. Inappropriate or unconventional social behavior

9. Impaired "executive" functions; self-awareness of strengths and weaknesses, goal setting, planning, self-initiating, self-inhibiting, self-monitoring, self-evaluating

Through the integral relationship between cognition and language, these disrupted processes affect the language processes of phonology, syntax, semantics, and pragmatics, and comprise the symptomatology after TBI, that is, the cognitive, language, and behavioral deficits.

COGNITIVE BASES
FOR COMMUNICATION DISORDERS

Neurobehaviorists have shown that cognitive, language, and behavior disorders result from TBI. Impairments can be classified into two categories: focal and generalized. Focal or specific deficits are clinically identified according to the location of the CNS damage and its severity and size. When a specific deficit is present after TBI, such as an aphasia, the assessment and remediation process should be tailored to the specific type of disorder, about which are numerous texts and publications. Generalized cognitive-language disorders typically present after TBI result from an array of underlying cognitive dysfunction and range from severe to mild (Malkmus, 1982; Hagen, 1984; Adamovich and colleagues, 1985).

The cognitive consequences following TBI should be viewed as an interwoven hierarchy, ranging from alertness and attention to integration. Although it is easiest to review aspects of impaired cognition in this manner, it is important to remember that the impaired dynamic interrelationships between these processes are the underlying cause of disrupted behavior, not any one process in isolation. The exact extent and nature of the injury determines which processes are more impaired. Several investigators have identified impaired processes following TBI: arousal and attention (vigilance, selective attention, and attention span); delayed and disordered information processing; thought disorganization; disorders of sequential analysis and problem solving; disorders of memory (particularly storage and retrieval of new information); impaired mental shifting; slowing of motor responses; and impaired reasoning and integration (Luria, 1980; Ben Yishay and colleagues, 1979; Levin and colleagues, 1982; Hagen, 1984; Prigatano and colleagues, 1984; Jacobs, 1984).

Performance will vary because the TBI individual is unable to focus on and filter relevant versus irrelevant stimuli; cannot organize, retain, and retrieve stimuli; and cannot integrate available information (Table 7-1) (Hagen et al, 1979a; Malkmus and colleagues, 1980; Luria, 1973; Jacobs,

Table 7-1. General behaviors associated with traumatic brain injury

Poor concentration	Incompleteness of activity
Poor mental shifting or perseveration	Poor reasoning
Disorientation	Poor impulse control
Reduced initiation	Impaired comprehension and use of
Confusion	humor
Confabulation	Impaired problem solving
Disorganized activity	Socially inappropriate behavior
Disorganized communication	Impaired planning and executing
Stimulus-bound responses	Limited insight
Impaired learning	
Incompleteness of thought	

1984). "The behavioral display of impaired cognitive function frequently is as fluctuating and random as the individual's perception of his internal and external environments" (Malkmus and Becker, 1983, p. 5). Each process or cluster of processes will be discussed, including the resulting impairments.

ATTENTION PROCESSES

Attention refers to a group of processes including alertness, selective attention, attention span, speed of processing, shifting attention, and sustained attention. As a group, these processes form the basis for other cognitive activity, being affected themselves, however, by abnormalities in other cognitive processes and by how familiar the stimulus is to the individual.

Alertness, selective attention, and rate of information processing have been discussed at length in the literature since Koppen first observed difficulties in concentration following TBI (Meyer, 1904). Later, Conkey (1938) made similar observations, documenting her findings on formal tests. Alertness, or arousal, has been referred to as a state of the CNS, which by its very nature fluctuates from low to high levels, influencing the reception of stimuli from the environment (Posner, 1975). Several authors have documented reduced alertness levels in individuals having sustained TBI (Rizzo and colleagues, 1978; Currey, 1981). Van Zomeren and colleagues (1984) found that sustained attention (ability to maintain attention to a specific activity over time) decreases significantly as measured by reaction times. In this study, the authors note that although there was a significant difference between overall performance time between the TBI group and the control group, the reaction times for the TBI group remained constant and did not become worse, as was anticipated.

Selectivity, or selective attention, is the ability to "select one stimulus over another or to differentially manipulate levels of arousal/alertness to specific stimuli" (Trexler, 1982, p.4). Early theories focused on the filtering of information entering the CNS (Treisman, 1964) and selection of a response (Broadbent, 1971). The theory of "automatic" versus "controlled" information processing (Shiffrin and Schneider, 1977) has received much acceptance because of its application to attention deficits. Van Zomeren and colleagues summarize this theory:

All information entering the system is processed automatically up till the highest level possible without conscious control. This processing is based on activation of a learned sequence of long-term memory elements; it is initiated by appropriate imputs, and then proceeds automatically. It is even possible that a complete stimulus-response chain occurs automatically, in particular in familiar situations. In other words, automatic processing happens without subject control, without stressing the capacity limitations of the system and without demanding attention (VanZomeren and colleagues, 1984, pp. 78–79).

After TBI, individuals demonstrate difficulty making adjustments in response to automatic tasks. This ability to "override" the automatic response requires monitoring and selection and is considered difficult even for uninjured populations. After TBI, the rate at which this occurs is significantly slower (Dencker and Lofving, 1958). Van Zomeren and colleagues (1984) found that when a distraction was imposed during a visual reaction task, decision-making time was significantly slower in the TBI group than in the control group. Again, these findings point to a "slowness" in the attention mechanism rather than actual impairment of selectivity.

Speed of processing, or information processing rate, has been shown to be delayed following TBI. Reaction time is influenced by two different variables in this population: the number of stimulus alternatives and the stimulus-response compatibility (Van Zomeren and Deelman, 1976, 1978; Gronwall and Sampson, 1974; Miller, 1970). For example, the more stimuli on which focusing is required, the more likely that reaction time will be slower for individuals after TBI. If the response required in a given situation is new, or different from the "routine" response, processing time will be slower. The implication here is that when placed in new or unpredictable situations or required to perform new tasks, the TBI individual will experience difficulty in rate of processing. Clinical observation supports this, since response to these situations are frequently slow and disorganized. For example, turn-taking rules are easily followed in structured and automatic conversations; however, if the conversation becomes open-ended, requiring the generation of creative responses, turn-taking skills become disordered. The effect of impaired attention on other cognitive processes is significant.

Linguistic processing deficits (auditory and visual) are present to varying degrees as the causes vary from attention deficits to visual perceptual deficits. Auditory processing and word retrieval deficits are believed to be the most common linguistic impairments associated with the TBI population (Hagen, 1984; Malkmus and Becker, 1983; Thomson, 1980). Because of the location and incidence of damage to the frontal-temporal and associated subcortical regions, this is not surprising.

Auditory processing deficits observed in individuals after TBI include an overall slowing of processing, inattentiveness, impaired selective listening, noise buildup phenomena, slow rise time, and intermittent auditory imperception. One explanation of these phenomena is that the impaired alerting or directing mechanism will interfere with the initial receipt, recognition, association, and categorization of the stimulus. Fitts and Posner (1973) proposed that expecting the presentation of a stimulus would optimize the processing of the stimulus. Because alertness and arousal mechanisms are impaired in the TBI population, a breakdown in processing may then occur at the initial presentation of the stimulus, as seen in inattentiveness or slow rise time.

Hagen (1984) suggests that the types of responses elicited during testing will assist in identifying the point of processing breakdown. Random errors that fluctuate at the beginning of a response indicate impaired selective attention, while errors that occur toward the end of a response suggest a reduced retention span or a noise buildup phenomenon. Intermittent errors during a language activity would indicate a fading of the attention mechanism.

Reduced inhibitory-control mechanisms also may result in nonparallel, temporal processing difficulty. Thus, the rate of processing cannot be controlled. As the rate increases, accuracy in processing decreases. Analysis-synthesis processes can be affected by impaired attentional mechanisms, organization, and integration, resulting in inaccurate conclusions and disordered part-whole analyses. For example, the individual will appear to have understood a humorous situation but will have only comprehended its "literal" interpretation (Malkmus and Becker, 1983).

Speed of processing affects daily communication, including comprehension, verbal and gestural expression, writing, and reading and the integrative use of these processes. Following TBI, individuals may be able to grasp only parts of messages and therefore interpret and integrate information inaccurately. Prigatano and Fordyce (1986) describe a study in which performance on the Trail Making Test (Part A) correlated highly with overall problem-solving skills, perceptual ability, tactual problem solving, and social withdrawal (using the Katz-R Adjustment Scale) (Katz and Lyerly, 1963). This again demonstrates the integration of language, analysis, and visuomotor speed and the effects on problem solving and psychosocial adjustment.

The processing of feedback is frequently impaired, as demonstrated by the TBI individual's difficulty in attending to and interpreting subtle changes in facial expressions, gestures, and body language in listeners (e.g. double meanings, sarcasm, humor) (Holland, 1982; Reimer and Tanedo, 1985; Malkmus and Becker, 1983). Prigatano and Pribram (1982) found that in individuals with reduced memory for affective facial expression, visuospatial deficits were also present.

PERCEPTION

Perception is highly dependent on attention processes and involves the interpretation of stimuli compared with what is already known (one's knowledge base or long-term storage). Differentiation of patterns, detail, and "gestalt" occur visually and auditorially, involving both hemispheres. Information that is considered to be new (whether it actually is, is not relevant) is more difficult to perceive because there exists no representational store with which to compare it (Flavell, 1977; Kirby and Biggs, 1980). The very nature of perception makes it impossible to separate it from other cognitive processes. This accounts for the sparsity of studies designed to investigate perceptual impairments in the TBI population. Visual perception has received some attention.

Visuoperceptual impairments following brain damage may be primary or secondary. Primary deficits include those which are specific, such as visual field cuts, visual neglects, agnosias, spatial or body neglects, topographic (environmental) disorientation, and inability to copy and synthesize shapes and images, and are associated with specific lesions (Cummings, 1975; Likavec, 1987; Whitely and Warrington, 1977). Secondary visuoperceptual deficits are the result of generalized cognitive disruption following TBI. "Perceptual inefficiency may result from generally weak organizing processes, from a shallow knowledge base or from impaired executive control" (Szekeres and colleagues, 1987, p. 93).

These generalized perceptual problems appear in various forms, depending on the other interfering processes. Facial recognition impairments, common in the early cognitive recovery stages, may be related to impaired visual discrimination, visual retention, or alertness and attention (Levin and Peters, 1976; Levin and colleagues, 1977). Visual inattentiveness to certain quadrants, observed in the nonspeaking TBI population, interferes with the use of communication boards, making positioning of the device important (DeRuyter and Becker, 1988).

ORGANIZATION

Adequate organization of information improves the likelihood that it will be encoded, stored, retrieved, and, as a result, learned. Therefore, it is difficult to discuss organization separately from memory. Retention and retrieval of information first depends on sufficient encoding capacity to associate what is presented with a linguistic symbol and to categorize the stimulus according to its salient features. A breakdown in sequencing, association, or categorization indicates a disturbance in the encoding phase of memory, affecting both immediate and recent recall (Malkmus and Becker, 1983). These internal organizational strategies are frequently impaired following TBI and are the result of impaired attentional and monitoring processes. For example, an individual may be unable to focus and direct his or her thoughts, so that only a portion of the stimulus is perceived and associated with the representational store. Or, due to delayed processing, the individual cannot select and retrieve from the representational store at a rate that allows for the association and categorization of the stimulus (Muma, 1978). The impact of impaired organization on input and output following TBI is presented in Table 7-2.

MEMORY AND LEARNING

Memory and learning impairments are of the most common complaints made by individuals and their family members following TBI (Brooks, 1984; Jacobs, 1984). The types and severity vary according to the site of injury, severity of injury, and concomitant cognitive dysfunction. Although it is not the purpose of this chapter to review memory theory, a brief overview is necessary to understand the relationship between impaired memory processes, learning, and language-communication impairment after TBI. Other sources are available for a more detailed review, including Chapter 6 in this book and the work of Baddeley (1984), Schacter and Crovitz (1977) and Levin and colleagues (1982).

Memory is composed of three parts—encoding, storage, and retrieval. Encoding of stimuli involves association with verbal and sensory representational stores. Storage, including short- and long-term stores, has recently been described in functional-clinical terms, such as semantic and episodic memory (Marshall and Newcombe, 1980). Semantic mem-

Table 7-2. Effects of impaired organization

Input (Encoding Memory)	Output (Formulation)
Unable to identify salient features	Impairs retrieval (word, thought)
Affects perceptual processes	Impairs sequencing
Impairs contrasting	Disorganized expression (sentence,
Impairs storage	conversation)
Impairs integration	Results in tangentiality

ory refers to our knowledge base, from which we retrieve linguistic and nonlinguistic symbols, as well as concepts, ideas, and relationships. Episodic memory refers to the recall of events and topographic (spatial) relationships. Prospective memory refers to knowledge of future events. Other types of "memory" include working memory (the coding and associating of information as it is presented) and procedural memory (recall of specific steps to complete a task). Retrieval includes recall (free and cued) and recognition.

Several types of memory disorders have been associated with TBI, although those most associated are found in studies of amnesia, retention span, and recall. Amnesia studies have found the presence of both retrograde and anterograde amnesia following TBI (Brooks, 1972; Russell and Smith, 1961; Lewin, 1966; Roberts, 1980). Roberts (1980) found that severe intellectual impairment was present ten years after injury in individuals whose post-traumatic amnesia (PTA) had exceeded 5 weeks. PTA has been used to "categorize" individuals for outcome studies under the assumption that the length of PTA is an indication of the severity of the injury (Brooks, 1983, 1984).

How long an individual retains information is described as immediate, recent, and remote memory. Although controversy exists over the nature of immediate memory (due to its dependency on attention and perceptual processes), recent memory impairment is well documented in TBI individuals (Levin and colleagues, 1979; Brooks et al, 1980; Brooks, 1972). Although remote memory remains relatively intact compared with recent memory, the presence of remote memory loss indicates the severity of the memory impairment. In general, the less the individual recalls from his or her past, the more severe the memory impairment and the worse the eventual prognosis for recovery of memory function. It is the authors' clinical experience that when an individual is unable to recall 1 to 2 years of his or her life (usually those just before the injury), the prognosis for improvement in recent memory processes is poor. The effects on learning can be so significant that daily living without someone else's assistance is not possible. Remediation for severe memory impairment must often be directed toward teaching compensatory strategies and using external cues (Gianutsos and Gianutsos, 1979; Harris, 1984).

Disordered or delayed recall of recent events and facts is also well documented in the literature (Hagen and colleagues, 1979a; Ben-Yishay and colleagues, 1982). Confusion and disorientation are the result of a severe impairment, whereas delayed responses and vague answers demonstrate a milder recall deficit. Ben-Yishay and colleagues (1982) concluded that the inability to remember events and facts was related to the lack of motivation to continue trying to remember. However, others have related recall impairment to disordered organizational strategies and recognition (Adamovich and Henderson, 1982; Brooks, 1972).

Disorders of memory (encoding, storage, and retrieval) are a common residual deficit that affect communication as well as vocational and psychosocial outcome (Brooks and colleagues, 1980; Jennett and Teasdale, 1981). The relationships between memory impairment, personality changes, and successful returning to work have been well substantiated (Bruckner and Randle, 1972; Weddell and colleagues, 1980; Jacobs, 1984). However, the relationship between memory impairment and language impairment has not received as much attention. Two aspects of memory and language will be discussed—disorders of retention and disorders of retrieval.

Reduced retention span for linguistic information has been identified in individuals with aphasia by documenting immediate recall for auditory items and verbal tones and impaired repetition (Gordon, 1983; Heilman and colleagues, 1976; Basso and colleagues, 1982). Long-term memory deficits have been reported in certain types of aphasia (Peach, 1978), although it appears that impaired retrieval and rehearsal mechanisms more commonly associated with aphasia are reponsible for the impairment in short-term storage (Loverso and Craft, 1982; Loverso, 1986). Thus, what may appear as a memory storage problem could actually be an inability to code and rehearse input.

Coding of information influences storage and retrieval. Adamovich (1978) found that aphasic adults demonstrated impaired coding abilities for short-term memory tasks. Cermak and Moreines (1976) determined that aphasic adults tended to use codes other than verbal ones. During free recall tasks, TBI individuals did not use any definable strategy, causing impaired recall (Adamovich and Henderson, 1982).

Word fluency–retrieval deficits have been identified as a residual problem after TBI by many (Levin and colleagues, 1976; Thomsen, 1976; Geschwind, 1964). In the absence of a focal lesion, a word retrieval impairment is related to other cognitive impairment, as noted by Kaye and colleagues (1984) in the correlation of word fluency impairment with poor initiation and impaired higher cognitive processing (planning, problem solving, executing, and abstraction). This supports the clinical observation that word retrieval deficits are most common during the highly confused stages of recovery, when other cognitive processes are severely impaired (Malkmus and Becker, 1983). Adamovich and Henderson (1982) demonstrated that TBI adults used fewer strategies to generate word lists than did the left cerebrovascular accident (CVA) group and changed strategies more often than did any group.

The recovery pattern of word retrieval impairments depends on the origin of the problem. If the individual is unable to inhibit and direct his or her thoughts because of severe attention impairment, then the recovery pattern will appear similar to the verbal patterns for Wernicke's aphasia (Becker, 1984). Neologistic jargon is the most severe form, resolving into the use of literal paraphasic errors. As monitoring improves, semantic substitutions will emerge, followed by the use of vague nouns and verbs. The TBI individual's word retrieval skills may resolve almost completely in conversation, except for slight disorganization in sentence structure or occasional delay in retrieval (Becker, 1984).

HIGHER COGNITIVE PROCESSES

Because of the required interplay of all cognitive, memory, and language processes, it is no surprise that higher cognitive processes are long-term residual deficits commonly associated with TBI. Impaired reasoning (inductive, deductive, and analytic), thinking processes (divergent and convergent), insight, and problem solving are documented as occurring in TBI during all stages of cognitive recovery. Difficulty with integration and part-whole relationships has been documented by several investigators (Hagen, 1984; Szekeres and colleagues, 1987; Mandleberg and Brooks, 1975).

Altered insight and self-perception result from the inability to attend to, retain, organize, synthesize, abstract, and integrate new information about oneself. The individual's perception of self following TBI is based on old knowledge of who he or she is (Kodimer and Styzens, 1980; Lezak, 1978). The individual may be able to identify isolated deficits, such as difficulty walking, trouble remembering, the presence of slurred speech, etc. but not be able to synthesize and integrate how these deficits will effect the future (i.e., returning to school or work). A classic example is the individual with significant physical or memory deficits, who on discharge from the rehabilitation facility attempts to return to work, despite counseling from numerous team and family members. Prigatano and Fordyce (1986) found that self-perception improved after "group" treatment in individuals with isolated frontal lobe involvement. However, if other brain structures were affected in the injury, such as the temporal lobes, the success rate for improving insight dropped. These individuals' altered ability to interpret "intent" and abstract information (double meanings, sarcasm, humor, etc.) affected reasoning and abstraction skills, so that very little improvement was observed.

Disorders of planning and execution reflect a range of deficits from basic to integrative. In the severe form, highly confused individuals demonstrate perseveration (motorically and verbally) as well as the disconnection of acts or responses. Each act is separate from the previous one, so that each step in an activity may require external assistance (verbal guidance or mediation) to become connected to the next step or part in the sequence (Yorkston, 1981). Prigatano and Fordyce (1986) noted that family members complained that TBI individuals required literal and step-by-step instructions to perform activities that they previously had performed independently. Deficits in abstract reasoning were present. Several authors have reported organizational difficulties leading to impaired planning and executing (Luria, 1973; Cummings, 1985; Hagen and colleagues, 1979a).

CHARACTERISTICS OF COGNITIVE-LANGUAGE DISORDERS

The basis for language impairment of a generalized nature is the same as for behavioral impairment, that is, the underlying cognitive dysfunction. Similarly, the results are random, fluctuating, and variable depending on the integrity of the cognitive system, the environment, and the effects of focal deficits (Malkmus, 1982). Incidence studies reporting language disorders following TBI should be reviewed first. Stages of recovery will be discussed next, followed by disorders of language use.

INCIDENCE STUDIES

Cognitive-language disorders following TBI have been identified in incidence studies for many years, with a higher incidence reported in the more recent studies. Several reasons explain this phenomena. Early studies did not distinguish between "aphasia" and "subclinical aphasia" symptoms. Also, investigators had different definitions of aphasia. Data were gathered at various points in recovery, and tests used were not sensitive to impairments of language use. Therefore, findings from studies vary.

Heilman and colleagues (1971) examined language in adults with closed head injuries. Of 750 individuals, they identified only 13 as having aphasia (nine with anomic and four with Wernicke's aphasia). Thomsen (1975) found that approximately 50 percent of the adults in his study demonstrated symptoms of aphasia, with the predominant features including naming errors and impaired self-monitoring. Halpern and colleagues (1973) found several language disorders in their sample of TBI adults. They noted that the distinguishing language characteristic in this population was the tendency to produce irrelevant responses. Levin and colleagues (1976) identified anomic aphasia as the predominant language impairment, although other language disturbances were present, such as auditory recognition and memory. Groher (1977) found similar results. His study was longitudinal and found that communication after TBI could best be described as "mildly" aphasic. He described such patients' communication as irrelevant, confused, and inappropriate. He noted that family members considered the individual's communication to be unimpaired, even though language deficits could be identified in traditional testing.

The presence of aphasia has also been associated with poor prognosis for functional recovery. Levin and colleagues (1979) found that the presence of aphasia correlated with low verbal intelligence quotient (IQ) scores on the Wechsler Adult Intelligence Scale (WAIS) (Wechsler, 1955). They noted that although conversational speech deficits and impaired comprehension resolved (as measured on standardized tests), other nonaphasic language disturbances prevailed (tangentiality and the presence of irrelevant topics). Later, Levin and colleagues (1982) found that the presence of aphasia or hemiparesis, oculovestibular problems, and intracranial hematomas negatively influenced intellectual recovery. Without these factors, good recovery could be predicted to at least a low average IQ higher or equal to 90 in individuals who had suffered a moderate coma. In general, the verbal IQ from the WAIS plateaued by 6 to 12 months following injury, while the Performance IQ improved for many years.

Recently, Filley and colleagues (1987) studied groups of children and adults with TBI. Three categories of brain injury were identified using computed tomography (CT) scan information—diffuse axonal injury, focal injury, and mixed injury categories. In children the classic syndromes of aphasia were more common in the mixed injury group; however, many more children (in the other two groups) displayed communication problems. Neuropsychological testing did not reveal any important differences among the children. The authors noted that many children who were identified as having good recovery on testing demonstrated behavioral problems stemming from either "overexcitability or underexcitability." In the adult groups, length of coma was related to PTA for both mixed and diffuse injury groups. The authors observations were as follows: (1) performance IQ was lower than verbal IQ due to reductions in speed, attention, motivation, and focal lesions; (2) memory quotients did not reflect actual new learning ability, since all adults had problems with learning; (3) word fluency was impaired in all the adults, although only five were considered "aphasic;" (4) all adults demonstrated reductions in concentration and problem solving, but the origin of the problem differed by groups; and (5) personality changes were noted in all. This study identifies and summarized the range of cognitive and language problems while highlighting the difficulty in identifying the causal relationships for the behaviors.

The Sarno studies (Sarno, 1980; Sarno, 1984; Sarno and colleagues, 1986) identified the presence and type of verbal impairment following TBI. The 1984 study reduplicated a study done in 1980, finding a higher incidence of verbal impairment than had been previously reported by other investigators. At 1 year after injury, 100 percent of the TBI individuals demonstrated some type of verbal dysfunction and could be categorized into one of three categories: those with "classic" aphasia, those with dysarthria accompanied by linguistic deficits on specific tests, and those demonstrating subclinical aphasia symptoms without dysarthria or classic aphasia (Sarno, 1984). Sarno and colleagues (1986) studied 125 adults with closed head injuries, finding the results similar to the earlier studies. Three groups of deficits again emerged. Of those in the "aphasia" category, 51 percent were considered fluent, 35 percent were considered nonfluent, and 14 percent were considered global. The dysarthria–subclinical aphasia group was characterized by a mean overall ranking in the 70th percentile on the Neurosensory Center Comprehensive Examination for Aphasia (Spreen and Benton, 1969), which includes visual naming, sentence repetition, word fluency, and the token test. In the subclinical aphasia group, sentence repetition was the most impaired (70th percentile), and 56 percent showed evidence of difficulty on two or more tasks (Sarno and colleagues, 1986). The authors concluded "that at least two thirds of all closed head injury (CHI) patients with a history of coma appear more linguistically intact than they actually are" Sarno and colleagues, 1986, p. 404).

STAGES OF RECOVERY

Several neurobehaviorists have organized behavior following TBI into stages of recovery. The most well-known and clinically useful tool is the Levels of Cognitive Functioning (LOCF) (Hagen and colleagues, 1979b). A summary of the LOCF is presented in Table 7-3. Linguistic components are presented also, corresponding with each level of cognitive-behavioral recovery (Malkmus, 1982) and will be discussed in the following section.

The LOCF (Hagen et al, 1979b) was developed as a behavioral rating scale to aid in the assessment process. It represents the progression of recovery of cognitive structures in the TBI population as demonstrated through behavioral change. Malkmus and colleagues (1980) describe its purpose as providing:

1. Assessment that does not require the individual's cooperation
2. Behavioral descriptions ranging from the most to the least severe, corresponding with cognitive recovery
3. A common and descriptive vocabulary for professionals
4. Improved understanding of behavioral recovery

Table 7-3. Levels of Cognitive Functioning and Associated Language Behaviors

General Behaviors	*Language Behaviors*
I. NO RESPONSE	
Patient appears to be in a deep sleep and is completely unresponsive to any stimuli.	Receptive and expressive: No evidence of processing or verbal or gestural expression.
II. GENERALIZED RESPONSE	
Patient reacts inconsistently and nonpurposefully to stimuli in a nonspecific manner. Responses are limited and often the same, regardless of stimulus presented. Responses may be physiologic changes, gross body movements, or vocalization.	Receptive and expressive: No evidence of processing or verbal or gestural expression.
III. LOCALIZED RESPONSE	
Patient reacts specifically, but inconsistently, to stimuli. Responses are directly related to the type of stimulus presented. May follow simple commands such as "Close your eyes" or "Squeeze my hand" in an inconsistent, delayed manner.	Language begins to emerge. Receptively: Patient progresses from localizing to processing and following simple commands that elicit automatic responses in a delayed and inconsistent manner. Limited reading emerges.
	Expressively: Automatic verbal and gestural responses emerge in response to direct elicitation. Negative head nods emerge before positive head nods. Utterances are single words serving as "holophrastic" responses.
IV. CONFUSED-AGITATED	
Behavior is bizarre and nonpurposeful relative to immediate environment. Does not discriminate among persons or objects; is unable to cooperate directly with treatment efforts; verbalizations are frequently incoherent or inappropriate to the environment; confabulation may be present. Gross attention to environment is very short, and selective attention is often nonexistent. Patient lacks short-term recall.	Severe disruption of frontal-temporal lobes, with the resultant confusion apparent. Receptively: Marked disruption in auditory and visual processing, including inability to order phonemic events, monitor rate, and attend to, retain, categorize, and associate stimuli. Disinhibition interferes with comprehension and ability to inhibit responses to self-generated mental activity.
	Expressively: Marked disruption of phonologic, semantic, syntactic, and suprasegmental features. Output is bizarre, unrelated to environment, and incoherent. Literal, verbal, and neologistic paraphasias appear with disturbance of logico-

Table 7-3. (continued)

General Behaviors	Language Behaviors
CONFUSED-AGITATED (continued)	sequential features and incompleteness of thought. Monitoring of pitch, rate, intensity, and suprasegmentals is severely impaired.
V. CONFUSED, INAPPROPRIATE, NONAGITATED Patient is able to respond to simple commands fairly consistently. However, with increased complexity of commands or lack of any external structure, responses are nonpurposeful, random, or fragmented. Has gross attention to the environment but is highly distractible and lacks ability to focus attention on a specific task; with structure, may be able to converse on a social-automatic level for short periods; verbalization is often inappropriate and confabulatory; memory is severly impaired, often shows inappropriate use of subjects; individual may perform previously learned tasks with structure but is unable to learn new information.	Linguistic fluctuations are in accordance with the degree of external structure and familiarity-predictability of linguistic events. Receptively: Processing has improved, with increased ability to retain temporal order of phonemic events, but semantic and syntactic confusions persist. Only phrases or short sentences are retained. Rate, accuracy, and quality remain significantly reduced. Expressively: Persistence of phonologic, semantic, syntactic, and prosodic processes. Disturbances in logicosequential features result in irrelevances, incompleteness, tangent, circumlocutions, and confabulations. Literal paraphasias subside, while neologisms and verbal paraphasias continue. Utterances may be expansive or telegraphic, depending on inhibition-disinhibition factors. Responses are stimulus bound. Word retrieval deficits are characterized by delays, generalizations, descriptions, semantic associations, or circumlocutions. Disruptions in syntactic features are present beyond concrete levels of expression or with increased length of output. Written output is severely limited. Gestures are incomplete.
VI. CONFUSED-APPROPRIATE Patient shows goal-directed behavior but depends on external input for direction; follows simple directions consistently and shows carryover for relearned tasks with little or no carryover for new tasks; responses may be incorrect due to memory problems but appropriate to the	Receptively: Processing remains delayed, with difficulty in retaining, analyzing, and synthesizing. Auditory processing is present for compound sentences, while reading comprehension is present for simple sentences. Self-monitoring capacity emerges.

Table 7-3. (continued)

General Behaviors	Language Behaviors
CONFUSED-APPROPRIATE **(continued)** situation; past memories show more depth and detail than recent memory.	Expressively: Internal confusion-disorganization is reflected in expression, but appropriateness is maintained. Language is confused relative to impaired new learning and displaced temporal and situational contexts, but confabulation is no longer present. Social-automatic conversation is intact but remains stimulus bound. Tangential and irrelevant responses are present only in open-ended situations requiring referential language. Neologisms are extinguished, with literal paraphasias present only in conjunction with an apraxia. Word retrieval errors occur in conservation but seldom in confrontation naming. Length of utterance reflects inhibitory-intiation mechanisms. Written and gestural expression increases. Prosodic features reflect the "voice of confusion," characterized by monopitch, monostress, and monoloudness.
VII. AUTOMATIC-APPROPRIATE Patient appears appropriate and oriented within hospital and home settings, goes through daily routine automatically, but is frequently robotlike with minimal-to-absent confusion; has shallow recall of activities; shows carryover for new learning but at a decreased rate; with structure, is able to initiate social or recreational activities; judgment remains impaired	Linguistic behaviors appear "normal" within familiar, predictable, structured settings, but deficits emerge in open-ended communication and less structured settings. Receptively: Reductions persist in auditory processing and reading comprehension relative to length, complexity and presence of completing stimuli. Retention has improved to short paragraphs but without the abilities to identify salient features, organize, integrate input, order, and retain detail. Expressively: Automatic level of language is apparent in referential communication. Reasoning is concrete and self-oriented. Expression becomes tangential and irrelevant when abstract linguistic concepts are attempted. Word retrieval errors are minimal. Length of utterance

Table 7-3. (continued)

General Behaviors	Language Behaviors
AUTOMATIC-APPROPRIATE (continued)	and gestures approximate normal. Writing is disorganized and simple at a paragraph level. Prosodic features may remain aberrant. Pragmatic features of ritualizing and referencing are present, while other components remain disrupted.
VIII. PURPOSEFUL AND APPROPRIATE Patient is able to recall and integrate past and recent events and is aware of and responsive to the environment, shows carryover for new learning and needs no supervision once activities are learned; may continue to show a decreased ability relative to premorbid abilities in language, abstract reasoning, tolerance for stress, and judgment in emergencies or unusual circumstances.	Language capacities may fall within normal limits. Otherwise, problems persist in competitive situations and in response to fatigue, stress, and emotionality, characterized in reduced effectiveness, efficiency, and quality of performance. Receptively: Rate of processing remains reduced but unremarkable on testing. Retention span remains limited at paragraph level but improved with use of retrieval-organization strategies. Analysis, organization, and integration are reduced in rate and quality. Expressively: Syntactic and semantic features fall within normal limits, while verbal reasoning and abstraction remain reduced. Written expression may fall below premorbid level. Prosodic features are essentially normal. Pragmatic features of referencing, presuppositions, topic maintenance, turn taking, and use of paralinguistic features in context remain impaired.

Source: Reprinted with permission from Hagen, C. (1984). Language disorders in head trauma. In A. Holland (Ed.), *Language disorders in adults* (pp. 245–281). San Diego, CA: College-Hill Press; Malkmus, D. (1982). Levels of cognitive functioning and associated linguistic behaviors. Presented at the Models and Techniques of Cognitive Rehabilitation-II, Indianapolis, Indiana.

5. Predictive information on cognitive-behavioral recovery;
6. Baseline information for establishing team treatment goals and objectives

Individual uniqueness should not be overlooked. Consideration must be given to the premorbid personality, intellect, and social skills as well as intrapersonal parameters (familiarity of task, emotional and health status, presence of focal injury).

Care should be taken when assigning a "level" to an individual. Behavior will fluctuate depending on the variables surrounding the activity being observed. When tasks are highly structured and predictable, the individual relies on remote memory and will perform better than during less predictable tasks (e.g., counting to 20 versus describing how two items are alike). The same principle should be applied to the type of environment in which the behavior is observed (quiet therapy room versus noisy physical therapy gym).

When assigning the cognitive level, behavior should be observed over time and in a variety of settings.

It is necessary to observe and note verbal and nonverbal performance across time in relation to the degree of structure and predictability present at any time as well as the type of behavior demonstrated, the stimuli precipitating the behavior and the frequency, consistency and duration of the behavior (Malkmus and colleagues, 1980, p. 2).

For a detailed description on the development and use of the LOCF in program planning, other sources are available (Malkmus and colleagues, 1980; Hagen 1984).

The nature of the language impairment reflects the cognitive processes that are impaired. Language behaviors may be inappropriate to the topic, include confabulation and confusion, or may be tangential, lacking the direction of attentional processes. For individuals who demonstrate severe attentional deficits, initiation of communication messages may be difficult. For individuals who are alert but confused, comprehending lengthy verbal and written messages can be impaired, reflecting slow processing as the amount of information increases. Processing becomes limited to only the briefest, most concrete information, creating an insufficient "store" from which to retrieve later.

The integrative functions of cognition and language are also manifested in expressive language. The individual lacks the capability to generate an internal response, retrieve appropriate vocabulary, organize and formulate the message, and transmit the message. Thus all linguistic levels are affected, including phonology, morphology, semantics, syntax, and pragmatics. Malkmus (1982) identified linguistic symptomatology with the LOCF (Hagen and colleagues, 1979b) in Table 7-3, showing how generalized receptive and expressive language recovers as cognition improves.

Early Stages of Language Recovery

During the early stages of cognitive recovery (LOCF II/III), language processing depends on alertness and arousal mechanisms. Bricolo and colleagues (1980) studied individuals who had been unresponsive for 2 weeks, finding that the ability to follow verbal commands was a significant turning point in their progressing out of coma to become responsive. Eighty-seven percent followed commands at 3 months after injury, and 98.5 percent did so within 6 months after injury.

Another study by Najenson and colleagues (1978) identified the recovery of communication skills in severely brain-injured individuals considered in coma (undefined). A consistent recovery pattern emerged. Gestural and verbal comprehension were recovered earliest (3 to 5 weeks after injury), while more integrative language functions (verbal expression, reading, and writing) requiring higher cognitive processing were recovered at a much slower rate or not at all. Eight of the nine who regained communication skills were dysarthric.

Although most investigators have reported on the incidence of general areas of language impairment, very little research has been done to identify the specific types of language deficits and their recovery patterns. In a recent study at Western Neuro Care, a rehabilitation center for individuals in the "slow to recover" category (LOCF II to V), Ansell and Keenan (1989) identified patterns of response behaviors using the Western Neuro Sensory Stimulation Profile (WNSSP). These preliminary results revealed the following communication recovery pattern after a structured sensory stimulation regimen:

1. If responses to auditory information (following commands) began to emerge, the individual had a 50 percent chance of attaining LOCF V (confused/inappropriate).
2. If responses to auditory and visual information returned simultaneously, the chances of reaching LOCF V were significantly better.
3. If responses to visual or tactile input were the only ones to emerge, chances for cognitive improvement were minimal.

These results are not surprising, given results of previous studies indicating that environmental and sensory deprivation leads to evidence of retardation of the development and recovery of CNS function (Finger and Stein, 1982). It also reemphasizes the importance of the integrity of the cognitive-language system in recovery of function following TBI.

Intervention at this stage often involves establishing basic communication approaches. DeRuyter and Becker (1988) identified the type and use of simple communication systems for individuals functioning at LOCF III (localized response). They observed that for individuals who were non-speaking, the success of yes-no systems depended on the most natural and automatic body movement. The most successful yes-no systems were head nods, with decreasing success with systems requiring other, less automatic movement and the use of other cognitive processes

Table 7-4. Hierarchy of yes-no response systems

Head nods
Gestures
Colored cards
Eye blinks
Buzzers

Source: DeRuyter, F., Becker, M.R., and Doyle, M. (1987). Assessment and intervention strategies for the nonspeaking brain injured. Presented at the American Speech-Language-Hearing Association, New Orleans.

(visual tracking and reading for the use of yes-no cards). Table 7-4 lists the type of yes-no systems used for individuals at LOCF III, starting with the most successful and ending with the least successful.

Middle Stages of Language Recovery

As alertness improves, language function becomes an avenue through which to view cognitive integrity. During this stage (see Table 7-3, LOCF IV, V and VI), it is not uncommon to observe severe disruption of all language processes. Comprehension and expression are affected by impaired attentional processes, including initiation-alerting, maintenance of attention, shifting, and inhibiting. Linguistically, these appear as expressive and ideational perseveration, verbal disinhibition, and impaired impulse control resulting in poor topic maintenance-shifting and stimulus-bound responses (Hagen and colleagues, 1979a; Adamovich and colleagues, 1985; Becker, 1984). Cummings (1985), Kapur and Coughlan (1980), Stuss and Benson (1984), Luria (1980), Stuss (1987), and Lezak (1976) all note that in patients with frontal lobe injuries, which are common after TBI, communication deficits result from inattentiveness to the listener, reduced self-monitoring, perseveration of thought, and lack of insight. These investigators have concluded that although the structural components of language may remain intact, the intent, semantics, and use of language concepts is significantly affected. Table 7-5 lists the language-communication behaviors associated with frontal lobe injuries.

During the period of severe cognitive disruption, disorders of sequencing are observed on a phonemic, semantic, and syntactic level in the highly confused individual. In both verbal and written forms, neologisms, paraphasias, and disorganized sentence structure occur with frequency. Compounded by the individual's inability to self-monitor and correct errors, expression is bizarre and unrelated to the task or environment. As attentional and monitoring processes improve, sequencing errors are observable in activities such as following multistage com-

Table 7-5. Behaviors associated with frontal lobe injury

Confabulation
Impaired word fluency
Inability to maintain ideas
Perseveration of thought or message
Disordered turn taking
Inattentiveness to listener
Disorganized messages
Repetition of information due to impaired memory
Inability to plan and execute functional communication activities
Aprosodic speech due to reduced self-monitoring
Social inappropriateness
Absence of nonverbal expression

Source: Adapted from Stuss, D.T. (1987). Contribution of frontal lobe injury to cognitive impairment after closed head injury: Methods of assessment and recent findings. In Levin, H.S., Grafman, J., and Eisenberg, H.M. (Eds.), *Neurobehavioral recovery from head injury* (pp. 166–176), New York: Oxford University Press.

mands and planning and executing activities of daily living in the later stages of cognitive recovery (LOCF VII and VIII).

Impaired organizational processes interfere with encoding and result in delayed or disordered information processing. A general slowing of thought processes is reflected in echolalic behavior, delayed mental operations of selecting and responding, and the inability to store rapidly presented information. Because the retrievability of a response depends on its proper association, categorization, and storage, highly confused individuals experience difficulty retrieving words and ideas in an organized manner. Thus the retrieval process may be delayed or disordered, resulting in slowed responses, word substitutions, disorganized sentence structure, and lack of fluidity in expressing ideas.

Later Stages of Language Recovery

As basic cognitive processes improve and provide a foundation for the reemergence of language and communication skills, the individual (at LOCF VI, VII, and VIII) is able to retrieve previously learned language rules (syntactic, semantic, pragmatic, phonologic, and morphologic). Therefore the language impairments observed in later stages of cognitive recovery reflect (1) any residual yet specific cognitive deficits (mildly impaired), (2) the integration of these deficits seen in "real life" activities, and (3) the impaired use of cognitive-language processes in social skills. For example, individuals who are slightly confused due to memory impairments will communicate using vague terminology while the message lacks meaningful content. Difficulty with making inferences will impair comprehension of abstract concepts and humor. Mild selective attention deficits can result in impaired interpretation of listener feedback during communication, which in turn impedes use of proper turn-taking rules. Difficulty with problem solving, planning, executing action, anticipating problems, and making decisions is common in the later stages of recovery. Psychological adjustment issues can have a reciprocal impact on cognitive-language processes. Denial, lack of insight, emotional liability, and anxiety interfere with the use of competent processes in stressful situations (Kodimer and Styzens, 1980; Lezak, 1983). The cognitive-language-psychological-social-environmental changes become intertwined, requiring the diagnostic skills of the speech-language pathologist, clinical psychologist, neuropsychologist, occupational therapist, social worker, and physician.

LANGUAGE USE; DISORDERS OF PRAGMATICS AND COMPETENCY

"Pragmatics, or the use of language in context, ties language and cognition to real situations, becoming a means of viewing the individual's social interactive capacities" (Malkmus and Becker, 1983, p. 32). Frequently, performance on standardized tests will appear adequate because of the insensitivity of such evaluation methods. Consequently, these communication deficits can be overlooked and not identified. Recently, however, we have become more observant and now identify altered pragmatic skills, the result of impaired integration of social, emotional, cognitive, and language components. Several authors have observed pragmatic disorders in conjunction with other linguistic disturbances, but few have described the nature and extent.

Pragmatic disturbances following TBI can be grouped into four categories; expressive disturbances, disorders of conversational rules or postulates, nonverbal aspects, and overall communication competence. Malkmus and Becker (1983) identified expressive disturbances as disorganization of the message, impaired message selection and modification, incomplete messages or absence of detail, or excessive information included in the message. Paralinguistic features of intonation, facial expression, gestures, proxemics, and eye contact can also be impaired or misused. Impaired use of conversational rules observed in TBI individuals includes (1) use of acknowledgements, (2) referencing and presupposing, (3) turn taking, and (4) topic selection, maintenance, expansion, shifting, termination. Others have alluded to pragmatic disorders, such as the use of irrelevant information (due to impaired selective filtering) (Geschwind, 1964) or to the presence of nonaphasic disturbances (i.e., disorganization, vague terminology, rambling) (Levin and colleagues, 1981; Holland, 1982).

Expressive Disturbances

Tangential communication, seen in both verbal and written forms, is described by Prigatano and colleagues as follows: "the surface structure of language output appears to be intact, conceptual confusion is obvious and is reflected in problems of poor word selection, loose connection of thoughts and ideas, impairment in abstract thinking and a strong tendency to stray from the core message or topic" (Prigatano and colleagues, 1986, p. 21). This type of output disorder indicates a lack of integration of many processes, including selective focusing of thoughts, retrieval of words and word order, and organization of ideas. An example of tangentiality is presented in Table 7-6, which is a paragraph written by an individual who was functioning at LOCF VII (automatic and appropriate).

The inclusion of excessive detail in messages or excessive talking has been documented by many investigators (Holland, 1982; Milton and colleagues, 1984). Prigatano and colleagues (1986) studied 48 TBI adults at a mean of 16 months after injury (range 1 to 18 months). Using the Katz-R Adjustment Scale (McSweeny and colleagues, 1982), they found that eight individuals were judged by family members as being "talkative." This group did not differ from the others on standard neuropsychological tests. However, they were perceived to be "emotional." The authors did not identify any premorbid personality comparison and did not administer language tests, yet they concluded that a relationship between "talkativeness" and affective disorders exists. Although excessive talking and psychopathology may coexist, this study does not show a cause-effect relationship.

Disorganization and lack of specificity in meaning are frequently the result of a combination of inattentiveness to the communication act and its parameters, a lack of attention to feedback given by the listener, and word retrieval problems. Weinstein and colleagues (1962) observed that amnesic individuals frequently used the third-person tense. They attributed this to a lack of sensitivity to the communication situation. Priga-

Table 7-6. Writing sample of tangentiality

When discussing the future. . .

But if I get to be an actress and get to be known all over the country someone will ask you about me or you might tell someone you know me and then someone will ask you about me. I really want to be an actress along the lines of Jane Fonda, Glenn Close, Kathleen Turner, Molly Ringwald. So at some point, in the future some one may ask you about me. Now that doesn't matter that everyone might ask you about me but there is a possibility that someone will. Then again someone may not. . .

tano and colleagues (1986) stated that disorders of phrasing reflect reductions in cognitive processing in that repetitions and revisions within messages actually serve to clarify the message for the speaker, not the listener. This conclusion supports the notion that verbalization of a message assists in focusing or structuring the speaker's own thoughts. Thus the speaker is attempting to compensate for his or her disorganization by imposing a self-generated strategy, similar to the use of echolalic speech in individuals who experience delays in processing.

Speirs and Dahlberg (1986) analyzed language performance in TBI adults using verbal and written descriptions of the Cookie Theft Picture (from the Boston Diagnostic Aphasia Examination, Goodglass and Kaplan, 1983a). The observed variables were number of concepts, number of syllables, and time. Two groups of TBI individuals were studied—low cognitive group (LOCF V and VI) and high cognitive group (LOCF VII and VIII). The TBI groups were also compared to normal, geriatric, and aphasia groups. The authors found that the TBI groups expressed fewer verbal concepts than the normal or mild aphasia groups. Speaker rate for the TBI groups were significantly lower than the normal and high-moderate aphasia group but did not differ from the mild aphasia group. Timed semantic units were used to assess communication efficiency, and findings, showed that TBI groups were much less efficient than normal and high-moderate aphasia groups. Between low and high cognitive groups, differences were noted on all measures. Verbal and written forms did not differ significantly from each other.

The findings of a study on discourse analysis supports the results of Speirs and Dahlberg (1986) and facilitates further questions regarding the "causes" of pragmatic disorders. Mentis and Prutting (1987) studied narrative and conversational discourse in TBI adults (N=3) using cohesion analysis (how semantic elements relate to each other) (for a detailed description of cohesion analysis, see Halliday and Hasan, 1976). They found that the TBI group used fewer cohesive ties in narratives but performed similarly to the control group in conversation. The authors noted that the TBI group did not complete the narrative without prompting. "Incomplete ties resulted in semantic confusions and ambiguities in the texts, which in turn resulted in requests for revision by their communication partners" (Mentis and Prutting, 1987, p. 93).

Most of the errors were in the category of referencing, due to poor topic maintenance and word finding deficits. The finding that TBI adults were less able to communicate meaning during narratives than during conversation is not surprising. Narratives require the use of many strategies and processes, including organization strategies, selection of appropriate items to include or exclude, word retrieval, deductive thinking, and drawing conclusions. These processes are integrated in a new manner for each narrative. Conversation, however, relies heavily on rules that are retrieved from past learning (remote memory) and are more reflective of the individual's premorbid social skills. Thus, conversation on a social, automatic level may occur without interruption. However, when the conversation becomes abstract or lengthy or requires detailed explanations, rules are often broken (Hagen and colleagues, 1979b; Malkmus and colleagues, 1980; Becker, 1984). Therefore, depending on the type of discourse, performance will vary because each type (narrative, conversation, procedural) has its own set of rules and requires the use of different processes (Becker, 1984; Wycoff, 1984; Mentis and Prutting, 1987).

In a study designed to identify pragmatic disturbances in individuals following TBI, Kennedy and colleagues (1989) have found that certain verbal expressive disorders are more likely to remain impaired than others. Using the Pragmatic Inventory for Brain Injury (see section on Pragmatics: Evaluation and Information Gathering, Figure 7-1), individuals were observed in two situations where verbal conversations were elicited. Ninety percent of the participants (N=12) demonstrated inconsistent ability to sequence ideas in an organized manner and communicate messages in a concise manner. Seventy percent of the sample exhibited impaired word finding skills, which affected overall fluency as observed in their difficulty with consistent use of pauses. Selecting accurate vocabulary (lexical choice) was indicative of the word finding problems, demonstrated in the 70 percent who used vague or inappropriate terminology. Sixty percent of the participants demonstrated impaired ability to presuppose accurately. The errors in these instances involved the individual's assuming that the listener already had the information. These findings are consistent with those of others described earlier, although they emphasize the interconnection between communication processes.

Disturbances in Conversation

Malkmus and Becker (1983), Milton and colleagues (1984), Mentis and Prutting (1987) and Britton-Hare and Hare (1987) have identified disturbances in conversation to include turn taking, topic maintenance and selection, excessive amounts of information, and redundancy. Milton and colleagues (1984) described pragmatic behavior in TBI adults compared with a control group of adults. Of 30 pragmatic behaviors judged, 76 percent were described as appropriate in the TBI group, compared with 99.4 percent in the control group. All individuals in the TBI group demonstrated problems with topic maintenance, and 50 percent demonstrated problems with topic initiation and selection, initiating turn taking, and giving the appropriate amount of information. Mentis and Prutting (1987) found similar results.

In the study currently in process, Kennedy and colleagues (1989) have found similar results, although analysis of trends in the reacquisition of conversational rules has demonstrated that patterns can be identified. For example, there is a clustering of "inappropriate" behaviors for individuals functioning at LOCF V (confused and inappropriate) in the areas of interaction and content) topic selection, initiation, maintenance, shifting, idea completion and organization, quality-conciseness, turn taking) and nonverbal communication (vocal and nonverbal aspects). More behaviors are identified as inconsistent but appropriate in individuals functioning at LOCF VI and VII (confused and appropriate, automatic and appropriate), as is expected. Second, several researchers have noted "topic maintenance" difficulties following TBI. In the Kennedy and colleagues (1989) study, topic maintenance was impaired in those individuals at LOCF V and VI. None of the individuals at LOCF VII exhibited problems with maintaining the topic, although topic initiation, expansion, and termination were impaired, reflecting initiation and inhibitory control problems. This more detailed analysis of conversational rules suggests that topic maintenance is more likely to reemerge than are the other topic-related rules.

Nonverbal Communication

The nonverbal aspects of communication are based on previously learned rules, sometimes unique to a specific culture. The vocal aspects, including intensity, pitch, rate, intonation, and quality, require selective monitoring for each specific communication situation, communication partner, and message. Individuals who have sustained a TBI are frequently unaware of and unable to monitor these suprasegmentals because of the profound effects of impaired attention, inhibition, disorientation, and initiation. However, it is not uncommon to observe these disturbances in individuals at "higher" functional levels (VII and VIII). Kennedy and colleagues (1989) found that five of seven individuals at LOCF VII displayed inconsistent ability to regulate and monitor rate, intonation, pitch, or intensity. The use of appropriate facial expression and eye contact continued to be problematic for three of the seven individuals at LOCF VII. Only the individuals at LOCF V and VI demonstrated inability to adjust body posture, monitor breathing, and maintain appropriate social distance.

Communication Competency

The notion of communication competency refers to the actual communication performance in the environment and requires identifying the individual's needs, deficit areas (processes and behaviors), the communication situation, and the compensatory strategies available to the individual. The individual's performance in "real-world" activities depends on the interplay of several variables, including the individual's goals and ability to carry out plans to accomplish them, the influence of the environment on the residual cognitive deficits, and the extent to which the individual is able to formulate and adjust responses quickly when the demands of the activity or the environment change (Szekeres and colleagues, 1985). Milton's (1987, 1988) "program-without-walls" takes a holistic yet functional approach to language therapy by addressing functional communication problems in a task-specific manner. Communication activities are defined (e.g., memo writing), with the individual's strengths and weaknesses outlined (a detailed list of functional communication tasks is provided in the section on nonstandardized assessment procedures). This focus on the dynamic relationship between cognitive-linguistic-environmental-psychological processes adds another dimension to our view of cognitive-language disturbances in the TBI population. Obviously, the impact of pragmatic and communication competency disorders on social and vocational success is great (Jacobs, 1984; Ben-Yishay and colleagues, 1982).

ASSESSMENT OF COGNITIVE-LANGUAGE DISORDERS

The assessment process, which identifies impaired processes (cognitive and language), and the resultant behaviors (verbal and nonverbal) can be problematic for the evaluator because of the range of possible deficits, the various stages of recovery, and the individual's fluctuating symptoms.

DILEMMAS IN ASSESSMENT

Assessment dilemmas that face the evaluator can be grouped into four areas: the population itself, assessment instruments, interdisciplinary issues, and the use of rating scales (Becker, 1986).

Population

The TBI population poses difficulty for the examiner. The type of injury varies, resulting in different types of recovery patterns and symptoms. For example, a generalized diffuse injury in one person may produce only temporary cognitive and language disorganization (Hagen, 1984), whereas the same type of injury in another may cause permanent cognitive and language dysfunction with focal symptoms. Depending on the severity and type of the injury, the nature of recovery may be rapid or slow. The examiner may assess the individual on one day and have invalid data the next day because of spontaneous neurologic improvement. In the "slow to recover" individual, evaluation tools must be adjusted and changed to assess very small increments of improvement.

As Hagen (1982) points out, it is not unusual to find that in the first 4 to 8 weeks after the injury, the language impairment may result from the combined effects of a global, temporary interruption of neural activity, from irreversible and diffuse damage, and from a specific or focal disorder. Also, due to the TBI individual's inability to cooperate with testing, nonstandardized methods must be employed. Finally, premorbid factors within the TBI population affect the assessment process. Epidemologic studies have indicated that learning disabilities, behavioral problems, and impaired judgment are present to a significant degree (Levin and colleagues, 1982). At Rancho Los Amigos Medical Center, an urban rehabilitation hospital, a review of the inpatient population from 1982 to 1988 indicated that 20 to 30 percent had a history of learning disabilities or had left school before the 11th grade. These findings imply that this population will have a negative "attitude" toward formal or academic testing and that testing must differentiate premorbid deficits from newly acquired ones.

Test Instruments

Traditional language test instruments are organized by expressive, receptive and integrative language skills. Because many of the communication disorders following TBI can be classified as generalized and pragmatic, these tests can lead to inaccurate and inappropriate diagnoses (Hagen, 1982). These tests are designed for and standardized on other populations, such as individuals with stroke and learning disabilities. Most aphasia batteries address only the specific parts of language and not language's integrative functions or pragmatics. Thus, the assessment process should include a "whole brain" approach, encompassing analysis of impaired communicative functions as well as those preserved (Malkmus and Becker, 1983).

Interdisciplinary Dilemmas

Interdisciplinary issues can arise when the clinician assesses the TBI population. The traditional view of the speech-language pathologist's role include the areas of aphasia, dysarthria, and dyspraxia. Therefore our role in cognitive-language disorders, pragmatics, and augmentative communication requires the reeducation of our colleagues. Territorial issues can occur due to the overlapping nature of cognition, language, and behavioral symptoms after TBI. Good working relationships with other disciplines and education regarding our emphasis on communication processes should resolve conflict in most situations.

Use of Rating Scales

Rating scales are an accepted part of the assessment process in this population, since they provide a common vocabulary, assist in viewing behavior in an organized manner, and provide baseline behavioral information with which progress can be compared. Several scales are used for a variety of purposes and at various stages in recovery. The Glasgow Coma Scale (Teasdale and Jennett, 1974) is the most commonly used tool to assess gross areas of change in comatose and semicomatose individuals. The Glasgow Outcome Scale (Jennett and Bond, 1975) is also useful but has come under criticism for its wide variability within each category. Rappaport, and colleagues (1982) scored performance in four categories on the Disability Scale. Hagen and colleagues (1979b) categorized behavioral recovery into eight levels, ranging from no response (I) to purposeful and appropriate (VIII) (see Table 7-3).

Although the usefulness of rating scales with the TBI population cannot be overemphasized, evaluators must consider the type of scale and its purpose. To be effective, a scale should be used for the designated population and specific period of recovery for which it has proved most useful. For example, the Glasgow Coma Scale is a rating scale sensitive to very small increments of change, and it should be used immediately following TBI (during the coma phase of recovery). The authors of the Glasgow Outcome Scale recommend its use at 1-, 3-, 6-, and 12-month intervals after TBI, although evidence from several studies has indicated that beginning at 6 months after injury, it is not likely that improvement will be significant enough to place the individual in the next category. However, the range of disability in the severe and moderate disability categories is so broad that improvement in specific deficit areas may be observed after this time frame. For example, in cases where a specific symptom is present, such as the status of nonspeaking, in conjunction with a mild generalized cognitive impairment, the disability level could likely improve once the individual is provided with a means of communication. The Glasgow Outcome Scale has recently come under criticism for its wide variability within the categories; however, its usefulness as a broad descriptor of disability cannot be overlooked (Jennett and colleagues, 1981).

Rating scales by nature tend to categorize individuals. Caution should thus be used to prevent "categorization." During the early phases of acute rehabilitation, the TBI individual frequently lacks the cognitive capacity to cooperate with standardized test procedures. Traditional means of assessment are not always successful in measuring and determining the nature and degree of cognitive impairment and subsequent recovery (Hagen and colleagues, 1979a). Therefore, clinical observation provides the only means of determining quality of response to environmental stimuli. In taking a critical view of the LOCF, Dowling (1985) found content validity and interrater reliability to be high, although for Level VII (Automatic and Appropriate) and Level VIII (Purposeful and Appropriate), content validity was slightly lower than for the other levels. This rating scale is more descriptive of behavior during acute rehabilitation. DeRuyter and colleagues (1987) found that nonspeaking TBI individuals are easily placed at a lower level of response because of their inability to communicate verbally and their frequently present "inappropriate" behaviors. In the "slow to recover" population, an assessment approach should be selected that will identify small increments of change, such as the WNSSP (Ansell and Keenan, 1989).

When using rating scales, one should be sensitive to the purpose of the scale (overall disability versus behavioral), the type of the individual with whom it is most valid (the semicomatose individual versus the alert, confused individual), and the interrater reliability and content validity.

ASSESSMENT ISSUES

Determining Processes versus Function

Given the dynamic nature of the consequences of TBI, that is, the cognitive, language, behavioral, and psychological deficits and the impaired relationship among them, the traditional "process" approach must be combined with a "functional" approach to identify communication disorders completely. By using a process approach to cognitive-language assessment, we are accepting Luria's (1967) idea that language is processed through systems (see the section on information processing theories). Many authors emphasized identifying "how" responses are generated (Luria, 1967; Kaplan, 1983; Lezak, 1983; Hagen, 1984). For example, difficulty in a naming task could result from impaired retrieval mechanisms, inability to associate the stimulus with its symbols, a loss of the stimuli's meaning (anomia), or an oral–motor planning impairment. A process analysis identifies the point of breakdown, indicating where remediation should begin (Hagen, 1988). Lezak (1983) warns that test scores in isolation are insufficient to identify overall performance. Observation of the individual's reactions to his or her responses, both within and outside the testing situation, will allow the evaluator to determine how emotional reactions and the absence of predictability adversely affect cognition and communication. These reactions will interfere with the integration of competent performance areas into activities of daily living.

Traditional assessment involves a process approach, but how well or effectively the individual communicates in the environment must also be addressed. This constitutes the "functional" portion of the assessment process (Beukelman and colleagues, 1984). Functional assessment is the identification of the individual's needs as well as measurement of actual performance in the environment. Both reflect the severity and type of injury as well as the velocity and period of recovery. Several examples are necessary. An individual who is at an acute rehabilitation facility and is highly confused or disoriented must communicate basic needs (e.g., "I am hungry" or "turn off the light") to hospital staff. At this period in recovery, communication with family members and familiar persons is also necessary (DeRuyter and colleagues, 1987). In the hospital environment, communication needs are very different from those in a transitional living center, vocational rehabilitation program, home, work environment, or school. Depending on the rate of recovery, the individual's communication needs will vary. For example, the individual who is recovering slowly will maintain the same needs for a longer time, assuming the environment does not change. Also, knowing the period of recovery will assist in determining whether the communication needs will change. The communication needs of an individual in a transitional living center whose injury was 3 years ago will be more determined by changes in the environment than by significant cognitive-language changes.

Milton (1988) organized the functional assessment by evaluating the individual's communication performance within the actual setting. This "program without walls" identifies performance of each communication activity and relates the individual's ability with the need (Milton, 1987). As Beukelman and colleagues state, "the magnitude of a communication disability can be defined as the gap between an individual's communication needs and his or her residual communication performance." (Beukelman and colleagues, 1984, p. 102). Therefore, by identifying the impaired process and the point of breakdown and assessing the actual performance in relation to speaker and environmental needs, the communication disorder can be remediated.

Pre-onset Factors

Obtaining a relevant and detailed social, vocational, educational, and medical history is vital to the assessment process but is frequently overlooked or not emphasized (Kodimer and Styzens, 1980; Doyle and colleagues, 1980). The pre-onset characteristics "set the stage" for symptoms that may be exacerbated following TBI. Knowledge of the individual's personality and learning style and ability to use self-appraisal strategies before the injury gives the evaluator a basis with which to compare current ability (Kodimer and Styzens, 1980). Interviews with family members as well as medical and school records should be used as sources of information. Historical information not only provides a basis for comparison but also indicates what will be of importance or priority to the individual following TBI. Finding out the individual's goals after the injury (even in the presence of decreased insight) and comparing them to his or her pre-onset goals assists in goal setting and treatment planning. It helps define what the individual perceives his-her own communication needs to be. Thus, gathering historical information and applying it to remediation will prevent "failure" or lack of follow-through during the remediation phase of recovery.

Assessment Variables

To identify the point of processing breakdown, the evaluator should be aware of two types of the variables—task variables and performance variables (Malkmus, 1980; Szekeres and colleagues, 1987; Hagen, 1984, 1988). Ever so slight changes in the activity itself or the environment will alter the response, sometimes puzzling the evaluator. Task variables are within the evalutor's control and include:

1. Amount of stimulus presented at one time or over time
2. Rate of presentation
3. Type of stimulus and response required (receptive modalities include visual, auditory, and tactile; expressive modalities include verbal, written, gestural, and facial)
4. Duration of the task itself and length of the testing session
5. Predictability or degree of familiarity of the task
6. Level of complexity
7. Context or situation in which the stimulus was presented

Performance variables are those aspects of the response that the evaluator observes while task variables remain constant or change. They include:

1. Endurance of the response during an isolated task or over time
2. Response delay or the amount of time that is required between presentation of the stimulus and the response
3. The length of time required for the individual to "recover" from one task and proceed to the next
4. How many times a stimulus must be repeated to elicit a response
5. Type of response
6. Overall pattern of responses

Hagen (1988) suggests that when task variables are held constant (task complexity), the type of errors identify the processing impairment. When errors occur at the beginning of a response, an alertness deficit should be suspected. Errors at the end of a task indicate an endurance problem, while errors that are commensurate with amount suggest a retention span problem.

ASSESSMENT METHODS

Methods used to assess cognitive-language disorders following TBI include rating scales, standardized instruments, and nonstandardized techniques. The methods chosen to obtain processing and functional performance information depend in part on the point of recovery, velocity of recovery, and the type and severity of injury. For example, the time immediately following a severe injury is often spent in intensive care units. The comatose or semicomatose individual is not alert enough to cooperate with testing, making the use of rating scales, such as the Glasgow Coma Scale (Teasdale and Jennett, 1974) and the Western Neuro Sensory Stimulation Profile (Ansell and Keenan, 1988), appropriate. A combined approach using rating scales (discussed earlier), standardized instruments, and nonstandardized methods should be used when individuals are progressing in an acute rehabilitation program. When recovery has stabilized and the individual's residual deficits are very subtle, nonstandardized methods that isolate performance on specific tasks are emphasized (Hagen, 1984; Milton, 1988). Thus, the choice and combination of methods depends on the individual's point in recovery and overall velocity of recovery.

Standardized Instruments

Standardized tests should become a part of the assessment process when the individual has adequate selective attention and inhibition to cooperate with testing (sometimes at Level V, confused and inappropriate, but usually at Levels VI through VIII). The information gathered from tests (1) provides baseline information to use as a comparison, (2) helps to differentiate between diffuse cognitive-language disorganization versus focal-specific symptoms, (3) identifies the primary and secondary processes responsible for the breakdown in communication, and (4) assists in determining the point at which remediation should begin (Malkmus and Becker, 1983).

"Any task the evaluator presents to the individual incorporates several cognitive processes and no single process can be clearly delineated from the others" (Malkmus and Becker, 1983, p. 22). However, at a minimum, formal assessment should attempt to identify the following interfering processes (Hagen, 1984; Malkmus, 1980; Adamovich and colleagues, 1985; Becker, 1986):

Attention processes: alertness, arousal, speed of processing, attention
  span, and selective attention
Discrimination and differentiation
Temporal ordering and Sequencing
Organizational abilities (association and categorization)
Memory processes (retention span, retrieval mechanisms, recent and
  remote versus episodic, prospective, procedural, semantic, and work-
  ing memory)
Analysis and synthesis
Higher level reasoning and abstraction
Integration
Maintenance of goal-directed activity over time (minutes, hours, days,
  weeks, months)

Because of the variability in responses to similar and dissimilar tasks,
and the wide range of symptoms following TBI, it is accepted practice
that portions from existing standardized batteries be used to gather information. Standardized tests designed for children, adolescents, and
adults in learning disabled and aphasia populations are commonly used.
However, there are potential psychometric dangers in using tests to
measure behavior of a population on which they have not been normed.
These include questionable content validity, poor reliability, and inappropriate application of norms and standardized data. No single test battery
currently exists to address the unique cognitive language problems encountered by the TBI population. Until a comprehensive battery is developed for TBI (at different stages of recovery), we have no choice but to
use standard tests in nonstandard procedures. Therefore, the collection
of subtests must include a variety of tasks that

Allow a comparison of modalities (both receptive and expressive)
Show a hierarchy of complexity among the tasks
Show a hierarchy of structure or predictability (ranging from automatic
  to open-ended tasks)
Provide a comparison of "processing" ability versus actual performance
  during functional tasks

Table 7-7 identifies several tests from which to choose. It is not finite,
and other sources are available (Hagen, 1984; Adamovich and colleagues, 1985; Lezak, 1983).

Nonstandardized Procedures

The use of nonstandardized procedures in evaluation of cognitive-
language disorders has been accepted practice for many years (Becker and
Malkmus, 1982; Beukelman and colleagues, 1985; Adamovich and col-

**Table 7-7. Standardized tests applicable to
the traumatic brain-injured population**

General Batteries Test and Author(s)	Description of Usefulness
Minnesota Test for Differential Diagnosis of Aphasia (Schuell, 1972)	Screening test of categorical areas, hierarchial tasks for complexity and predictability
Boston Diagnostic Aphasia Examination (Goodglass and Kaplan, 1983a)	Provides a range of language tasks for comprehension, expression in multimodalities
Clinical Evaluation of Language Functions (Semel and Wiig, 1980)	Visual and verbal subtests test word fluency, verbal retention, associations, reasoning
Detroit Tests of Learning Aptitude-2 (Hammill, 1985)	Specific subtests evaluate verbal-visual sequencing, visual analysis, conceptual thinking
Woodcock-Johnson Psychoeducational Battery: Tests of Cognitive Ability (Woodcock and Johnson, 1977)	Specific subtests evaluate visual analysis, problem solving, reasoning, concept formation
Illinois Test of Psycholinguistic Abilities (Kirk and colleagues, 1968)	Visual and auditory subtests test closure, differentiation, memory, analysis-synthesis
Wechsler Adult Intelligence Scale (Wechsler, 1955)	Verbal subtests test attention, recall (immediate and remote), knowledge, abstract comprehension, reasoning, fluency; performance subtests test visual attention, speed of response, organization, scanning, eye-hand coordination
Wide Range Achievement Test (Jastak and Jastak, 1978)	Reading section is useful for measuring reading rate and single word recognition
Word Test (Jorgenson and colleagues, 1981)	Tests word retrieval, association-categorization, similarities-differences
Revised Visual Retention Test (ed. 4) (Benton, 1974)	Sensitive to visual attention, recall span, visuospatial organization
Raven Coloured Progressive (1965)	A nonlinguistic test identifying visual abstract reasoning and visuospatial analysis
Reporter's Test (DeRenzi and Ferrari, 1978)	Tests verbal formulation and organization (verbal counterpart to the Token Test)
Galveston Orientation and Amnesia Test (Levin and colleagues, 1982)	Tests general orientation to person, place, time, and purpose
Test of Problem Solving (Zachman and colleagues, 1984)	Tests visual attention and synthesis, reasoning, deductive and inferential processing
Ross Test of Higher Cognitive Processes (Ross and Ross, 1979)	Tests complex abstract reasoning and problem solving
Fullerton Language Test for Adolescents (Thorum, 1979)	Subtests test retention, verbal formulation, association, retrieval, abstract reasoning

Table 7-7. (continued)

General Batteries Test and Author(s)	Description of Usefulness
Goldman-Fristoe-Woodcock Auditory Skills Test Battery (Goldman and colleagues, 1974)	Tests auditory processing including discrimination, attention, figure-ground
Wechsler Memory Scale-Revised (Wechsler, 1985)	Tests visual and auditory retention for verbal and nonverbal input at varying levels of complexity; useful for testing processes of attention, organization, analysis-synthesis, learning with repetition
Boston Naming Test (Goodglass and Kaplan, 1983b)	Tests confrontation naming, word retrieval with or without cuing
Revised Token Test (McNeil and Prescott, 1978)	Tests auditory comprehension for increasingly complex and lengthy instructions; tests auditory attention and retention
Rivermead Behavioural Memory Test (Wilson and colleagues, 1985)	Functional memory test for immediate and delayed recall for stories, faces, objects, and multistep procedures
Reading Comprehension Battery for Aphasia (LaPointe and Horner, 1979)	Subtests range from word to picture-sentence, to functional reading tasks, for factual-inferential paragraphs
Peabody Picture Vocabulary Test (Dunn and Dunn, 1981)	Receptive vocabulary test that evaluates visual attention, scanning, and knowledge base

leagues, 1985). As with other populations, their use with the TBI individual augments formal assessment (Malkmus, 1980), provides actual or functional performance information, and can be collected and organized easily. When the individual is unable to cooperate due to severely decreased alertness or attention (LOCF II to IV or V), or when the deficits are mild, nonstandardized activities must be used. Tasks designed to determine similarities and differences, verbal opposites, scrambled sentences, verbal absurdities, sentence construction, problem solving, synonyms, and antonyms all provide useful information when identifying the underlying impaired processes (Malkmus and Becker, 1983). Adamovich and colleagues (1985) outline several activities in a hierarchy, ranging from low-level (arousal and alertness) to high-level (reasoning and abstraction) cognitive tasks. Other materials are found in Kilpatrick and colleagues (1977), Kilpatrick (1979), Brubaker (1983), and Chapey (1986).

Assessing functional communication skills employs a nonstandardized approach. The impact of mildly impaired selective attention, memory, organization, reasoning, abstraction, and integration on communication may be observable in situations where performance is stressed to its maximum limit, such as environments that are noisy and distracting or environments in which rapid decision making and problem solving are demanded or when subtle adjustments must be made because of communication breakdowns. Nonstandardized tasks designed to evaluate the use of processes (cognitive-language-pragmatic) help in "bridging the gap" between performance of structured test items and the individual's performance in the environment. For example, the individual who cannot organize and recall visual shapes on formal testing will also be unable to organize and integrate visual retention skills functionally (e.g., making a grocery list). Or the inability to comprehend and retain detailed paragraphs will be demonstrated functionally by the inability to comprehend and retain short newspaper articles.

Collecting information on communication needs involves systematic clinical observation using nonstandardized data collecting. Determining the individual's communication needs involves identifying the environmental needs, the communication partners, what types of messages must be communicated and how communication occurs. (Table 7-8).

Some literature is available on the interaction needs of nonspeakers (Light, 1988); however, little has been written on the communication needs for the adult neurogenic population. Beukelman (1987) suggests that the interaction processes required for communicating one's needs change over one's life span. For example, the predominant interactions of a young preschooler are used to obtain basic needs and wants and to facilitate social closeness (mostly with the parents). As the child matures and has his or her needs met, interaction patterns change to that of sharing information and promoting social closeness because of the emphasis on education and vocation.

DeRuyter and colleagues (1987) applied this concept to the adult, nonspeaking TBI individual. They suggest that as cognitive recovery occurs, as observed in improvements in the level of functioning, interaction needs also change. For example, the individual functioning at LOCF III (localized response) must communicate basic needs, being cognitively unable to filter and attend to the external environment. However, as basic processes improve, as in individuals at LOCF IV (confused and appropriate), the need to share information increases as these individuals become more aware of their disabilities. Although this notion has yet to be quantified, it provides a clinical framework from which to obtain baseline information on interaction status and track improvement.

PRAGMATICS: EVALUATION AND INFORMATION GATHERING

Evaluation of pragmatic or social communication skills should include analysis of conversational rules, discourse, and the use of communication skills in "real-life" activities. Several authors have designed and

Table 7-8. Communication needs of the traumatic brain-injured population

ENVIRONMENTAL NEEDS
   Hospital: hospital room, therapy room, unit
   Home
   Job setting
   School
   Stores or restaurants
   Outdoors/indoors
   Noisy or quiet setting
   Time of day when communication is best

COMMUNICATION PARTNERS
   Hospital or center personnel
   Familiar individuals (family and friends)
   General public
   Teachers, supervisors
   One or more listeners at a time

COMMUNICATION MESSAGES
   Answers yes and no
   Conveys wants and needs
   Social greetings
   Makes requests and answers questions
   Leaves messages
   Converses with others in organized manner
   Conveys, comprehends, and retains lengthy information
   Conveys and comprehends humor
   Reads, comprehends, and retains functional items (signs, maps, messages,
      lists, newspapers, books, magazines)
   Uses integrative skills for money management, planning and organizing
      daily activities, telephone skills, coordinating transportation

COMMUNICATION MODES (what is needed)
   Gestural-facial expression
   Verbal expression (identify level)
   Written expression (identify level)
   Telephone skills
   Alternative communication system type
   Use of computer (with or without printed output)
   Typewriter

Source: Adapted from Beukleman, D.R., Yorkston, K.M., and Dowden, P.A. (1985). *Communication augmentation: A casebook of clinical management.* Boston, MA: College-Hill Press.

organized assessment checklists that include pragmatic aspects applicable to the behaviors observed following TBI. Prutting and Kirchner (1983) designed a pragmatic protocol consisting of 30 aspects of communication that are organized into the following categories: (1) verbal-paralinguistic, (2) nonverbal, (3) lexical selection and use, (4) stylistic variations, (5) speech acts, (6) topic aspects, and (7) turn taking. This protocol is currently under revision. Mentis and Prutting (1987) and Milton and colleagues (1984) used this protocol, finding that TBI individuals demonstrated reduced performance in topic maintenance and selection as well as turn taking.

There are few protocols specifically designed for use with the TBI population. Reimer and Becker (1986) developed the Rancho Pragmatic Inventory: Revised, which identified pragmatic behaviors in correspondence with the LOCF. Britton-Hare and Hare (1987) developed the Assessment of Interpersonal/Communication Skills for the TBI population and included categories of expressive organization (topic, turn taking, lexical selection and use), prosody (intonation, stress, loudness, pitch), intelligibility (articulation, vocal quality, intensity, rate), and nonverbal behaviors (facial expression, eye contact, and posture). The authors recommend that each behavior be assigned given a score of either severely reduced, occurring inconsistently, or within normal limits. Scores are then added, and the individual is given one of five severity ratings ranging from severe to minimal-normal limits. Neither of these inventories included the necessary verbal, conversational, semantic, and nonverbal aspects of impaired pragmatics after TBI.

Pilot data have been collected, and field testing is currently underway at Rancho Los Amigos Medical Center for the Pragmatic Inventory for Brain Injury (Kennedy and colleagues, 1989) (see Figure 7-1). In developing this inventory, the authors included behaviors known to be impaired by cognitive language dysfunction in adults with TBI, as documented in the literature and from many years of clinical experience. The categories were chosen and revised from Penn (1986), since her inventory was behaviorally oriented yet retained the pragmatic aspects of fluency and sociolinguistic differences. Given the word findings–word generation problems and the cultural differences in the TBI population, these two categories are believed to include important clinical information.

Each of the behaviors, having been observed in the identified communication situation, is rated as being consistent (and appropriate), inconsistently present and appropriate, inappropriate, or not present (not observed). The "inappropriate" category refers to a behavior that either by its absence is socially unacceptable or by its impairment or misuse is socially unacceptable. For example, the use of conjunctions in connecting semantic units is acceptable, except when the use is excessive, as in tangential or "run-on" speech. The absence of conjunctions may be illustrated in the example of the individual who begins each sentence in the same manner because of word finding problems (also categorized as a impairment in lexical choice). Field tests of this inventory indicate that behaviors cluster together based on the impaired underlying processes. For example, highly confused and disinhibited individuals have more inappropriate behaviors in the semantics and response categories than do individuals with subtle processing deficits. Higher-level individuals (LOCF VI to VIII) demonstrate more inconsistent and appropriate behav-

---

PRAGMATIC INVENTORY FOR BRAIN INJURY

NAME _____ DATE_____

ETIOLOGY_____ COGNITIVE LEVEL_____

SITUATION #1 _____

SITUATION #2 _____

SPECIFIC PROBLEMS_____

Instructions: indicate the category with a checkmark. Mark
only one for each behavior.
  C= consistent   INP= inappropriate
  INC= inconsistent   NO= no opportunity to observe

INTERACTION/CONTENT	C	INC	INP	NO
Requests	—	—	—	—
Acknowledges	—	—	—	—
Repair strategies:				
Asks for clarification	—	—	—	—
Modifies/shifts when partner asks	—	—	—	—
Turn-taking	—	—	—	—
Shift when partner introduces new topic	—	—	—	—
Topic selection	—	—	—	—
Topic initiation	—	—	—	—
Topic maintenance	—	—	—	—
Topic expansion	—	—	—	—
Topic termination	—	—	—	—
Lexical choice (vocabulary)	—	—	—	—
Idea sequencing/organization	—	—	—	—
Quality/conciseness	—	—	—	—
Other:_____	—	—	—	—

COHESION

	C	INC	INP	NO
Use of Conjunctions	—	—	—	—
Presupposes	—	—	—	—
References	—	—	—	—

Figure 7-1

iors in specific categories depending on their individual residual processing deficits.

Discourse analysis through a cohesion analysis approach has provided clinically useful information (Mentis and Prutting, 1987). It is important to remember that this detailed analysis is most useful in analyzing discourse in individuals who have subtle communications deficits,

	C	INC	INP	NO
COHESION (continued)				
Use of Pronouns	—	—	—	—
Word order (syntax,phrasing)	—	—	—	—
Other:_____	—	—	—	—
FLUENCY (Motor function)				
Interjections (fillers)	—	—	—	—
Repetitions	—	—	—	—
Revisions (whole word, restarts)	—	—	—	—
Phrasing (completeness of)	—	—	—	—
False starts	—	—	—	—
Pauses	—	—	—	—
Word-finding	—	—	—	—
Other:_____	—	—	—	—
SOCIOLINGUISTIC SENSITIVITY				
Polite forms	—	—	—	—
Placeholders, fillers, stereotypes	—	—	—	—
Sarcasm/humor	—	—	—	—
Adjustments in style	—	—	—	—
Other:_____	—	—	—	—
NONVERBAL COMMUNICATION				
Vocal aspects:				
Intensity				
Pitch	—	—	—	—
Rate	—	—	—	—
Intonation	—	—	—	—
Quality:_____	—	—	—	—
Nonverbal aspects:	—	—	—	—
Facial expression				
Body posture	—	—	—	—
Breathing	—	—	—	—
Social distance	—	—	—	—
Gesture/pantomine	—	—	—	—
Eye contact	—	—	—	—
	—	—	—	—

Portions adapted from Penn,C. (1986). Pragmatic Inventory. Unpublished manuscript. Santa Barbara, CA: University of California, Santa Barbara.

Figure 7-1 (continued)

having recovered many of the more basic cognitive-language processes. This type of analysis assists in determining therapy goals specific to the individual and the communication situation. It would not be the most efficient method for determining therapy goals with highly confused, rapidly improving individuals, although the collection of baseline information is important.

Milton (1988) describes an analytic approach identifying communication competency in specific tasks and environments. For individuals at LOCF VII (automatic and appropriate) and LOCF VIII (purposeful and appropriate), this approach should be emphasized, since the impaired processes now require compensation or retraining rather than "reorganization" at this latter point in recovery (see Table 7-13 for a list of functional communication skills).

PLANNING INTERVENTION AT VARIOUS STAGES OF RECOVERY

Intervention changes as the individual's cognitive-language processes improve. A variety of assessment procedures are used to determine goals, including the ones discussed in the preceding sections. Which procedures are used at any one time depends on the stability of the recovery phase (fluctuating or static), the individual's ability to cooperate, the initial processes and behaviors impaired, and the individual's communication needs. Assessment can be divided into three categories depending on the cognitive-language recovery phase. Each will be discussed separately.

ASSESSMENT FOR INDIVIDUALS AT LEVELS II AND III (GENERALIZED AND LOCALIZED RESPONSE LEVELS)

With the advent of improved life-sustaining techniques, many TBI individuals are surviving who would otherwise have died 10 years ago. Jennett and Teasdale (1981) found that 7 percent of their severe TBI population was considered in a persistent vegetative state (PVS) at 1 month after injury. Thirteen percent demonstrated some attention and arousability at 1 month, for which the category PVS was uncertain. These individuals reached the moderate disability or good recovery outcome categories on the Glasgow Outcome scale. This is a significant number who showed improvement. Thus it appears that although some early measures are useful in identifying outcome for those in the "severe" category, for many the prognosis is unpredictable (Whyte and Glenn, 1986; Bartkowski and Lovely, 1986). Therefore, assessment tools must be sensitive enough to provide prognostic information.

Assessment of cognitive-language function utilizes nonstandardized procedures with a interdisciplinary team approach. The team (including speech-language pathology, physical therapy, nursing, occupational therapy, the family, social work, psychology, physician) provides discipline-specific information on the individual's cognitive status. There are several reasons for a team approach. Logistically, these individuals are considered "total care," requiring positioning, lifting, ranging, and assistance in activities of daily living. Thus, assessment actually requires two or more therapists. Also, because of the variability, inconsistency, and delay in responses, checklists and record sheets must be kept by all persons having contact with the TBI individual to identify patterns of behavior over time. Last, integrated knowledge from all treating disciplines also provides different perspectives on how to elicit responses during the evaluation. For example, physical therapists know the effects of positioning, muscle tone, and head positioning on facilitating movement and therefore behavioral responses. By having one therapist position the individual while another observes changes in responses, the evaluation becomes more efficient and effective (Reimer and Donoghue, 1987).

The evaluation of cognitive-language function in individuals at Levels II and III involves the nonstandardized yet systematic presentation of stimuli. The evaluator presents stimuli from various sensory modalities in isolation first while altering the rate, complexity, duration, repetition, and amount. Then performance in each of the modalities is compared with and contrasted to other modalities (Reimer and Donoghue, 1987; Malkmus and colleagues, 1980). Observations in performance variables are made and recorded (type of response, endurance, response delay, recovery time, repetitions). Table 7-9 identifies the most common stimuli used to elicit responses.

Table 7-10 identifies processes, areas, and methods applicable to individuals functioning at LOCF II and III. The speech-language pathologist is often the team member primarily responsible for defining alertness and

Table 7-9. Commonly used stimuli for evaluating individuals at LOCF II and III

TACTILE	OLFACTORY
Shapes (cubes, balls)	Extracts
Surfaces (cloth, Velcro, cotton ball)	Perfumes and colognes
Fur	Spices
Brushes and combs	Soap
Firm touch	Vinegar
KINESTHESIA	VISUAL
Range of motion	Objects from home
Positioning (extremities and body)	Pictures of family and individual
AUDITORY	Mirror
Bells	Colorful items
Chimes	ADL items
Clapping	GUSTATORY
Music	Extracts
Voice (familiar and unfamiliar)	Lemon
Snapping fingers	Vinegar

Table 7-10. Evaluation process for individuals at LOCF II and III

Processes/areas	Methods
Alertness: amount, frequency timing, activities, body positions	Team evaluation
Arousability: types of stimulation and responses	Systematic presentation of hierarchial tasks
Sensory modalities: tactile, kinesthetic, olfactory, gustatory, auditory, visual	Observe at various times and during various tasks
	Interview family members
Communication: following commands, type of response, communication system, basic reading	Observe individual with family, note responses
	Use familiar items: music, pictures
Presence of reflexes: oral chewing, defensiveness, whole body reflexes	Record frequency, rate, duration, variety and quality of responses
Balance: posture, head control limb alignment, sitting, standing	Observe responses with cuing (manual, verbal, gestural, nonverbal)
Arm and hand function: reaching, grasping, gestures	
Tone: overall, at rest, in motion, various positions	

Adapted from Reimer, T.J. and Donoghue, K. (1987). The speech pathologist's role in the stimulation of the low level brain injured patient. Presented at the California Speech-Language-Hearing Association Convention, San Diego, CA.

attention, arousability, responses to sensory modalities, receptive, and expressive communication.

A particularly useful tool recently developed to access cognitive and communication changes in this population is the WNSSP (Ansell and Keenan, 1989). It consists of 33 items selected from a range of commonly associated behaviors in individuals functioning at LOCF II to V (generalized to confused and inappropriate). Six subscales have been delineated to identify patterns of behavior. These include:

Arousal and attention
Auditory comprehension
Visual comprehension
Visual tracking
Object manipulation
Expressive communication
Olfactory response

The WNSSP is sensitive to small increments of change and has predictive value for cognitive recovery for extremely severely impaired individuals (Ansell and Keenan, 1989). Other sources that describe assessment of slow-to-recover individuals and those at LOCF II and III are Malkmus and colleagues (1980), Bartkowski and Lovely (1986), Jennett and Teasdale (1981), and Teasdale and Jennett (1976).

ASSESSMENT FOR INDIVIDUALS AT LEVELS IV AND V (CONFUSED AND AGITATED, CONFUSED AND INAPPROPRIATE)

Because individuals functioning at LOCF IV and V are unable to focus and maintain their attention to specific task, to discriminate, and to sequence and organize their responses, the speech-language pathologist must employ nonstandardized procedures to obtain assessment information. As discussed earlier, these individuals frequently appear "unmotivated" and display uncooperative and agitated behavior. Use of standardized tests is at times not practical, although baseline data (gathered as early as possible) can clarify the pattern of recovery and provide prognostic information. Table 7-11 outlines processes and methods specifically applicable to these individuals.

This is frequently a time of frustration for the therapist who believes that baseline information must be obtained through traditional methods. It is important to remember that this phase of recovery is organically based and is actually a sign of improvement from the lower levels of cognitive response (LOCF II and III). As soon as standardized methods can be used, they should be incorporated into the evaluation.

Table 7-11. Evaluation process for individuals at LOCF IV and V

Processes/areas	Methods
Hyper attentiveness of hypo-attentiveness	Team evaluation
Selectivity, attention span	Systematic presentation of hierarchical tasks
Orientation or confusion: time, place, persons, objects	Use standardized tests if able
Sequencing: in expression, thought, activity	Present simple, motor, functional activities
Inhibition or disinhibition	Evaluation sessions 15 to 30 minutes long
Organization: associating, categorizing	Vary tasks to allow for attention and disinhibition
Agitation: causes, frequency, duration, what reduces it	Include behavioral reinforcements for reducing agitation
Communication: modalities, content, generalized versus focal, comprehension, use of social skills	Include familiar persons to elicit best response

Source: Adapted from Becker, M. (1986). Cognitive-linguistic assessment protocol: Revised. Presented at the Ninth Annual Conference, "Coma to Community." Santa Clara Valley Medical Center, San Jose, CA.

ASSESSMENT FOR INDIVIDUALS AT LEVELS VI, VII AND VIII (CONFUSED AND APPROPRIATE, AUTOMATIC AND APPROPRIATE, PURPOSEFUL AND APPROPRIATE)

The evaluation process is tailored to the individual and his or her type, severity, and location of injury as well as his or her communication needs. Individuals who are disoriented and confused and have difficulty learning new tasks (LOCF VI) require investigation of impaired processes and a comparison with the actual performance during functional activity. Individuals who display mild to minimal cognitive deficits (LOCF VII and VIII) but demonstrate impairment in higher thought processes require a more detailed task-specific evaluation, although attempts at determining impaired processes should be made (using standardized tests). Thus, processes, performance, needs, and capacity to learn must be identified to provide prognostic information, both in general and task-specific evaluation.

The interdisciplinary team approach to cognitive-language-behavioral evaluation for individual functioning at LOCF VI to VIII is vital. The neuropsychologist can determine subtle attention deficits and speed of performance through rigorous testing, while the occupational therapist analyzes the individual's behavior during activities of daily living. Having the training in task analysis and processing, the speech-language pathologist frequently assumes the role of analyzing the effects impaired processes have on performance in daily activities and communication. Table 7-12 identifies the areas needing evaluation and the methods for gathering the information.

The task of organizing and recording data from nonstandardized activities can be time consuming and cumbersome. Tefft and colleagues (1986) developed a Functional Skills Profile that includes checklists for cognitive-communication skills in individuals who are beyond the spontaneous recovery period (Table 7-13). Each area includes activities arranged in a hierarchy from basic to complex and from predictable to unpredictable. A detailed example of this is presented in Table 7-14. This hierarchy allows for an organized approach to the presentation of stimuli and a useful method for recording data over time.

THE EFFECTS OF COGNITIVE-LANGUAGE IMPAIRMENT ON OUTCOME

It is evident that the cognitive, language, behavioral, and psychological consequences of brain injury have reciprocal relationships with communication. In turn, the impact of impaired communication on functional

Table 7-12. Evaluation process for individuals at LOCF VI, VII or VIII

Processes/areas	Methods
Identify processes: from attention to integration	Team evaluation
Focus on speed of processing, memory retrieval, problem solving, attention to detail, endurance, reasoning, organization	Administer standardized test
Performance for functional communication: reading, writing, humor, retention, retrieval, money skills, school and work skills, planning and executing tasks	Administer nonstandardized tasks
Pragmatics: conversational rules and cohesion	Use checklists for recording and organizing
Communication needs: environmental and listener demands, content, type of message	Interview individual and family to find out their goals
Analyze relationship between processes, performance, and communication needs	Observe "real-life" situations
	Observe performance during "stressful" tasks and situations
	Simulate communication situations

outcome (vocational, educational, familial, and social) constitutes a difficult and complex problem. It is difficult to compare and contrast the results of outcome and overall adjustment studies due to (1) variability on populations (acute hospital studies have shown a higher incidence of returning to work than rehabilitation-center-based studies), (2) the variability between studies in the time after onset in which the data were gathered, (3) various forms of assessment or data gathering, (4) the various ages included, obviously clouding certain issues involving younger individuals (Oddy, 1984), and (5) the usual lack of information about premorbid intellect and psychological status (Levin and colleagues, 1982). Therefore, drawing conclusions across studies is difficult. For example, Heilman and colleagues (1971) found that only 2 percent of closed head injury individuals exhibited aphasia. Later studies report a much higher incidence (Levin and colleagues, 1976; Sarno, 1980, 1984; Sarno 1986)).

However, in light of these problems, some useful information about the long-term effects of cognitive, memory, and language disorders has been gathered through the use of specific neuropsychological and linguistic assessment. Levin and colleagues (1979) found that the presence of aphasia correlated with low verbal performance IQs on the Wechsler Adult Intelligence Scale (WAIS) (Wechsler, 1955). Conversational speech deficits and impaired comprehension "resolved" (as measured on stan-

Table 7-13. Functional cognitive and language skills

Functional communication: Verbal and written expression, spelling, auditory and reading comprehension

Functional memory: Orientation (time, space, and community), recall of schedule and events, learns instructions and new skills, retains directions over time, use of recall for planning

Functional reading: Signs, coupons, menus, advertisements, labels, schedules, maps, pamphlets and brochures, applications, order forms, newspapers, magazines, books

Money management: Coins and paper money, calculations, purchases, banking (checkbook, automatic teller, bank statements, etc.), budgeting (itemizing, checks and balances, paying bills), credit cards, investments, tax forms

Study and testing skills (for school): Follows schedule, behavior in class, initiates asking for help, concentration, study habits (time organization, completion of work)

Telephone skills: Places a call, records information, includes pertinent information, initiates use of the phone, uses telephone book, makes emergency calls

Transportation: Basic planning for public transportation (bus, taxi, subway, etc.), organizes and executes trips, obtaining driver's license, use of maps, problem solving for auto breakdowns

Source: Reprinted with permission from Tefft, D., Briggs, D., and Stone, D. (1986). Functional Skills Profile. Downey, CA: Professional Staff Association of Rancho Los Amigos Medical Center, Inc.

Table 7-14. Sample of functional skills: Banking and telephoning

BANKING
Completes checks
Fills out deposit and withdrawal slips
Balances checkbook
Manages savings record
Opens, closes, and transfers accounts
Uses "ready-cash" card
Records computerized transactions
Uses back statements to verify records

TELEPHONING
Initiates use of telephone
Dials phone and holds receiver
Calls information and records number
Uses telephone directories (white and yellow)
Can place emergency calls
Communicates on phone in a concise, organized, and complete manner
Records or retains information
Connects or disconnects telephone service
Solves common telephone problems (inaccurate bills)

Source: Reprinted with permission from Tefft, D., Briggs, D., and Stone, D. (1986). Functional Skills Profile. Downey, CA: Professional Staff Association of Rancho Los Amigos Medical Center, Inc.

dardized tests), but Levin's group reported that pragmatic deficits were present in the moderate and severe disability groups. There is an obvious discrepancy in reporting that speech deficits had resolved. Klove and Cleeland (1972) concluded that variation in the duration of coma was reflected in the performance IQ on the WAIS 7 months following the injury but no sooner. Many studies have supported the theory that the longer the PTA, the more severe the intellectual impairment. Roberts (1980) found that severe intellectual impairment was present at 10 years after injury in individuals whose PTA had exceeded 5 weeks. Levin and colleagues (1982) concluded that in general, the verbal IQ of the WAIS plateaus by 6 to 12 months following injury, while the performance IQ may improve for many years.

Specific deficits influence outcome also. The presence of oculovestibular problems, intracranial hematomas, aphasia, or hemiparesis negatively affects intellectual outcome. Without these factors, Levin and colleagues (1982) found that good recovery can be predicted to at least a low average IQ (> 90) in individuals who had a moderate coma. A surprising result of this study was that the presence of oculovestibular deficits correlated higher with significant cognitive and memory impairment than did prolonged coma.

VOCATIONAL OUTCOME

The ability to return to work has received much attention. Although early studies indicated a higher percentage of individuals returning to work after TBI (McIver and colleagues, 1958; Steadman and Graham, 1970), more recent reports indicate that the percentage returning to work can range from 8 to 30 percent (Thomsen, 1974; Oddy and colleagues, 1978; Weddell and colleagues, 1980; Jacobs, 1984, 1988). As Jacobs concluded, the reasons for being unable to work included deficits in communication, cognition, perception, and behavior, as identified by family members. Seventy-two percent of the injured population had been the primary source of income for the family before the injury, while only 15 percent remained so after the injury. In this report on individuals who had participated in local rehabilitation programs in the greater Los Angeles area, of those working after the injury, "54% had returned to their previous employer while the remainder had to find new opportunities. An additional 20% of the total population had found employment since their injury only to subsequently lose their jobs and federal aid had become the primary source of extra-family support for 75% of the unemployed survivors" (Jacobs, 1984, p. 14).

The presence of aphasia and impaired word fluency are generally poor prognostic indicators for successfully returning to work (Ben-Yishay and colleagues, 1982; Kaye and colleagues 1984). Prigatano and colleagues (1984) found that performance on the Digit Symbol subtest of the WAIS (Wechsler, 1955) was a powerful discriminator between those who will return to work successfully. The Digit Symbol subtest measures learning with practice and speed of new learning for nonlinguistic information. Poor visual reaction time scores as measured on computer-based tasks have been correlated with reduced speed and accuracy and can be associated with poor performance in work-related situations. Kaye (1986) reported preliminary results of one study that indicated that low scores on reading rate from the Wide Range Achievement Tests (WRAT) (Jastak and Jastak, 1965), and performance on the logical memory subtest of the Wechsler Memory Scale (Wechsler, 1985) correlated with employment status.

SOCIAL OUTCOME

Resuming leisure and social activities following TBI has received far less attention by researchers, although recently this trend is changing. As Oddy (1984) indicates, those who experienced social isolation are more likely to be a part of the population who required a rehabilitation program. "Confusion" and "verbal expansiveness" as measured by the Katz Adjustment Scales (Katz and Lyerly, 1963) were related to social isolation. Similarly, Jacobs found that the quality of social activities had decreased significantly and that the family had become the source of "social-leisure stimulation, instead of friends and coworkers" (Jacobs, 1984, p. 13)

EFFECTS ON FAMILY RELATIONSHIPS

Family relationships frequently change when one member sustains a brain injury. Family members are confronted with the added responsibility of caring for the person, emotionally, physically, and financially (Jacobs, 1984, 1988; Oddy and Humphrey, 1980; Rosenbaum and Najenson, 1976). Roles within the family structure are altered due to cognitive and communication impairments as well as reductions in self-esteem and financial power, resulting in increased levels of stress and tension in families. Bond's (1975) work has shed light on predicting the variables that become burdensome on families. These variables are the presence of personality changes, mental changes, and PTA longer than 4 weeks. McKinlay and colleagues (1981) had family members fill out questionnaires on their own "stress" level. At 3, 6, and 12 months after injury, families became increasingly discouraged when emotional control and disturbances of language and memory remained the same in the injured individual. The families viewed the basis of their anxiety to be the disinhibited and socially inappropriate behaviors of the injured person. By 12 months after injury, family members perceived these behaviors as personality traits, making statements such as "he could control that behavior if he wanted." Thus over time, families lose perspective on the organicity of the behavior and begin to "blame" the injured person. Clearly, this highlights the importance of identifying and treating cognitive, language, and pragmatic disturbances early in the recovery phase as well as continual education to family members and treatment of residual deficits in later recovery phases.

PSYCHOSOCIAL ADJUSTMENT OF INDIVIDUALS WITH COMBINED GENERAL AND FOCAL LANGUAGE IMPAIRMENT

As described earlier, two specific types of language disorders common after brain injury are processing disorders and word retrieval disorders associated with frontal and temporal lobe contusions (Heilman and colleagues, 1971; Levin and colleagues, 1979; Groher, 1977). It has been the experience of these authors that certain psychosocial behaviors are commonly associated with these language disorders, even when the language disorder has resolved or was present to a mild degree during the early phase of recovery. These associated behaviors are described below:

Paranoia and fear of people, places, and situations

Because of misinterpretation of auditory and visual information, the individual can become suspicious and accusatory. Impaired word retrieval skills produces awkward communication situations. The individual "learns" to associate communication with fear and avoidance (Becker, 1984).

Exacerbation of denial of deficits and lack of insight

The individual is able to identify obvious problems, but lacks the ability to identify consistently more subtle cognitive and language problems (Kodimer and Styzens, 1980).

Reduced stress tolerance

With an accompanying language impairment, frustration is observed more frequently than in those individuals with only generalized communication impairment. During communication acts, as well as during activities that are perceived as too difficult or too easy, a limited tolerance for "perceived" stress is accentuated. These moments of frustration are usually short lived but are often expressed as aggressiveness. By reducing the demands of the situation and environment and redirecting the individual, these situations can be managed easily.

IMPLICATIONS FOR FUTURE RESEACH

The cognitive-language-communication impairment is a complex problem. Understanding the problem requires knowledge of normal processing and development as well as neuropathologic and neurobehavioral relationships. Impaired processes, viewed in isolation and within the period of recovery, are observable in verbal and nonverbal behavior.

Although incidence studies have identified the presence of specific deficits, long-term studies are needed to identify recovery patterns. It is only through the knowledge of how an impairment began that the eventual outcome can be determined. Outcome studies have been general and descriptive but lack the detailed attention to specific cognitive-language disorders, such as verbal recovery patterns in TBI individuals with frontal lobe injury. Although some research has begun, more studies are needed to identify the subtle communication deficits associated with mild injuries, attempting to differentiate between cognitive-language-psychological symptoms. However, until sensitive evaluation tools are developed that target specific types of cognitive language impairments (such as subtle pragmatic disorders) and certain populations within the TBI population (such as the "slow to recover" individual for which the WNSSP is designed, by Ansell and Keenan, 1989), we are unable to gather precise data on the various combinations of communication disorders.

Acknowledgments. The authors want to express appreciation to Terry Jennings-Reimer, Ronald L. Kaufman, MD, Patricia Joseph, and Rhonda Pollard for their assistance in preparing the manuscript and to Paul Kennedy for his support and encouragement.

REFERENCES

Adamovich, B.B. (1978). A comparison of the processes of memory and perception between aphasia and non-brain injured adults. *Proceedings from clinical aphasiology conference.* Minneapolis: BRK Publishers.
Adamovich, B.B., and Henderson, J.A. (1982). An investigation of the cognitive

changes of head trauma patients following a treatment period. Presented at the American Speech-Language-Hearing Association Convention, Toronto.

Adamovich, B.B., Henderson, J.A., and Auerbach, S. (1985). *Cognitive rehabilitation of closed head injured patients: A dynamic approach.* San Diego, CA: College-Hill Press.

Adams, R.D., and Victor, M. (1981). *Principles of neurology.* New York: McGraw-Hill.

Adams, J.H., Graham, D.I., Murray, L.S., and Scott, G. (1982). Diffuse axonal injury due to nonmissile head injury in humans: An analysis of 45 cases. *Annuals of Neurology, 12,* 557–563.

Alexandar, M.P. (1987). The role of neurobehavioral syndromes in the rehabilitation and outcome of closed head injury. In H.S. Levin, J. Grafman, and H.M. Eisenberg, (Eds.), *Neurobehavioral recovery from head injury* (pp. 191–205). New York: Oxford University Press.

Ansell, B., and Keenan, J., (1989). The Western Neuro Sensory Stimulation Profile: a tool for assessing slow-to-recover head-injured patients. *Archives of Physical Medicine and Rehabilitation, 70(2),* 104–108.

ASLHA report of the Subcommittee on Language and Cognition. (June 1987). The role of the speech-language pathologist in the habilitation and rehabilitation of cognitively impaired individuals. *ASHA Journal,* 53–55.

Atkinson, R.C., and Shiffrin, R.M. (1968). Human memory: A proposed system and its control processes. In K.M. Spence and J.N. Spence (Eds.), *The psychology of learning and motivation: Advances in research and theory* (Vol. 2). New York: Academic Press.

Baddeley, A.D. (1984). Memory theory and memory therapy. In B. Wilson and N. Moffatt (Eds.), *Clinical management of memory problems* (pp. 5–27). Rockville, MD: Aspen Publications.

Bartkowski, H.M., and Lovely, M.P. (1986). Prognosis in coma and the persistent vegetative state. *The Journal of Head Trauma Rehabilitation, 1,* 1–6.

Basso, A., Spinnler, H., Vallar, G., and Zanobia, M.E. (1982). Left hemisphere damage and selective impairment of auditory verbal short-term memory. A case study. *Neuropsychologia, 20,* 263–274.

Becker, M.R. (1984). Profile of the language disordered head injured. Paper presented at Interdisciplinary Management of the Head Injured Patient. Champaign, IL: Burnham Hosptial.

Becker, M.R. (1986). Cognitive-linguistic assessment protocol: revised. Paper presented at the Ninth Annual Conference, "Coma to Community." Santa Clara Valley Medical Center, San Jose, CA.

Becker, M.R., and Malkmus, D. (1982). Non-standardized cognitive-linguistic assessment of the adult. Paper presented at Rehabilitation of the Head Injured Child and Adult: Selected Problems, Palm Springs, CA.

Benton, A.L. (1974). *Revised visual retention test* (ed. 4). New York: Psychological Corporation.

Ben-Yishay, Y., Rattock, J., and Diller, L. (1979). A clinical strategy for the systematic amelioration of attentional disturbances in severe head trauma patients (monograph). New York: Institute of Rehabilitation Medicine.

Ben-Yishay, Y., Rattock, Ross, B., Lakin, P., Ezrachi, O., Silver, S., and Diller, L. (1982). Rehabilitation of cognitive and perceptual deficits in people with traumatic brain damage: A five-year clinical research study. In *Working approaches to remediation of cognitive deficits in brain damaged persons* (Rehabilitation Monograph No. 64), New York University Medical Center, Institute of Rehabilitation Medicine, 127–176.

Beukelman, D.R. (1987). Augmentative communication. . .working together. Paper presented to the American Speech-Language-Hearing Foundation Conference, Denver, CO.

Beukelman, D.R., Yorkston, K.M., and Dowden, P.A. (1985). *Communication augmentation: A casebook of clinical management.* San Diego, CA: College-Hill Press.

Beukelman, D.R., Yorkston, K.M., and Lossing, C.A. (1984). Functional communication assessment of adults with neurogenic disorders. In A.S. Halpern and M.J. Fuhrer (Eds.), *Functional assessment in rehabilitation* (pp. 101–115). Baltimore: Paul H. Brookes Publishing.

Bloom, L., and Lahey, M. (1978). *Language development and language disorders.* New York: Wiley.

Bond, M.R. (1975). Assessment of psychosocial outcome after severe head injury. In *Outcome of severe damage to the central nervous system,* CIBA Foundation Symposium 344 (pp. 141–158). Amsterdam: Elsevier.

Bricolo, A., Turazzi, S., and Feriotti, G. (1980). Prolonged posttraumatic unconsciousness. *Journal of Neurosurgery,* 52, 625–634.

Britton-Hare, C., and Hare, S. (1987). *Assessment of interpersonal communication skills.* Sunnyview Hospital and Rehabilitation Center (unpublished manuscript).

Broadbent, D.E. (1958). *Perception and communication.* London: Pergamon Press.

Broadbent, D.E. (1971). *Decision and stress.* London: Academic Press.

Brooks, D.N. (1972). Memory and head injury. *Journal of Nervous and Mental Diseases,* 155, 350–355.

Brooks, D.N. (1983). Disorders of memory. In M. Rosenthal, E.R. Griffith, M.R. Bond, and G.D. Miller (Eds.), *Rehabilitation of the head injured patient.* Philadelphia: Davis.

Brooks, N. (1984). Cognitive deficits after head injury. In N. Brooks (Ed.), *Closed head injury: Psychological, social and family consequences* (pp. 44–73). New York: Oxford University Press.

Brooks, D.N., Aughton, M.E., Bond, M.R., Jones, P., and Rizvi, S. (1980). Cognitive sequelae in relationship to early indices of severity of brain damage after severe blunt head injury. *Journal of Neurology, Neurosurgery and Psychiatry, 43,* 529–534.

Brubaker, S.H. (1983). *Workbook for reasoning.* Detroit, MI: Wayne State University Press.

Bruckner, F.E., and Randle, A.P.H. (1972). Return to work after severe head injuries. *Rheumatology and Physical Medicine, 11,* 344–48.

Bruner, J.S. (1964). The course of cognitive growth. *American Psychologist, 19,* 1–15.

Cermak, L.S., and Moreines, J. (1976). Verbal retention deficits in aphasic and amnesic patients. *Brain and Language,* 3, 16–27.

Chapey, R. (1986). Cognitive intervention: Stimulation of cognition, memory, convergent thinking, divergent thinking and evaluative thinking. In R. Chapey (Ed.), *Languge intervention strategies in adult aphasia* (ed. 2) (pp. 215–238). Baltimore: Williams & Wilkins.

Clifton, G.L., Grossman, R.G., Makela, M.E., Miner, M.E., Handel, S., and Sadhu, V. (1980). Neurological course and correlated computerized tomography findings after severe closed head injury. *Journal of Neurosurgery,* 52, 611–624.

Conkey, R.C. (1938). Psychological changes associated with head injuries. *Archives of Psychology, 33,* 232.

Courville, C.B. (1937). *Pathology of the central nervous system*. Mountain View, CA: Pacific Press.

Cummings, J. (1985). Behavioral disorders associated with frontal lobe injury. In *Clinical neuropsychiatry*. Orlando, FL: Grune & Stratton.

Currey, S.H. (1981). Event-related potentials as indicant of structural and functional damage in closed head injury. *Progressive Brain Research, 54*, 507–515.

Dencker, S.J., and Lofving, B. (1958). A psychometric study of identical twins discordant for closed head injury. *Acta Psychiatry Neurological Scandinavia (Suppl.), 122*, 119–126. In Levin, H.S., Benton, A.L., and Grossman, R.G. *Neurobehavioral consequences of closed head injury*. New York: Oxford University Press.

Denny-Brown, D., and Russell, W.R. (1941). Experimental cerebral concussion. *Brain, 64*, 93–164.

DeRenzi, E., and Ferrari, C. (1978). The Reporter's Test: A sensitive test to detect expressive disturbances in aphasic. *Cortex, 14*, 279–293.

DeRuyter, F., and Becker, M.R. (1988). Augmentative communication: Assessment, system selection, and usage. *The Journal of Head Trauma Rehabilitation, 3*, 35–44.

DeRuyter, F., Becker, M.R., and Doyle, M. (1987). Assessment and intervention strategies for the nonspeaking brain injured. Presented at American Speech-Language-Hearing Association Convention, New Orleans, LA.

Dodd, D., and White, R.M. Jr. (1980). *Cognition: mental structures and processes*. Boston: Allyn and Bacon.

Dowling, G.A. (1985). Levels of cognitive functioning: Evaluation of interrater reliability. *Journal of Neurosurgical Nursing, 17*, 129–134.

Doyle, M., Kauss, P., and Smith, R. (1980). The art of societal re-entry. In *Rehabilitation of the head injured adult: Comprehensive management* (pp. 106–109). Downey, CA: Professional Staff Association of Rancho Los Amigos Hospital, Inc.

Dunn, L.M., and Dunn, L.M. (1981). *Peabody Picture Vocabulary Test-Revised*. Circle Pines, MN: American Guidance Service.

Filley, C.M., Cranberg, L.D., Alexander, M.P., and Hart, E.J. (1987). Neurobehavioral outcome following closed head injury in childhood and adolescence. *Archives of Neurology, 44*, 194–201.

Finger, S., and Stein, D.G. (1982). *Brain damage and recovery* (pp. 153–173). New York: Academic Press.

Fitts, P.M., and Posner, M.I. (1973). *Human performance*. London: Prentice-Hall.

Flavell, J.H. (1977). *Cognitive development*. Englewood Cliffs, NJ: Prentice-Hall.

Galin, D. (1974). Implication for psychiatry of left and right cerebral specialization. *Archives of General Psychology, 1*, 572–583.

Gazzaniga, M.S. (1979). The frontal lobes. *Handbook of behavioral neurobiology: Neuropsychology* (Vol. 2). New York: Plenum Press.

Gazzaniga, M.S., and Hillyard, S.A. (1971). Language and speech capacity of the right hemisphere. *Neuropsychologia, 9*, 273–280.

Gennarelli, T.A., Adams, J.H., and Graham, D.J. (1981). Acceleration induced head injury in the monkey. II. The model, its mechanical and physiological correlates. *Acta Neuropathologica (Berlin), Suppl. 7*, 23–25.

Gennarelli, T.A., Thibault, L.E., Adams, J.H., Graham, D.I., Thompson, C.J., and Marcincin, R.P. (1982). Diffuse axonal injury and traumatic coma in the primate. *Annals of Neurology, 12*, 564–574.

Geschwind, N. (1964). Non-aphasic disorders of speech. *International Journal of Neurology, 4*, 207–214.

Gianutsos, R., and Gianutsos, J. (1979). Rehabilitating the verbal recall of brain-injured patients by mnemonic training: An experimental demonstration using single-case methodology. *Journal of Clinical Neuropsychology, 1,* 117–135.

Goldman, R., Fristoe, M., and Woodcock, R. (1974). *Goldman-Fristoe-Woodcock Auditory Skills Test Battery.* Minnesota: American Guidance Service, Inc.

Goodglass, H., and Kaplan, E. (1983a). *Boston Diagnostic Aphasia Examination.* Philadelphia: Lea & Febiger.

Goodglass, H., and Kaplan, E. (1983b). *The Boston Naming Test.* Philadelphia: Lea & Febiger.

Gordon, W.P. (1983). Memory disorders in aphasia: I. Auditory immediate recall. *Neuropsychologia, 21,* 325–339.

Groher, M. (1977). Language and memory disorders following closed head trauma. *Journal of Speech and Hearing Research, 20,* 212–223.

Gronwall, D., and Sampson, H. (1974). *The psychological effects of concussion.* Auckland: Auckland University Press.

Guilford, J.P. (1967). *The nature of human intelligence.* New York: McGraw-Hill.

Hagen, C. (1981). Language disorders secondary to head injury: Diagnosis and treatment. *Topics in Language Disorders, 1,* 73–87.

Hagen, C. (1982). Language-cognitive disorganization following closed head injury: A conceptualization. In L. Trexler (Ed.), *Cognitive rehabilitation: Conceptualization and intervention* (pp. 131–149). New York: Plenum Press.

Hagen, C. (1984). Language disorders in head trauma. In A. Holland (Ed.), *Language disorders in adults: Recent advances* (pp. 245–282). San Diego, CA: College-Hill Press.

Hagen, C. (1988). Treatment of aphasia: A process approach. *The Journal of Head Trauma Rehabilitation, 3,* 23–34.

Hagen, C., Malkmus, D., and Burditt, G. (1979a). Intervention strategies for language disorders secondary to head trauma. Read before the American Speech-Language-Hearing Association Convention, Atlanta, GA.

Hagen, C., Malkmus, D., and Durham, P. (1979b). Levels of cognitive functioning. In *Rehabilitation of the head injured adult: Comprehensive physical management.* Downey, CA: Professional Staff Association of Rancho Los Amigos Hospital.

Halliday, M.A.K., and Hasan, R. (1976). *Cohesion in English.* London: Longman.

Halpern, H., Darley, F. L., Brown, J.R. (1973). Differential language and neurologic characteristics in cerebral involvement. *Journal of Speech and Hearing Disorders, 38,* 162–173.

Hammill, D.D. (1985). *Detroit Tests of Learning Aptitude-2.* Austin, TX: Pro-Ed.

Harris, J.E. (1984). Methods of improving memory. In B. Wilson and N. Moffatt (Eds.), *Clinical management of memory problems* (pp. 46–62). Rockville, MD: Aspen Systems Corporation.

Heilman, K., Safron, A., and Geschwind, N. (1971). Closed head trauma and aphasia. *Journal of Neurology, Neurosurgery, and Psychiatry, 34,* 265–269.

Heilman, K., Scholes, R., and Watson, R.T. (1976). Defects of immediate memory in Broca's and conduction aphasics. *Brain and Language, 3,* 201–208.

Holland, A. (1982). When is aphasia aphasia? The problem of closed head injury. Presented at the Clinical Aphasiology Conference Proceedings, University of Pittsburgh, PA.

Jacobs, H. (1984). The family as a therapeutic agent: Long-term rehabilitation for traumatic head injury patients. Final Report, National Institute of Handicapped Research.

Jacobs, H.E. (1988). The Los Angeles head injury survey: Procedures and initial findings. *Archives of Physical Medicine and Rehabilitation, 68,* 425–431.

Jastak, J., and Jastak, S. (1965). *The Wide Range Achievement Test manual* (revised edition). Wilmington: Jastak Association.

Jennett, B. (1984). The measurement of outcome. In N. Brooks (Ed.), *Closed head injury: Psychological, social and family consequences* (pp. 37–43). New York: Oxford University Press.

Jennett, B., and Bond, M. (1975). Assessment of outcome after severe brain damage. *Lancet, 1,* 480–487.

Jennett, B., Snoak, J., Bond, M., and Brooks, N. (1981). Disability after severe head injury: Observations on the use of the Glasgow Outcome Scale. *Journal of Neurology, Neurosurgery, and Psychiatry, 44,* 285–293.

Jennett, B., and Teasdale, G. (1981). *Management of head injuries.* Philadelphia: Davis.

Jorgenson, C., Barrett, M., Huisingh, R., and Zachman, L. (1981). *The word test.* Moline, IL: Lingui Systems, Inc.

Kaplan, E. (1983). Process and achievement revisited. In S. Wapner and Kaplan, B. (Eds.), *Toward a holistic developmental psychology.* Hillsdale, NJ: Erlbaum.

Kapur, N., and Coughlan, A.K. (1980). Confabulation and frontal lobe dysfunction. *Journal of Neurology, Neurosurgery, and Psychiatry, 43,* 461–463.

Katz, M.M., and Lyerly, S.B. (1963). Methods for measuring adjustment and social behavior in the community. I. Rationale, description, discriminative validity and scale development. *Psychological Reports, 13,* 503–535.

Kaye, T.E. (1986). National Research and Training Centers: Current research in head injury. Presented at the Fifth Annual National Symposium, National Head Injury Foundation, Chicago, IL.

Kaye, T.E., Walsh, P.M., Ezlachi, O., and Ben-Yishay, Y. (1984). Word fluency after head injury: More than a language test. Presented at the American Speech-Language-Hearing Association Convention, San Fransisco, CA.

Kennedy, M.R., Reimer, T.J., and Lawson, A.C. (1989). Disorders of pragmatics and communication competency following traumatic brain injury. Presented at the American Speech-Language-Hearing Association Annual Convention, St. Louis, MO.

Kilpatrick, K. (1979). *Therapy guide for the adult with language and speech disorders: Advanced stimulus materials, II.* Akron, Ohio: Visiting Nurse Service, Inc.

Kilpatrick, K., Jones, C.L., and Reller, J. (1977). *Therapy guide for the adult with language and speech disorders: A selection of stimulus materials, I.* Akron, Ohio: Visiting Nurse Service, Inc.

Kirby, J.R. (1980). Individual differences and cognitive processes: Instructional application and methodological difficulties. In J.R. Kirby and J.B. Biggs (Eds.), *Cognition, development, and instruction.* New York: Academic Press.

Kirby, J.R., and Biggs, J.B. (1980). *Cognition, development and instruction.* New York: Academic Press.

Kirk, S.A., McCarthy, J.J., and Kirk, W.D. (1968). *Illinois Test of Psycholinguistic Abilities.* Urbana, IL: University of Illinois Press.

Klove, H., and Cleeland, C.S. (1972). The relationship of neuropsychological impairment to other indices of severity of head injury. *Scandinavian Journal of Rehabilitation Medicine, 4,* 55–60.

Kodimer, C., and Styzens, S. (1980). The psychology of the head injured adult. In *Rehabilitation of the head injured adult: Comprehensive management* (pp. 53–57). Downey, CA: Professional Staff Association of Rancho Los Amigos Hospital, Inc.

La Pointe, L., and Horner, J. (1979). *Reading comprehension battery for aphasia.* Tigard, Oregon: C.C. Publications, Inc.

Levin, H.S., and Peters, B.H. (1976). Neuropsychological testing following head injuries: Prosopagnosia without visual field defect. *Disorders of the Nervous System, 37,* 68–71.

Levin, H.S., Benton, A.L. and Grossman, R.G. (Eds.) (1982). *Neurobehavioral consequences of closed head injury.* New York: Oxford University Press.

Levin, H.S., Grossman, R.G., and Kelly, P.J. (1976). Aphasic disorder inpatients with closed head injury. *Journal of Neurology, Neurosurgery, and Psychiatry, 39,* 1062–1070.

Levin, H.S., Grossman, R.G., and Kelly, P.J. (1977). Impairment of facial recognition after closed head injuries of varying severity. *Cortex, 13,* 119–130.

Levin, H.S., Grossman, R.G., Rose, J.E., and Teasdale, G. (1979). Long-term neuropsychological outcome of closed head injury. *Journal of Neurosurgery, 50,* 412–422.

Levin, H.S., Grossman, R.G., Sarwar, M., and Meyers, C.A. (1981). Linguistic recovery after closed head injury. *Brain and Language, 12,* 360–374.

Lewin, W. (1966). *The mangement of head injuries.* Baltimore: Williams & Wilkins.

Lezak, M. (1976). *Mechanisms of neurological disease.* Boston: Little, Brown.

Lezak, M. (1978). *Living with characterologically altered brain injured patient.* Framingham, MA: National Head Injury Foundation, Resource Materials.

Lezak, M. (1983). *Neuropsychological assessment* (ed. 2). New York: Oxford University Press.

Light, J. (1988). Interaction involving individuals using augmentative communication systems: State of the art and future directions for research. *Augmentative and Alternative Communication* 4, 66–82.

Likavec, J. (1987). The interdisciplinary management of the right-cva patient. Presented at the California Speech-Language-Hearing Association Convention. San Francisco, CA.

Loverso, F.L. (1986). Rehabilitation of language-related memory disorders in aphasia. In R. Chapey (Ed.), *Language intervention strategies in adult aphasia* (ed. 2) (pp. 239–250). Baltimore: Williams & Wilkins.

Loverso, F.L., and Craft, R.B. (1982). Memory performance as a function of stimulus input characteristics for both aphasic and normal adults. In R. Brookshire (Ed.), *Clinical aphasiology conference proceedings.* Minneapolis, MN: BRK Publishers.

Luria, A.R. (1967). *Higher cortical functions in man.* New York: Basic Books.

Luria, A.R. (1973). *The working brain: An introduction to neuropsychology.* New York: Basic Books.

Luria, A.R. (1980). *Higher cortical functions in man* (ed. 2). New York: Basic Books.

Malkmus, D. (1980). Cognitive assessment and goal setting. In *Rehabilitation of the head injured adult: Comprehensive management* (pp. 1–11). Downey, CA: Professional Staff Association of the Rancho Los Amigos Hospital, Inc.

Malkmus, D. (1982). Levels of cognitive functioning and associated linguistic behaviors. Presented at Models and Techniques of Cognitive Rehabilitation—II. Indianapolis, Indiana.

Malkmus, D., and Becker, M.R. (1983). Assessment of cognitive-linguistic functions. In D. Garland (Ed.), *Management of head injury* (unpublished manuscript).

Malkmus, D., Booth, B.J., and Kodimer, C. (1980). *Rehabilitation of the head injured adult: Comprehensive cognitive management.* Downey, CA: Professional Staff Association of Rancho Los Amigos Medical Center, Inc.

Mandleberg, I.A., and Brooks, D.N. (1975). Cognitive recovery after severe head injury. I. Serial testing on the Wechsler Adult Intelligence Scale. *Journal of Neurology, Neurosurgery, and Psychiatry, 38,* 1121–1126.

Marshall, J.C., and Newcombe, F. (1980). The structuring of language by biological and neurological processes. Group report. In U. Bellugi and M. Studdert-Kennedy (Eds.), *Signed and spoken language: Biological constraints on linguistic form*. Report at the Dahlem Workshop, Berlin.

McIver, I.N., Lassman, L.P., Thomson, C.W., and McLeod, I. (1958). Treatment of severe head injuries. *Lancet* 2, 544–550.

McKinlay, W.W., Brooks, D.N., Bond, M.R., Martinage, D.P., and Marshall, M.M. (1981). The short-term outcome of severe blunt head injury as reported by the relatives of the injured person. *Journal of Neurology, Neurosurgery, and Psychiatry, 44*, 527–33.

McNeil, M.R., and Prescott, T.E. (1978). *Revised token test*. Baltimore: University Park Press.

McSweeney, A.R., Grant, I., Heaton, R.K., Adams, K.M., and Timms, R.M. (1982). Life quality of patients with chronic obstructive pulmonary disease. *Archives of Internal Medicine, 142*, 473–478.

Mentis, M., and Prutting, C.A. (1987). Cohesion in the discourse of normal and head-injured adults. *Journal of Speech and Hearing Research, 30*, 88–98.

Meyer, A. (1904). The anatomical facts and clinical varieties of traumatic insanity. *American Journal of Insanity, 60*, 373–441.

Miller, E. (1970). Simple and choice reaction time following severe head injury. *Cortex, 6*, 121–127.

Milton, S.B. (1987). A program-without-walls treatment model: What's it all about. Presented at the Sixth Annual National Head Injury Foundation Symposium, San Diego, CA.

Milton, S.B. (1988). Subtle cognitive communication deficits. *Journal of Head Trauma Rehabilitation, 3*, 1–11.

Milton, S.B., Prutting, C.A., and Binder, G.M. (1984). Appraisal of communicative competence in head injured adults. In R. Brookshire (Ed.), *Proceedings from the Clinical Aphasiology Conference*. Minneapolis, MN: BRK Publishers.

Muma, J.R. (1978). *Language handbook: Concepts assessment and intervention*. Englewood Cliffs, NJ: Prentice-Hall.

Najenson, T., Mendelson, L., Schechter, I., Davis, C., Mintz, N., and Groswasser, Z. (1974). Rehabilitation after severe head injury. *Scandinavian Journal of Rehabilitation Medicine, 6*, 5–14.

Najenson, T., Sazbon, L., Fiselzon, J., Becker, E., and Schechter, I. (1978). Recovery of communicative functions after prolonged traumatic coma. *Scandinavian Journal of Rehabilitation Medicine, 10*, 15–21.

Nebes, R.D. (1974). Hemispheric spatialization in commissurotomized man. *Psychological Bulletin, 81*, 1–14.

Neisser, V. (1976). *Cognition and reality: Principles and implications of cognitive psychology*. San Francisco, CA: W.H. Freeman.

Oddy, M. (1984). Head injury and social adjustment. In N. Brooks (Ed.), *Closed head injury: Psychological, social and family consequences* (pp. 108–122). New York: Oxford University Press.

Oddy, M., and Humphrey, M. (1980). Social recovery during the year following severe head injury. *Journal of Neurology, Neurosurgery, and Psychiatry, 43*, 798–802.

Oddy, M., Humphrey, M., and Uttley, D. (1978). Stresses upon the relatives of head-injured patients. *British Journal of Psychiatry, 133*, 507–513.

Parrill-Burnstein, M. (1981). *Problem solving and learning disabilities: An information processing approach*. New York: Grune & Stratton.

Peach, R.K. (1978). On long term memory deficits: A clinical procedure designed to stimulate memory recall in an aphasic patient. In R. Brookshire (Ed.), *Proceedings from clinical aphasiology conference,* Minneapolis, MN: BRK Publishers.

Penn, C. (1986). *Pragmatic inventory.* Santa Barbara, CA: University of California, Santa Barbara (unpublished manuscript).

Piaget, J. (1969). *The child's conception of the world.* Patterson, NJ: Littlefield, Adams.

Piaget, J., and Inhelder, B. (1969). *The psychology of the child.* New York: Basic Books.

Posner, M. (1975). Psychobiology of attention. In M. Gazzaniga and C. Blakemore (Eds.), *Handbook of psychobiology.* New York: Academic Press.

Prigatano, G.P., and Fordyce, D.J. (1986). Cognitive dysfunction and psychosocial adjustment after brain injury. In G.P. Prigatano (Ed.), *Neuropsychological rehabilitation after brain injury* (pp. 1–17). Baltimore: Johns Hopkins University Press.

Prigatano, G.P., and Pribram, K.H. (1982). Perception and memory of facial affect following brain injury. *Perceptual and Motor Skills, 54,* 859–869.

Prigatano, G.P., Roueche, J.R., and Fordyce, D.J. (1986). Nonaphasic language disorders after brain injury. In G.P. Prigantano (Ed.), *Neuropsychological Rehabilitation after brain injury* (pp. 18–28). Baltimore: Johns Hopkins University Press.

Prigatano, G.P., Fordyce, D.J., Zeiner, H.K., Roueche, J.R., Pepping, M., and Wood, B.C. (1984). Neuropsychological rehabilitation after closed head injury in young adults. *Journal of Neurology, Neurosurgery, and Psychiatry, 47,* 505–513.

Prutting, C., and Kirchner, D.M. (1983). Applied pragmatics. In T.M. Gallagher and C. Prutting (Eds.), *Pragmatic Assessment and Intervention Issues in Language* (pp. 29–64). San Diego, CA: College-Hill Press.

Rappaport, M., Hall, K.M., Hopkins, K., Belleza, T., and Cope, N. (1982). Disability rating scale for severe head trauma: Coma to community. *Archives of Physical Medicine and Rehabilitation, 63,* 118–123.

Raven, J.C. (1965). *Guide to using the coloured progressive matrices.* London: H.K. Lewis.

Reimer, T., and Becker, M.R. (1986). *The Rancho Pragmatic Inventory: Revised.* Downey, CA: Professional Staff Association of Rancho Los Amigos Medical Center, Inc.

Reimer, T., and Donoghue, K. (1987). The speech pathologist's role in the stimulation of the low level brain injured patient. Presented at the California Speech-Language-Hearing Association Convention, San Diego, CA.

Reimer, T., and Tanedo, T. (1985). Assessment and treatment of pragmatic disorders in the adult head trauma population. Videotape presentation at the American Speech-Language-Hearing Association Convention, Washington, DC.

Rimel, R.W., Giordani, B., Barth, J.T., and Jane, J.A. (1982). Moderate head injury: Competing the clinical spectrum of brain trauma. *Neurosurgery, 11,* 344–351.

Rizzo, P.A., Amabile, G., Caporali, M., Spadaro, M., Sanasi, M., and Morocutti, C. (1978). A CNV study in a group of patients with traumatic head injuries. *Electroencephalography Clinical Neurophysiology, 45,* 281–285.

Roberts, A.H. (1980). *Severe accidental head injuries: An assessment of long-term prognosis.* Baltimore: University Park Press.

Rosenbaum, M., and Najenson, T. (1976). Changes in life patterns and symptoms of low mood as reported by wives of severely brain-injured soldiers. *Journal of Consulting Clinical Psychology, 44,* 881–888.

Ross, D. (1986). *Ross Information Processing Assessment.* Princeton Junction, NJ: The Speech Bin.

Ross, J.P., and Ross, C.M. (1979). *Ross Test of Higher Cognitive Processes.* Novato, CA; Academic Therapy Publications.

Russell, W.R., and Smith, A. (1961). Post-traumatic amnesia in closed head injury. *Archives of Neurology, 5,* 4–17.

Sarno, M.T. (1980). The nature of verbal impairment after closed head injury. *Journal of Nervous and Mental Disease, 168,* 685–692.

Sarno, M.T. (1984). Verbal impairment after closed head injury. *Journal of Nervous and Mental Disease, 172,* 475–479.

Sarno, M.T., Buonaguro, A., and Levita, E. (1986). Characteristics of verbal impairment in closed head injured patients. *Archives of Physical Medicine and Rehabilitation, 67,* 400–405.

Schacter, D., and Crovitz, H. (1977). Memory function after closed head injury: A review of the quantitative research, *Cortex, 13,* 105–76.

Schuell, H. (1972). *Minnesota Test for Differential Diagnosis of Aphasia; Revised.* Minneapolis, MN: University of Minnesota Press.

Semel, E.M., and Wiig, E. (1980). *Clinical evaluation of language functions.* Columbus, OH: Charles Merrill Publications.

Shiffrin, R.M., and Schneider, W. (1977). Controlled and automatic human information processing. II. Perceptual learning, automatic attending and a general theory. *Psychological Review, 84,* 127–190.

Speirs, J., and Dahlberg, C. (1986). Analysis of verbal and written output in closed head injury. In R. Brookshire (Ed.), *Proceedings from the clinical aphasiology conference.* Minneapolis: BRK Publishers.

Spreen, O., and Benton, A.L. (1969). *Neurosensory center comprehensive examination for aphasia: Manual of directions.* Victoria, BC: Neuropsychology Laboratory, University of Victoria.

Springer, S.P., and Deutsch, G. (1981). *Left brain, right brain.* San Francisco: W.H. Freeman.

Steadman, J.H., and Graham, J.G. (1970). Head injury: Analysis and follow-up study. *Proceedings of the Royal Society of Medicine, 63,* 23–28.

Strich, S.J. (1961). Shearing of nerve fibres as a cause of brain damage due to head injury. *Lancet, 2,* 443–448.

Stuss, D.T. (1987). Contribution of frontal lobe injury to cognitive impairment after closed head injury: methods of assessment and recent findings. In H.S. Levin, J. Grafman, and H.M. Eisenberg (Eds.), *Neurobehavioral recovery from head injury* (pp. 166–176). New York: Oxford University Press.

Stuss, D.T., and Benson, D.F. (1984). Neuropsychological studies of the frontal lobes. *Psychology Bulletin, 95,* 3–28.

Szekeres, S., Ylvisaker, M., and Holland, A. (1985). Cognitive rehabilitation therapy: A framework for intervention. In M. Ylvisaker (Ed.), *Head injury rehabilitation: Children and adolescents* (pp. 219–246). San Diego: College-Hill Press.

Szekeres, S., Ylvisaker, M., and Cohen, S. (1987). A framework for cognitive rehabilitation therapy. In M. Ylvisaker and E.M.R. Gobble (Eds.), *Community re-entry for head injured adults* (pp. 87–136). San Diego: College-Hill Publication.

Teasdale, G. and Jennett, B. (1974). Assessment of coma and impaired consciousness. A practical scale. *Lancet, 2,* 81–84.

Teasdale, G., and Jennett, B. (1976). Assessment and prognosis of coma after head injury. *Acta Neuochirugie 34,* 45–55.

Tefft, D., Briggs, D., and Stone, D. (1986). *Functional skills profile.* Downey, CA: Professional Staff Association of Rancho Los Amigos Medical Center, Inc.

Thomsen, I.V. (1974). The patient with severe head injury and his family—a follow-up study of 50 patients. *Scandinavian Journal of Rehabilitation Medicine, 6,* 180–183.

Thomsen, I.V. (1975). Evaluation and outcome of aphasia in patients with severe closed head trauma. *Journal of Neurology, Neurosurgery, and Psychiatry, 38,* 713–718.

Thomsen, I.V. (1976). Evaluation and outcome of aphasia in patients with severe verified focal lesions. *Folia Phoniatrica, 28,* 362–377.

Thomson, N.J. (1980). Residual language disorders: assessment and intervention. In *Rehabilitation of the head Injured Adult: Comprehensive management* (pp. 66–69). Downey: CA: Professional Staff Association of Rancho Los Amigos Hospital, Inc.

Thorum, A. (1978). *Fullerton Language Test for Adolescents.* Palo Alto, CA: Consulting Psychologists Press.

Treisman, A.M. (1964). Verbal cues, language and meaning in attention. *American Journal of Psychology, 77,* 206–219.

Trexler, L. (1982). The neuropsychology of arousal and attention. In *Models and techniques of cognitive rehabilitation-II: Second annual international symposium* (pp. 4–9). Indianapolis, Indiana.

Van Zomeren, A.H., and Deelman, B.G. (1976). Differential effects of simple and choice reaction after closed head injury. *Clinical Neurology, and Neurosurgery, 79,* 81–90.

Van Zomeren, A.H., and Deelman, B.G. (1978). Long-term recovery of visual reaction time after closed head injury. *Journal of Neurology, Neurosurgery, and Psychiatry, 41,* 452–457.

Van Zomeren, A.H., Brouwer, W.H., and Deelman, B.G. (1984). Attentional deficits: The riddles of selectivity, speed and alertness. In N. Brooks (Ed.), *Closed head injury: Psychological, social and family consequences* (pp. 74–107). New York: Oxford University Press.

Vygotsky, L.S. (1962). *Thought and language.* Cambridge, MA: The MIT Press.

Wechsler, D. (1955). *Manual for the Wechsler Adult Intelligence Scale.* New York: Psychological Corporation.

Wechsler, D. (1985). *Wechsler Memory Scale-Revised.* San Diego: The Psychological Corporation/Harcourt Brace Jovanovich.

Weddell, R., Oddy, M., and Jenkins, D. (1980). Social adjustment after rehabilitation: a two year follow-up of patients with severe head injury. *Psychological Medicine, 10,* 257–263.

Weinstein, E.A., Marvin, S.L., and Keller, N.A. (1962). Amnesia as a language pattern. *Archives of General Psychiatry, 6,* 259–270.

Whitely, A.M., and Warrington, E.K. (1977). Prosopagnosia: a clinical, psychological, and anatomical study of three patients. *Journal of Neurology, Neurosurgery, and Psychiatry, 40,* 395–403.

Whyte, J., and Glenn, M.D. (1986). The care and rehabilitation of the patient in a persistent vegetative state. *Journal of Head Trauma Rehabilitation, 1,* 39–54.

Wilson, B., Cockburn, J., and Baddeley, A.D. (1985). *The Rivermead Behavioural Memory Test.* Reading, England: Thames Valley Test Company.

Woodcock, W., and Johnson, M.B. (1977). *Woodcock-Johnson Psychological Educational Battery: Tests of cognitive ability.* Allen, TX: DLM Teaching Resources.

Wycoff, L.H. (1984). Narrative and procedural discourse following closed head injury. Unpublished doctoral dissertation, University of Florida. In M. Mentis, and C.A. Prutting (1987). Cohesion in the discourse of normal and head injured adults. *Journal of Speech and Hearing Research, 30,* 88–89.

Yorkston, K. (1981). Treatment of right hemisphere damaged patients: A panel discussion. *Proceedings from Clinical Aphasiology Conference.* Minneapolis: BRK Publishers.

Zachman, L., Jorgensen, C., and Huisingh, R. (1984). *Test of problem solving.* Moline, IL: Lingui Systems, Inc.

CHAPTER 8

Reading and Writing Disorders

NICKOLA W. NELSON
BARBARA A. SCHWENTOR

David walked into the clinic and sat down to talk about his past therapies and future hopes. He had not completely given up on the possibilities of returning to his job as an insurance agent, he said, and he wanted to participate in a program that would help him determine whether he would ever be able to read and write well enough again to be able to do so. His problem was that, since his automobile accident, he could not read for any length of time without being bothered by the noise in his head so much that he had to stop. He had not tried to write much, but he could not seem to remember how to spell most words. A sample of his writing appears in Fig. 8-1. Either they were "there" or they were not. He also demonstrated some expressive oral language problems. Many planning pauses occurred, both for formulating sequences of sounds in words and words in sentences, and the results of his efforts were not always quite accurate. Pragmatic problems got in the way of effective communication as well. A lack of informativeness often caused his conversational partners to try to guess what David meant, and he almost always followed by shaking his head and saying, "No, no," when they tried to check their understanding of his meanings.

It was not very easy or pleasant to try to communicate with David, but his communicative problems were mild compared with those of Chris. Chris was pushed into the clinic in his wheelchair by his mother. Another time his adult brother brought him in. Chris was a big strapping fellow even in his wheelchair and not easy to push, but his hands were not working much better than his legs, so he could not propel himself. He had to use the bathroom often and tended to forget that he had just gone. Chris would have been just about to graduate from high school, but he had dropped out before his accident, because he had always had trouble learning and school was not very rewarding for him. His family had to guess about what had happened to him when he was hit as a pedestrian by a motor vehicle, because Chris could not remember anything about it. He could not remember much about his life before either, or at least he could not talk about it so that anyone could understand. Chris did not initiate much of anything, movements or conversation, unless he was specifically prompted. Then, slow moving and minimal response of either articulation or gesture conveyed that Chris was processing more than it appeared. His family wanted to know how they could help Chris occupy his time now in fairly independent pursuits that might help him gain further recovery. The possibility that use of a microcomputer might provide one means of doing so was being considered, but it was not clear whether Chris could read well enough to run through the routines of software when they required written language use.

These two men, David and Chris, were very different in their life stories and their rehabilitation needs. They shared the one experience of

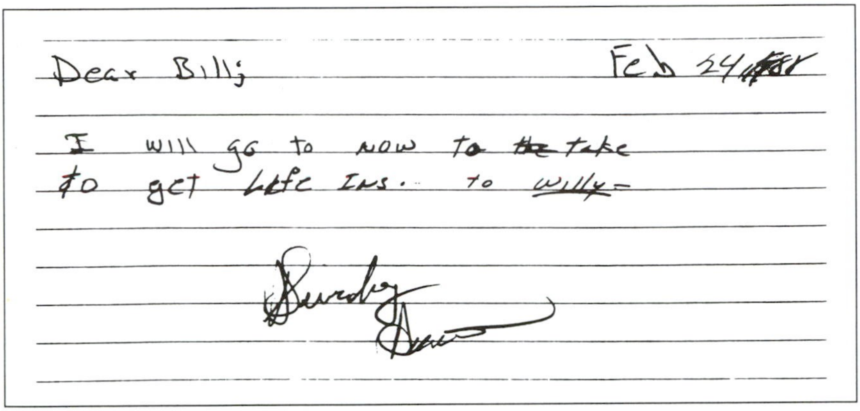

Figure 8-1. David's attempt when asked to write a letter like one he might have produced in the insurance business. The date was added with prompting. He recognized that he had misspelled "Sincerely," but he did not know how to correct it. When questioned about the meaning of the letter, he had difficulty explaining who "Willy" was. Eventually, he explained that the policy was *on* Willy.

having suffered a traumatic brain injury (TBI) that changed their lives dramatically, and each had many needs for communicative and cognitive rehabilitation. One of those needs, for both men, was the assessment of, and possible intervention for, their written language abilities. The techniques to be used for doing so would have to be very different. After all, their pretrauma backgrounds were different, their pretrauma skills were different, their current abilities were different, and their immediate and long-term needs were different.

Any time a clinician faces a clinical problem, issues of commonality and distinction arise. A frequent question is, how can one apply knowledge regarding the predictable expectations for a particular population to this one individual, who may exhibit some of the expected characteristics, but certainly not all? That question is an implicit part of every clinical decision, but never is it more pertinent than when providing assessment and intervention for persons who have experienced TBI. The details of their etiologies, their backgrounds, their retained abilities, and their life goals are all so different that the common ground one can rely on in making clinical decisions is fairly sparse. It is the purpose of this chapter to try to provide greater clarity to one portion of the landscape—the area of reading and writing disorders.

Part of the problem is that little is currently known about the expected characteristics of reading and writing disorders associated with TBI. The research literature, with a few exceptions, is almost silent on this topic. Much of what has been reported will be reviewed here. Another source of information is clinicians who are learning through experience how to work with reading and writing disorders of their TBI clients. The results of a survey of the current scope of practice within major rehabilitation facilities (Surges and Nelson, 1988) will be shared. Finally, direct suggestions for the assessment and intervention of reading and writing disorders based on the authors' own clinical experience and review of the clinical literature will be presented.

CHARACTERISTICS OF WRITTEN LANGUAGE ASSOCIATED WITH TRAUMATIC BRAIN INJURY

Comprehension and production of written language require the integration of a number of cognitive and linguistic skills. Reading and writing are complex acts that involve auditory and visuoperceptual ability, reasoning and organizing ability, access to linguistic and nonlinguistic knowledge, and the ability to draw on past experiences (Singer and Ruddell, 1985). In a society that is dominated by written language, this higher level of cognitive processing is necessary for academic and vocational success as well as for effective social communication.

Investigations of recovery processes following TBI have identified specific cognitive functioning deficits that influence written language processing. Several studies have shown intelligence test score reductions (e.g., Becker, 1975; Chadwick and colleagues, 1981; Levin and Eisenberg, 1979; Levin and colleagues, 1979; Mandleberg and Brooks, 1975; Richardson, 1963), cognitive and memory impairments (e.g, Brooks, 1974, 1976; Levin and colleagues, 1982), learning difficulties (e.g., Brink and colleagues, 1970; Heiskanen and Kaste, 1974; Klonoff and colleagues, 1977), information processing and behavior problems (e.g., Brown and colleagues, 1981; Gronwall and Wrightson, 1974; Rutter, 1981), visuomotor and visuospatial functioning difficulties (e.g., Chadwick and colleagues, 1981c; Levin and Eisenberg, 1979; Klonoff and colleagues, Clark, 1977), and expressive and receptive language deficits (e.g., Brown and colleagues, 1981; Groher, 1977; Heilman and colleagues, 1971; Sarno, 1980; Smith, 1974).

READING AND WRITING DISORDERS IN ADULTS WITH TRAUMATIC BRAIN INJURY

In contrast to the extensive literature on cognitive and oral language disturbance after TBI, few studies have specifically addressed the effects of TBI on written language processing. Those studies that have been reported are difficult to interpret. Some interpretation problems relate to subtest data for written language measurements being reported within tables and figures that do not always correspond directly to subject numbers and discussions of results. Others concern the definitions of reading and writing implicit in many of the studies or definitions of such things as "deficit," "reading backwardness," or "good recovery." For example, the ability to read, match, copy, or write single words may be taken as evidence that a person has no difficulty processing written language. Most professionals who are concerned with the development and use of literacy by children and adults now recognize that being literate involves much more than just being able to transform words and sentences from one modality to another. However, studies of written language processing among people with TBI have not yet begun to reflect this view. It will be important for future studies to address the abilities of persons with TBI to read and write for various purposes, to manage different types of text, to relate written language to broader concepts of the world, and to perform adequately in varied contexts (not just on standardized tests).

Studies reported thus far have involved varied approaches. Some have used reading and writing subtest scores from batteries testing broad cognitive processing abilities as criterion measures of long-term outcome. This type of approach was used by Levin and colleagues (1979), who studied long-term recovery of 27 persons with severe closed head injury between 16 and 50 years of age. A series of neuropsychological tests and interview sessions provided data that were used to rate the subjects' levels of recovery in accordance with the Glasgow Outcome Scale (Jennett and Bond, 1975). Selected subtests from the Multilingual Aphasia Examination (Benton, 1977), the Neurosensory Center Comprehension Examination for Aphasia (Spreen and Benton, 1969), and the Wide Range Achievement Test (Jastak and Jastak, 1978) were administered to evaluate linguistic disturbance. Tests that assessed written language processing included such tasks as reading words from flashcards, matching written words and phrases to pictures, and writing to dictation. Test scores falling below the second percentile of scores obtained for normally functioning adults were used to define deficits. Of the 27 subjects studied, 10 subjects attained a good recovery status. Test results for the good recovery group (interpolated from the authors' data presented in figures) indicated that one subject had a deficit in writing to dictation, and none of the subjects in this group had deficits in reading comprehension or sentence copying. Of the 12 persons who were identified as moderately disabled, the test results indicated that one subject had a deficit in copying sentences, two subjects had deficits in reading comprehension, and none of the subjects had deficits in writing to dictation. Of the five subjects identified as severely disabled, three had deficits in writing to dictation, two had deficits in sentence copying, and three had deficits in reading comprehension.

Levin and colleagues (1979) concluded that their findings showed that residual intellectual level, memory storage and retrieval, linguistic deficit, and personal social adjustment all corresponded to overall outcome. They reported that the results related specifically to written language showed that, according to the measures they selected, reading comprehension recovered within their series of patients and impairment of writing was essentially confined to the severely disabled patients. However, it should be remembered that the "reading comprehension" task in this study required only matching of words and phrases to pictures and that the "writing" tasks required only copying and writing to dictation. Also, individuals were compared with norms that were developed either for normally functioning or aphasic individuals, not for those with TBI.

Groher (1977) evaluated memory and language skills at 1-month intervals for 4 months after 14 adult males had suffered closed head trauma. All the individuals had histories of normal sensory, motor, and intellectual skills. Groher compared the initial scores and recovery patterns of these individuals on the "Gestural," "Verbal," and "Graphic" subtests of the Porch Index of Communicative Ability (PICA; Porch, 1967) by using mean scores (16 being the highest possible score) and percentile data. The percentile data were based on the mean scores "achieved by other individuals with language disability secondary to brain damage" (p. 215) (presumably individuals with aphasia). Groher's results showed that the brain-injured group initially evidenced reductions in gestural, verbal, and graphic skills, with gestural the poorest (mean 6.6; 6th percentile), verbal the strongest (mean 6.6; 33rd percentile), and graphic in between (mean 4.9; 12th percentile). After 4 months, percentile scores for the Graphic subtests (mean 10.1; 75th percentile) were superior to Verbal (mean 13.2; 67th percentile) and Gestural (mean 13.5; 70th percentile) performances. Although graphics skills received the highest percentile ranking at the end of the 4-month assessment period, Groher reported that writing by the individuals with TBI continued to be characterized by spelling errors, incomplete sentence construction, and poor syntax.

Groher's (1977) results also must be interpreted with care in light of the methods of comparison he used. The relative changes in percentile rankings for the three sets of subtests were based on comparisons with scores of individuals with aphasia, who could be expected to have different patterns of recovery from those of persons with TBI. For example, aphasic persons as a group might be expected to score relatively higher on gestural measures (thus requiring a higher mean score to place relatively higher in the percentile rankings) than on verbal and graphic measures (with the result that a lower mean score would place higher in the percentile rankings). In fact, if one simply compares mean scores, smaller gains were made by the individuals with TBI on the Graphics subtests (increase of 5.2) than on either the Verbal (increase of 6.6) or the Gestural (increase of 6.9) subtests. It is questionable whether comparisons between subtest changes would be significant. In the study, statistical tests were only performed on the differences within subtest areas. Perhaps the best conclusion to be drawn from Groher's study is that although individuals with TBI made gains in all three areas without treatment during the 4 months following their closed head injuries, they continued to demonstrate some difficulty with complex and accurate processing of tasks, including those involving written language. Groher also concluded that no significant correlations existed between the length of unconsciousness and initial and final language and memory scores.

The problems inherent in using test instruments standardized for other purposes, and in identifying tests that provide valid measures of written language, were underscored in a study by Rand (1988). Rand investigated the use of reading subtests from standard aphasia batteries with individuals with closed head injury when she replicated a study that had originally been conducted by Nicholas and colleagues (1986) with aphasic adults. Nicholas and colleagues studied the passage dependency of the reading comprehension tests from five aphasia assessment batteries by asking aphasic and non-brain-damaged adults to answer comprehension questions first without the reading passages and then with the passages available. Because more than half the test items could be answered without reading the passage by both normal and aphasic subject groups at a level significantly greater than chance, Nicholas and colleagues concluded that the tests did not provide a valid estimate of the ability to comprehend information from printed texts. Rand (1988) found similar results for individuals with closed head injury. Of the three tests used in Rand's investigation, the Boston Diagnostic Aphasia Examination (BDAE; Goodglass and Kaplan, 1983), the Western Aphasia Battery (WAB; Kertesz, 1982), and the Reading Comprehension Battery for Aphasia (RCBA; LaPointe and Horner, 1979), Rand found that only the RCBA resulted in significantly improved scores when the individuals with closed head injury were able to read the passages before answering comprehension questions. Rand also concluded that "there is a great need for standardized language assessment tools designed specifically for the unique deficits displayed by the head injured population" (p. 25).

Jacobs (1988) used not standardized tests, but functional outcome measures, to study the long-term rehabilitation needs of 142 patients in the Los Angeles area who agreed to participate in in-depth interviews. Although some children between the ages 10 and 19 were included in the study (27.3% of the total sample), the majority of Jacobs' subjects were above age 20. Reading and writing were included as major areas of interest in the survey questions that were addressed to family members regarding the brain-injured individuals' long-term adjustments 1 to 6 years after trauma. Analysis of the results showed a wide range of needs and deficits among the brain-injured participants, with survivors exhibiting problems in every life skills area that was addressed but showing greater deficits among higher-order and more complex skills. Reading and writing deficits were identified as playing a role in difficulties with several higher-order skills. For example, "some persons had problems arranging for medical services because they could not write or talk clearly, sometimes got lost on the way to the office, or would forget their appointments" (p. 428). Problems in the demonstration of independent mobility were sometimes attributed to such factors as "getting lost, problems, reading or following directions, or an inability to use transportation" (p. 428).

Because the average age of survivors in Jacobs' (1988) study was 22 years, most had already completed their educational careers. Of the 25 percent still in school at the time of injury, one third had returned to their studies after approximately 1 year. Approximately half of those who had begun school again after the injury were still in at the time of the study; 13.6 percent had graduated, and 37.8 percent had dropped out before completing their programs. Cognitive, physical, and financial problems were listed as reasons for dropping out.

READING AND WRITING DISORDERS IN CHILDREN WITH TRAUMATIC BRAIN INJURY

Characteristics of reading and writing performance following TBI have also been investigated specifically for school-age children. Fuld and Fisher (1977) were concerned that the use of simplistic tests to quantify intellectual deficits in brain-injured survivors had given the impression that intellectual deficits among children with closed head injury were self-limited and of brief duration. In contrast, Fuld and Fisher reviewed data regarding several children who were recovering from closed head injury but who showed persistent deficits and academic difficulties. They identified complex diagnostic tests of such higher-order cognitive skills, and especially reading comprehension tests, as being particularly useful because (1) they measure the kind of cognitive activity that is most highly correlated with both general intelligence and success in school, (2) they are sensitive to disruption by either diffuse or focal brain damage, and (3) performance can often be compared with information about premorbid functioning in the same area at school. Fuld and Fisher (1977) reported that, in their experience, if premorbid test scores were not available, a reading comprehension score based on a test of reading single words could be used to estimate premorbid ability (because they assumed that single-word reading was less vulnerable to mild to moderate organic brain dysfunction) unless there was a posterior focal lesion.

Shaffer and colleagues (1980) investigated reading abilities of school-age children who sustained closed head injury producing a depressed skull fracture. The Neale Analysis of Reading Ability (Neale, 1958) was administered to assess reading abilities. In this test, children are required to read aloud six prose passages of increasing length and complexity. Reading difficulties were defined for this study as "backward" if the child's chronologic age exceeded reading accuracy age by at least 2 years. The minimum reading age on this test is 6 years; therefore, children younger than 8 years at the time of testing were excluded from the analysis. Of the 88 children included in this portion of the study, 55 percent had reading ages 1 or more years behind their chronologic ages, 33 percent were 2 or more years behind in their reading skills, and similar prevalence was observed for girls and boys. However, the authors pointed out the difficulties in interpreting the results of their within-group, retrospective study because of their inability to assess the effects of such confounding variables as low intelligence, social disadvantage, inadequate or interrupted schooling, and interfering behavioral or physical difficulties, all of which are known to be higher in populations at risk for head injury.

In a similar investigation (possibly involving the same subjects), Chadwick and colleagues (1981a) studied the reading performance of brain-injured children who were 8 years of age or older at the time they sustained unilateral compound depressed fractures of the skull. The authors selected subjects with depressed fractures because they wanted to study laterality effects associated with TBI, and they viewed the contrecoup effect (i.e., trauma to the brain contralateral to the point of impact) to be less of a factor in such individuals than in those with closed head injury. In this study, reading backwardness, as identified by 2-year discrepancy between chronologic age and reading age on the Neale Analysis of Reading Ability (Neale, 1958) was compared with several neurologic characteristics associated with TBI, one of which was duration of unconsciousness. Results were compared for those children who remained unconscious for less than 72 hours and those who were unconscious for more than 72 hours. Of those children who remained unconscious for up to 72 hours, 29 percent (19/66) were reading at least 2 years behind their chronologic age. Of those children who remained unconscious for 72 hours or more, 47 percent (9/19) were behind in their reading skills.

Effects of hemisphere of injury and age of injury on reading scores were also considered by Chadwick and colleagues (1981a). The investigators found that results regarding hemisphere of injury showed no significant differences in scores on any of the cognitive tests between those with left-sided and those with right-sided fractures. However, there was a slight, but consistent, tendency for all tests of scholastic attainment (including tests of reading and spelling) to show greater impairment in individuals with left hemisphere lesions. The effect of age at injury also was nonsignificant in that when reading scores were compared with the child's age at injury, a strong age effect was not found. Of the 56 children who were younger than 5 years of age at the time of injury, 19 (35%) had reading difficulties. Of the 41 children who were 5 years of age or older at the time of injury, 13 (30.8%) were identified as being backward in reading. However, when the subgroup of children with clear left hemisphere damage was studied, 8 of the 12 children (68%) who were under the age of 5 years at the time of injury were backward at reading, whereas none of the 44 children aged 5 years or over was backward at reading. The authors considered, as a possible explanation for this finding, that brain injury is more likely to impair the acquisition of new skills than to cause the loss of well-established skills.

To reduce some of the problems associated with the earlier retrospective studies, Chadwick and colleagues (1981b) conducted a prospective followup study of children who were between the ages of 5 and 14 at the time of injury. The Neale Analysis of Reading Ability (Neale, 1958) again was used to evaluate children who were at least eight years of age at the time of testing. Reading performance was assessed shortly after recovery from posttraumatic amnesia (PTA) and at 4 months, 12 months, and 27 months after injury. Subjects were divided into groups of severe and mild brain injury according to the duration of PTA. The severe brain-injury group consisted of 25 children. Of this group, 16 children had PTA persisting 1 to 3 weeks and 9 children had PTA persisting more than 3 weeks. The mild brain-injury group consisted of 29 children who had PTA durations ranging from 1 hour to less than 1 week. In this study, a control group of 28 children with hospital-treated orthopedic injuries was included to attempt to control for other risk factors (e.g., socioeconomic level and behavior disorder) that might make a child who already exhibits academic problems more prone to head injury or other types of accidents.

In the final assessment, Chadwick and colleagues (1981b) found that 14 of the 29 children (43%) with a PTA of less than 1 week exhibited reading backwardness, but only one of the 15 children (7%) in the severe group with a PTA of 1 to 3 weeks had reading problems. This surprising result was interpreted by focusing on the finding that throughout the duration of the followups, the reading scores of the children in the mild group did not progressively improve. Based on this evidence, and on the general rule that intellectual deficit will show progressive improvement during the months following acute damage to the brain, the authors hypothesized that the poor performance shown by the children with mild head injuries on the reading tests may not have been the result of head injury but of some prior condition. However, Chadwick and colleagues (1981b) concluded that some of the children with a PTA that exceeded 3 weeks did show reading difficulties as a result of brain injury. In this case, the proportion of children (6/9; 67%) who showed reading backwardness at the time of the initial assessment was significantly higher than the proportion of matched controls (1/7; 14%) who showed such difficulties. At the time of final assessment, when four of the severely brain-injured children showed backwardness and only two of their nine matched controls showed problems, the differences were less marked.

In addition to standardized testing, Chadwick and colleagues (1981b) sought to determine the effects of TBI on school performance of the children in the severe brain-injury group by interviewing their classroom teachers. It was reported that 7 of the 25 children, all of whom had had PTA for at least 3 weeks, were either experiencing difficulties with school-work or were placed in special schools because of their inability to maintain progress in the classroom. The authors emphasized the need for considering real-life effects when attempting to study outcome following TBI. They pointed out the limitations of psychometric tests for demonstrating the performance of individuals when confronted with intellectual tasks in everyday life. Psychometric tests are constructed to assess what individuals can accomplish under optimal, temporally controlled circumstances. Real-life time pressures and contextual demands are often considerably greater.

This factor was also noted by Levin and Eisenberg (1979), who commented that, in their experience a child's capability merely to attend school "does not necessarily imply a good recovery, as learning problems may be overlooked" (p. 401). In their study of recovery of motor and intellectual functioning in children who had sustained severe brain injuries, Brink and colleagues (1970) reported that 34 of 52 survivors who were injured between 2 and 18 years of age were eventually placed in school after they returned home from Rancho Los Amigos Hospital. However, the majority of the children were in special classes. Even those eight children who were able to be placed in regular classes demonstrated impaired academic performance and were not able to perform to the standard expected from their intelligence scores.

A departure from large group studies that also offers promise for developing understanding of reading and writing and TBI is the publication of individual case studies. Herzog (1988) contributed one such case report of the acute care and initial rehabilitation phases for a 14-year-old girl. Herzog focused on the girl's initial mutism, described as absent verbalization and alternate means of communication in the presence of relatively good comprehension and intact cranial nerves. About five weeks after onset, however, the girl began to vocalize a few words when heavily prompted. At 8 weeks after onset, she began to respond in

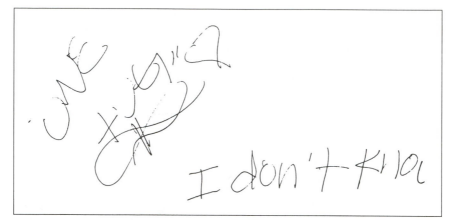

Figure 8-2. Sample of Herzog's (1988) patient's writing, approximately 8 weeks after injury. The words "one hug" were accompanied by a heart and a premorbid characteristic flourish. "I don't know" was printed with the "w" partially off the right side of the page.

writing, writing both her name and short phrases (Fig. 8-2), but during the ninth and tenth weeks she no longer verbalized, refused to write, and began to use gestures more frequently to communicate. At 13 weeks after onset, her verbalizations again increased, and during the 14th week, she began to eat. At that point, it was also possible to administer formal tests for the first time. Several tests of oral and written language were administered. The results showed that marked cognitive deficits affected all areas of communication. For example, "Auditory and reading comprehension were affected by her reduced ability to attend and poor memory, and she was quite concrete in her interpretation of any material" (p. 16). Herzog also noted that her written language deficits were similar to her oral language deficits, demonstrating such traits as poor organization, difficulty with abstraction, and tangential writing. At the time of her release from acute care (at 17 weeks after onset), she had begun to attempt to use simple spelling rules, verbalizing as she wrote. It was also commented that she block printed almost exclusively at the time of discharge, even though much of her writing when she was mute was done in cursive. It was reported that she continued to demonstrate good improvement in outpatient therapy.

A SURVEY OF CURRENT PRACTICE

To benefit from the experiences of individuals who work clinically with the TBI population, a survey was conducted by Surges and Nelson

(1988). The study had two major purposes. First, it was designed to gather information about reading and writing problems experienced by persons with TBI. Second, it was intended to result in a "state of the art" review of assessment procedures and intervention techniques currently being used with such individuals in rehabilitation facilities.

METHODS

Survey Procedures

A 30-question survey was constructed to obtain data in four areas: (1) the nature of the facilities being surveyed, (2) characteristics of TBI clients served in those facilities, (3) assessment of the clients' reading and writing skills, and (4) intervention involving the clients' written language. The participating professionals were requested to answer the survey questions based on an informal review of their clinical caseloads within the past 12-month period. They were not expected to pull individual client records. Many of the survey questions requested participants to estimate proportions of their caseloads who exhibited a particular characteristic as 0 to 10 percent, 10 to 25 percent, 25 to 50 percent, 50 to 75 percent, 75 to 100 percent, or "unknown."

The survey was mailed to 131 representatives from rehabilitation centers in the United States that serve TBI individuals. The sites were selected by sampling every third facility (except for those providing only coma treatment) from the list of 366 facilities in the *National Directory of Head Injury Rehabilitation* (National Head Injury Foundation, 1988). Of the 131 surveys mailed, 61 were returned, yielding a response rate of 47 percent. Frequency and percentage data for the coded responses from the 58 facilities who responded to the survey were obtained using the SPSSX statistical software program (SPSS Inc., 1988).

Survey Respondents

The data regarding survey respondents indicated that nearly three fourths of the surveys included responses made by speech-language pathologists (42; 72%) and that approximately one third of them included contributions by administrators (11; 19%) or neuropsychologists (10; 17%). It was also found that the majority of the clinical facilities represented in this study were acute rehabilitation centers (29; 50%), long-term rehabilitation centers (17; 29%), or community reentry centers (16; 28%). Participants from 53 facilities responded to the question about the number of clients served at their facilities during a 12-month period, with a range of 2 to 600 clients. Analysis showed that a mean of 65 clients, a median of 30, and a mode of 40 clients (8 facilities) with TBI were served. Because the size of caseloads varied widely (ranging from 2 to 600 clients), it is important to remember that a percentage range selected by one facility may only represent a small number of clients; the same percentage range, when reported by another facility, may represent a large number of clients.

Clinical Caseload Characteristics

The data from this study showed that, in many respects, the caseloads surveyed matched characteristics reported in the literature for the TBI population in general. For example, the age group of 18 to 30 years is often reported to be the most prevalent, the duration of coma frequently exceeds 24 hours, and PTA usually lasts a minimum of 1 to 7 days (Rimel and Jane, 1983). These also were the most frequent categories noted by the participants in this survey. That is, most of the clinics reported the largest proportions of their caseloads to be between 18 and 30 years of age and few of their clients to be between birth and 12 years of age or over 60 years of age. Additionally, most facilities reported that the majority of their clients had experienced coma of over 24 hours.

The categories for duration of PTA used in this survey were suggested by Bever (1975) as being important in determining prognosis. However, research regarding the relationship of PTA and subsequent cognitive impairment has shown equivocal results (Brooks and colleagues, 1980; Mandleberg and Brooks, 1975; Smith, 1974). The levels Bever (1975) suggested were less than 5 minutes, less than 1 hour, 1 to 24 hours, 1 to 7 days, longer than 7 days, and longer than 4 weeks. In this study, more than one third (20; 36%) of the participants reported that they did not know the percentage of the clients in their clinics' caseloads who had experienced PTA at the indicated duration levels. Of those participants who reported percentage information, analysis showed that most clinical caseloads included primarily clients who experienced PTA that lasted either 1 to 7 days or longer than 4 weeks.

Because the data were obtained from specialized rehabilitation facilities, the survey results would be expected to be more representative of persons with more severe head injuries than of persons with mild or minor head injuries. To estimate levels of functioning of the caseloads, respondents were asked to provide information about patients' levels of functioning at admission and at discharge using the *Rancho Los Amigos Scale* (RLA; Hagen, 1981). Considerable variable was found in response to these questions. However, the greatest proportion of clients was reported to be functioning at RLA levels V, VI, and VII at the time of admission to the facilities. At the time clients were discharged, the greatest proportion was reported to be functioning at RLA levels VI, VII, and VIII.

The results of questions about educational history showed that most of the facilities had access to information about their clients' education. Many participants (23; 44%) reported that more than half the individuals in their clinics' caseloads had no history of premorbid learning or reading problems. However, when this question was asked in reverse, almost three fourths of the participants (38; 70%) reported that between 10 and 75 percent of the individuals in their clinic's caseloads did show evidence of learning or reading problems before injury. In agreement with previous researchers (Shaffer and colleagues, 1980; Chadwick and colleagues, 1981b; Fuld and Fisher, 1977), these data support the need to consider whether individuals may have experienced problems before TBI that might impede their ability to use written language during the recovery process.

RESULTS AND DISCUSSION

Current Assessment Practices

The results of this survey had a number of implications regarding assessment, both for rehabilitation facilities and for professional preparation programs. In these rehabilitation facilities, speech-language pathologists, followed by neuropsychologists, were the professionals most frequently responsible for directly assessing reading and writing abilities. In 52 (90%) of the facilities responding, speech-language pathologists were responsible for conducting such assessments. Additionally, 25 (43%) facilities reported that neuropsychologists, and 16 (28%) reported that educational specialists, conducted reading and writing assessments. Other professionals mentioned were occupational therapists (10; 17%), vocational counselors (2; 3%), and reading specialists (1; 2%). Certainly, professional preparation programs for the disciplines most frequently reported should include some preparation for conducting written language assessments for persons with TBI. Indeed, one concern raised by participants in this study was the limited knowledge of reading and writing among professionals most often responsible for its assessment and intervention.

The data also indicated that, at the time of initial assessment in rehabilitation facilities, a majority of the clients were functioning at a level that made it appropriate to administer formal tests of written language skills (Fig. 8-3). However, the data also indicated that assessing written language skills was the *primary* interest for only a small percentage of indi-

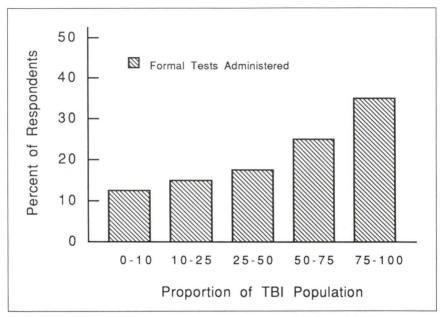

Figure 8-3. Percentage of respondents to Surges and Nelson (1988) survey who reported varied proportions of their client caseloads to be functioning at such a level that it was appropriate to administer formal tests of reading and writing.

viduals in the participating clinics' caseloads. These results suggest that reading and writing assessments are performed on a regular basis for clients with TBI in rehabilitation facilities but that the assessments are usually a part of more comprehensive evaluation procedures.

A wide range of published tests of reading and writing was reported as currently being used to establish performance levels. Table 8-1 includes a listing of the tests reported by two or more of the facilities in order of frequency. As indicated, many of the participants (21; 38%) reported using informal testing procedures to assess reading skills. Of the formal tests used, the most frequently reported was the RCBA (LaPointe and Horner, 1979), followed by the Gates-MacGinitie Reading Test (Gates and MacGinitie, 1969) and the BDAE (Goodglass and Kaplan, 1983).

The tests used to assess writing skills that were reported by at least two survey participants are shown in Table 8-2. When questioned in this area, even more of the participants (31; 58%) reported that their facilities use informal testing procedures to assess writing than to assess reading. Of the formal tests used, the most frequently mentioned were the BDAE (Goodglass and Kaplan, 1983) and the Test of Written Language (TOWL; Hammill and Larsen, 1983).

**Table 8-1. Tests administered to assess reading skills
(reported by at least two survey respondents)**

Name of test	*N=56* Frequency
Informal testing	21
Reading Comprehension Battery for Aphasia (LaPointe and Horner, 1979)	22
Gates-MacGinitie Reading Test (Gates and MacGinitie, 1969)	16
Boston Diagnostic Aphasia Examination (Goodglass and Kaplan, 1983)	16
Wide Range Achievement Test-Revised (Jastak and Wilkenson, 1984)	13
Woodcock-Johnson Psycho-Educational Battery (Woodcock and Johnson, 1977)	12
Peabody Individual Achievement Test-Revised (Dunn and Markwardt, 1988)	11
Woodcock Reading Mastery Tests-Revised (Woodcock, 1987)	10
Western Aphasia Battery (Kertesz, 1982)	7
Minnesota Test for Differential Diagnosis of Aphasia (Schuell, 1965)	6
The Nelson-Denny Reading Test (Brown and colleagues, 1976)	5
Wechsler Adult Intelligence Scale—Revised (Wechsler, 1981)	5
Slosson Intelligence Test (Slosson, 1985)	4
Frostig Developmental Test of Visual Perception (Frostig and Horne, 1964)	3
Peabody Picture Vocabulary Test-Revised (Dunn and Dunn, 1981)	3
Gray Oral Reading Tests-Revised (Wiederholt and Bryant, 1986)	3
Bender Visual Motor Gestalt Test (Bender, 1946)	2
Durrell Analysis of Reading Difficulty (Durrell, 1955)	2
Stanford Achievement Test (Gardner and colleagues, 1987)	2
Test of Reading Comprehension (Brown and colleagues, 1986)	2

In response to open-ended questions, a number of survey participants commented on the need for standardized instruments that provide normative data specific to the TBI population. Until such instruments are available, clinicians have little choice but to adapt currently available

**Table 8-2. Tests administered to assess writing skills
(reported by at least two survey respondents)**

Name of test	N=53 Frequency
Informal Testing	31
Boston Diagnostic Aphasia Examination (Goodglass and Kaplan, 1983)	18
Test of Written Language (Hammill and Larsen, 1983)	12
Wide Range Achievement Test-Revised (Jastak and Wilkenson, 1984)	8
Minnesota Test for Differential Diagnosis of Aphasia (Schuell, 1965)	6
Western Aphasia Battery (Kertesz, 1982)	6
Bender Visual Motor Gestalt Test (Bender, 1946)	2
Porch Index of Communicative Ability (Porch, 1967)	2
Woodcock-Johnson Psycho-Educational Battery (Woodcock and Johnson, 1977)	2
Test of Adolescent Language-2 (Hammill and colleagues, 1987)	2

tools. When they do so, however, they should be aware of the psychometric dangers of using bits and pieces of tests or of using tests to measure the behavior of individuals who differ from the population on which the tests were standardized (Duffy and colleagues, 1988).

The findings of this survey also suggested that routine evaluation procedures should include the assessment of such specific difficulties as visuoperception and visuomotor impairments. This need is supported, as well, by the research of such groups as Chadwick and colleagues (1981b), who found that timed measures of visuospatial and visuomotor skills tended to show more impairment than verbal skills. In the survey, most of the participants (45; 79%) reported that testing of such skills was performed at their facilities. Of those participants who reported that their facilities did not perform visuoperception or visuomotor testing routinely, 13 (23%) reported that they have a referral source when such testing is warranted. Of those, four (31%) indicated that they refer to an occupational therapist, three (23%) to a neuro-opthalmologist, and the remaining to an optometrist, neurologist, or psychologist.

The majority of the participants reported that problems involving visuoperception and motor control or limb apraxia occur among some members of their clinics' caseloads. Of these difficulties, visuoperception impairments were reported as occurring most frequently, but many of the participants (31; 55%) reported that more than one fourth of the TBI persons on their clinics' caseloads had motor control or limb apraxia problems. Visuomotor difficulties also were reported for more than one fourth of TBI clients by 22 (45%) of the survey participants.

In addition, it was found that assessments of auditory comprehension and the potential to use an augmentative communication device are usually performed if a client's visual or motor impairment precludes written language processing. When visual problems do preclude reading, a majority (50; 89%) of the participants reported that their facilities perform assessments of auditory comprehension of written language read aloud. However, only a small percentage of the clinics' caseloads appeared to fall into this category. Specifically, 38 (71%) participants reported that fewer than one fourth of the individuals in their clinics' caseloads needed this type of an assessment procedure.

For clients who have motor problems that interfere with writing, most of the survey participants (46; 81%) reported that an assessment is performed to determine the client's potential to use an augmentative communication device. However, many of the participants also reported that few individuals in their clinics' caseloads fall into this category. Thirty-six (54%) participants reported that fewer than one fourth of the individuals in their clinics' caseload have motor difficulties that suggest the need to assess the use of an augmentative device to assist writing. On the other hand, 20 facilities (36%) reported that more than 10 percent of the individuals on their caseloads did need this kind of assessment.

Current Intervention Practices

Survey findings indicated that the professional most often responsible for implementing treatment goals addressing reading and writing is the speech-language pathologist. Such professionals were listed as interventionists by 50 (86%) of the facilities surveyed. Other professionals mentioned in this category were educational specialists (16; 28%), occupational therapists (15; 28%), neuropsychologists (3; 5%), program coordinators (2; 3%), and reading specialists (1; 2%).

Data for percentages of the clinics' caseloads that have treatment plans addressing written language skills are shown in Figure 8-4. As illustrated, slightly more of the treatment plans include goals to improve reading skills than to improve writing skills. Twenty-nine of the participants (52%) reported that a majority of the individuals in their clinics' caseloads have intervention goals that focus on improvement of reading skills, and 24 (43%) reported that a majority of the treatment plans for TBI individuals on their caseloads include writing skills.

Types of intervention goals also were surveyed. Results showed that written language is commonly used as a compensatory strategy (e.g.,

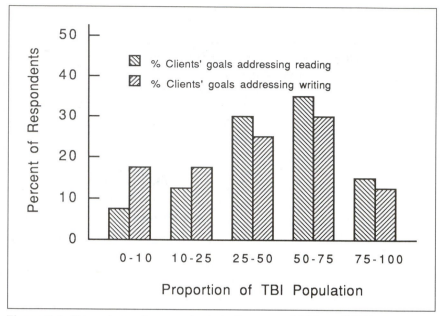

Figure 8-4. Percentage of respondents to Surges and Nelson (1988) survey who reported varied proportions of their client caseloads whose intervention plans included goals to address reading and writing.

writing daily logs, reading memory charts) to enhance other memory and cognitive skills that are impaired due to TBI. Most of the participants (43; 77%) reported that the majority of individuals in their clinics' caseloads use written language in this way. Many of the participants also reported that improvement of reading and writing is often targeted in management programs for personal, social, behavioral control, or entertainment purposes. Specifically, 30 (51%) participants indicated that more than half the individuals in their clinics' caseloads have reading and writing treatment goals aimed at one or more of these areas.

Academic development was less frequently selected as a purpose for improving literary skills. Only seven facilities (13%) indicated that a majority of their clients have reading and writing treatment goals for academic development, and only 20 (36%) indicated that a majority had such goals for vocational development. The results regarding academic goals possibly reflect the fact that most of the clients in the facilities surveyed were past the academic age or that they exhibited serious enough cognitive impairments to make it difficult for them to attend college. As noted previously, only one third of the TBI individuals in families surveyed by Jacobs (1988) who were in school at the time of their injuries were able to return to school within approximately 1 year after the trauma. The level of impairment exhibited by individuals in the rehabilitation facilities surveyed by Surges and Nelson (1988) also may have made it unlikely that they would be able to return to work. It is impossible to project, based on these survey results, how many individuals with milder TBI might need intervention to improve their abilities to function in academic or vocational environments.

In response to open-ended questions regarding intervention, several participants noted that a frequent problem in rehabilitation facilities is lack of client motivation for using written language. Reading and writing therapy was reported to be more successful, and to be given higher priority as a treatment goal, for clients who needed to restore these skills to participate in pretraumatic activities that were important to them (e.g., school, work, pleasure reading). For increasing clients' motivation related to reading and writing intervention, some participants reported success in using group therapy activities that incorporated reading and writing skills.

Surges and Nelson (1988) concluded from the survey of current practice that written language is an important part of the management programs of many TBI persons. In view of this fact, they reaffirmed the need for further research to contribute to a better understanding of written language processing abilities and problems associated with TBI. Also apparent was a need for professional degree programs to include academic coursework and clinical practicum experiences in written language processing among persons with TBI.

MANAGEMENT STRATEGIES

INITIAL ASSESSMENT

General Guidelines for Test Selection and Administration

The purposes of the initial assessment are to identify reading and writing abilities and problems, facilitating strategies used, and goals for intervention. When planning and implementing this process, the clinician must consider pretrauma factors, the nature and severity of the injury, treatment, progress to date, and the expected outcomes of rehabilitation. Assessment instruments are then selected and administered to obtain current levels of skills and abilities. The information gathered and results of testing are organized and analyzed. Goals for intervention are developed.

The desired outcome of the assessment process is the understanding of the client's present abilities and limitations relative to the client's and family's stated goals for long-term recovery. Although few neuropsychological batteries address written language skills directly, many published tests of reading, and a few of writing, are available for establishing performance levels. However, when administering these tests, the clinician must keep in mind that they were not standardized for use with individuals with TBI. In addition, published tests vary considerably in length, complexity, and the skills that they are designed to assess. It is up to the clinician to decide which tests are most appropriate for the client and most relevant to the stated goals. This decision is guided by the client's "literacy history," which is discussed in a subsequent section.

Generally, goals for improving literacy skills fit into one of three categories: (1) functional literacy skills for the necessary environment, (2) recreational literacy skills, and (3) literacy skills for learning and independence in the home, school, workplace, and community (Table 8-3). The complexity, amounts, and types of skills required for successful performance in each of these categories differ. For example, many basic living skills can be carried out effectively if the client has functional reading skills at the single word or simple sentence level. These include ordering from a menu, locating a specific street sign, and following simple package directions. Reading for pleasure from magazines and newspapers requires the ability to maintain comprehension for passages of one to several paragraphs long and to identify main ideas and supporting details. Writing for pleasure (e.g., notes, letters, or journal entries) requires memory and recall strategies and a sense of audience. Reading and writing for learning and independence requires a complex repertoire of skills that allows the individual to integrate new information with that which is familiar as well as to retain information over time. To ensure that the tests and subtests administered measure the skills that an individual needs for goal attainment, the clinician should preview and analyze the content and tasks of prospective test instruments (not just their labels).

Assessment of reading skills should be accompanied by assessment of writing abilities, because disorders in these two areas rarely occur in isolation. The evidence from studies of brain injury of varied etiologies (e.g., Benson, 1979, 1981; Kaplan and Goodglass, 1981; Lezak, 1983) supports that alexia and agraphia are most often found together and in association with parallel disorders of oral language processing. When discussing the TBI population specifically, Lezak (1983) pointed out that impairments of speaking and writing are generally more common and severe than are impairments of reading and speech comprehension.

In addition to establishing performance levels for reading and writing skills, it is important to observe for facilitating strategies used by the client. The strategies that clients select spontaneously, or retain from previous intervention efforts, provide clues to understanding the impact

Table 8-3. Types of literacy skills

FUNCTIONAL LITERACY SKILLS
Communication
Writing identifying information
Filling out forms
Recording and reading appointment planner
Reading and interpreting schedules
Reading and writing simple messages
Reading and responding to notes regarding children
Reading and writing letters and social notes
Handling mail
Using a telephone directory
Consumer-related activities
Reading basic instructions
Reading package directions
Writing checks
Reading and writing shopping lists
Home management
Following recipes
Writing and reading menu plans
Paying bills
Assisting children with homework
Mobility
Reading or recognizing directional signs
Reading or recognizing safety words and symbols
Basic map skills
Reading and writing directions
RECREATIONAL LITERACY SKILLS
Reading newspapers
Reading magazines
Reading stories and novels for entertainment
Reading nonfiction books for entertainment
Reading instructions for recreational games
Maintaining hobbies
Keeping a journal or diary
LITERACY SKILLS FOR INDEPENDENT LEARNING
Reading textbooks and other printed material for content
Comprehending new or unfamiliar subject matter
Recording and comprehending lecture notes
(in writing or on tape)
Reading information from chalkboard or other visual aids
Reading and writing fictional or personal narratives
Critical reading and writing skills
Reading and completing workbook pages and other homework
Reading and writing essays or expository pieces
Taking tests
Library usage skills
Study skills

of underlying deficits on reading and writing processes. For example, repeated reading of a short paragraph before attempting to respond to comprehension questions often indicates difficulties with memory or concentration. Readers who use this strategy demonstrate some awareness of their failure to comprehend, even though they may not be able to talk about it. Recognition of such strategies provides a way for the clinician to identify instructional needs and potentials. To make the information most useful, the clinician should observe for any approach the individual selects to facilitate task completion, the frequency of its use, and its impact on task performance.

Information Gathering

Information gathering is the first step of a comprehensive assessment. It is accomplished through review of available records, interviews with the client and family, and consultation with other professionals working with the client.

If possible, the clinician should review all available medical, educational, and rehabilitation records before meeting with the client. Knowledge of the client's history alerts the clinician to factors that may affect prognosis, such as the presence of a preexisting learning disability. It also provides a framework for determining a starting point for assessment and expected outcomes for intervention. In addition to a history of learning problems, the clinician should note other significant educational factors, such as the client's level of formal educational attainment, course grades obtained, pretrauma results of standardized testing, any grade levels or courses that were repeated, any remedial or special education services that were received, participation in extracurricular activities, and types of elective courses taken.

The neuropsychological report is particularly important because it provides information regarding current levels of cognitive and perceptual abilities as well as recovery patterns and prognosis. Cognitive and perceptual deficits are both known to affect reading and writing performance directly (Lezak, 1983). The clinician should therefore be aware of general difficulties with the cognitive aspects of attention, memory, and reasoning, as well as specific difficulties with visual processing skills involving acuity, scanning, recognition, and organizing and auditory processing skills involving acuity, discrimination, sequencing, retention, and comprehension.

Interviews with the client and family help to fill information gaps noted after reviewing the records. When interviewing clients, it is important to identify their pretrauma literacy skills, interests, and experiences as well as their perceptions of current personal strengths, limitations, and effects of their disability in terms of their reading and writing capabilities. Their prior use and the level of competency of such specialized skills as typing, word processor use, and Morse Code communication should be ascertained. Clients' goals for improving their reading and writing skills also should be discussed. Obtaining this "literacy history" is essential to the treatment of reading and writing disorders, particularly for adults, because it is usually not possible to teach adults reading skills that they did not have before TBI (Webb, 1987). Later in the management program, this information can aid the clinician in selecting intervention materials with content that is likely to be interesting and familiar to the client.

The family and significant others provide an important additional source of information for estimating the survivor's pretrauma and current functioning levels. Spordone (1987) found that most TBI survivors tend to deny or minimize their deficits, especially during the first year. Discrepancies in information obtained from clients and their treatment records can often be explained by family members who have had frequent, long-term contact with them.

Input is also sought from other professionals working with the client. This should be in addition to information documented in the records. TBI results in deficits that may have a lasting adverse effect on the survivor's ability to live independently, to work, and to relate to others (Jacobs, 1988). Meeting the broad range of need TBI survivors face usually requires the services of several professionals from various disciplines (Surges and Nelson, 1988), and it is important for efforts to be coordinated and directed toward the same general outcomes. Consultation with other professionals is essential to a coordinated effort. The clinician should find out what treatment approaches requiring the use of reading and writing skills are planned, and what successes and difficulties the client experiences with these approaches. These data are used to inform the clinician of the client's performance in various settings and under differing conditions with varied types of materials and content.

Reading and Writing Assessment

Most published reading batteries include subtests that address the major components of the reading process, such as word attack, vocabulary, comprehension, and reading rate. The subtests of these batteries have advantages in certain applications. However, just as no single reading battery is appropriate in all situations, it is frequently the case that only some of the subtests of a particular reading battery are suitable for an individual TBI client. In these situations, selective testing is necessary so that the clinician can obtain performance levels that reflect the client's present abilities and can identify patterns of errors. However, in such instances, the clinician must keep in mind the psychometric limitations of using bits and pieces of standardized tests in nonstandard ways (Duffy and colleagues, 1988).

Although formal test batteries for assessing writing are less prevalent, subtests are available for assessing most of the major components involved in the process of producing written language, including handwriting (or typing); spelling; use of conventions for punctuation, spacing, and capitalization; grammatical formulation and word choice; and the use of organizational strategies for expressing ideas, conveying information, or telling stories. In addition to assessing skills in each of the component areas of reading and writing processes, the clinician may need to examine the client's letter recognition skills. To supplement formal tests that are designed to assess some or all of these components, a variety of informal techniques can be used.

In this section, a discussion is provided for each of the individual components of reading and writing processes. Suggestions are made for subtests that may prove useful in particular situations. The subtests chosen for presentation here are those that have been helpful in the authors' own clinical experiences and those that were reported frequently in the Surges and Nelson (1988) survey of major rehabilitation centers. The list is not intended to be exhaustive, nor is it intended that anyone would ever use all the tests discussed here with a particular client.

A better approach would be to gather some informal preliminary information about a client's reading and writing abilities. By combining that information with findings from information-gathering activities, hypotheses can be formulated about the individual's areas of strength and impairment in written language processing. These hypotheses can then be tested by selecting appropriate tasks from among those discussed here or by designing unique tasks. The depth and breadth of the assessment will be determined by a variety of factors that relate to the client, the facility, the professionals involved, the time that can be devoted to it without detracting from other needs, and the prognosis and value of written language processing for the individual.

Letter Identification and Production. Street signs, business signs, and printed reading material differ in the style of print used. The ability to recognize and name the letters of the alphabet printed in a variety of sizes and common styles of type is generally considered to be an essential foundation skill for any type of reading activity. If it appears warranted, assessment of letter identification skills can be accomplished using materials designed by the clinician, including handwritten stimuli. Some published test batteries also contain subtests to address this area. The Letter Identification subtest of Form G of the Woodcock Reading Mastery Tests-Revised (WRMT-R; Woodcock, 1987) contains 45 items designed to measure the client's ability to name isolated upper- and lower-case letters in a variety of type styles. The Letter-Word Identification subtest of the Woodcock-Johnson Psycho-Educational Battery (WJPEB; Woodcock and Johnson, 1977) also measures letter naming skills, but it contains only seven items for this purpose. The prereading section of the Wide Range Achievement Test-Revised (WRAT-R; Jastak and Wilkenson, 1984) requires individuals to name 13 letters.

A caveat in the assessment of letter identification (as in other areas) with TBI persons is that, although such a skill may appear to be a prerequisite to all other levels of reading, assessment activities should take place on higher linguistic levels even when "lower" ones appear to be impaired. This is because of the multilevel nature of reading and writing processes and the possibility that brain damage may have spared some skills while impairing others. Such was the case for the 14-year-old girl, described by Herzog (1988), who wrote the phrase (see fig. 8-2) "one hug" (accompanied by a heart and a premorbid characteristic flourish) and "I don't know," at a point when she was verbalizing only infrequently and before she had recovered sufficiently to be given standardized tests.

Although not yet proved by research, it seems plausible that the older the client is at the time of injury (perhaps up to a point when aging begins to enter as a factor), the greater the likelihood that word level and text level strategies for obtaining meaning might be available to help compensate for perceptual and decoding level deficits. Younger children who have been taught to read with multilevel strategies that stress meaning as well as decoding may also have an advantage for using more sophisticated strategies, even when their TBI is acquired during their elementary school years. Children who sustained TBI during their preschool years may have difficulty acquiring and retaining the ability to associate letters, letter names, and phonologic patterns and yet be able to access written language meaning at higher levels. Therefore, even if letter naming appears to be impossible, the clinician should present writing materials and written language stimuli to the client, at least at the word level, and possibly at the sentence and paragraph levels, to determine whether other access pathways to word and text meaning (either for reading or writing) might be available.

If letter naming is impossible, it may also be helpful to determine if the client can match letters of the same and different types to sort out possible distinctions among perceptual, association, retention, recall, and naming problems. The Symbol and Word Discrimination subtest of the BDAE (Goodglass and Kaplan, 1983) requires letter and word matching. The prereading section of the WRAT-R (Jastak and Wilkenson, 1984) also includes a matching task for ten letters.

For persons who are nonspeaking and nonwriting due to posttrauma physical disabilities, it may be possible for them to indicate their letter recognition abilities by striking the keys on a computer or typewriter keyboard to copy letters or by using some other kind of access method that does not require them to talk or point (e.g., eye gaze or electronic scanning with a single switch). Typing may also be an option for other persons who do have some retained hand use, particularly if they could type before their brain trauma occurred, but who have reduced handwriting ability.

To determine such need, the ability to write letters to dictation should be assessed. The ability to form letters and to write legibly may have been affected by visual and motor deficits associated with TBI. Direct observation and evaluation of writing samples provides information about letter formation, spacing, size, and rate of production. When possible, it is helpful to obtain a sample of the individual's writing before the brain injury for comparison. Visuoperception and visuomotor skills should be assessed if disabilities in these areas are suspected of playing a role in reading or writing difficulties.

Published evaluation scales for rating handwriting directly are available as well. For example, the Test of Written Language (TOWL; Hammill and Larsen, 1983) and the Test of Written Language-2 (TOWL-2, Hammill and Larsen, 1988) include various graded writing samples. However, such scales have limited use with TBI adults because most adults have developed their own styles of handwriting that do not necessarily match the styles found in published evaluation scales. In most cases, legibility, rather than style, should be the criterion of greatest concern during written language assessments. If the clinician is uncertain whether the TBI individual has retained the ability to integrate the visuoperceptual and visuomotor aspects of the process of forming written symbols, Level I of the WRAT-R (Jastak and Wilkenson, 1984) includes a subtest that assesses the ability to copy nonletter symbols. The Minnesota Test for Differential Diagnosis of Aphasia (Schuell, 1965) also includes some tasks in this area, as does the BDAE (Goodglass and Kaplan, 1983). When scoring the mechanics of writing with the BDAE, a five-level scale is used that includes judgments of (1) no legible letters, (2) occasional success on single letters (block printing), (3) block printing with some malformed letters, (4) legible but impaired cursive writing or upper- and lower-case printing, and (5) the same as premorbid writing, with allowance made for use of the nonpreferred hand. Herzog's (1988) case study was informative in this area as well. During the early stages of recovery when Herzog's 14-year-old client was mute, much of her writing was done in cursive. However, at the time of discharge she wrote in block printing almost exclusively.

Word Attack and Spelling. Assessment in the area of word attack focuses on the individual's ability to decode isolated and nonsense words by applying knowledge of phoneme-grapheme relationships, rules of syllabication, and rules relating to affixes and root words. Some subtests, such as the Phonetic Analysis and Structural Analysis subtests of the Stanford Diagnostic Reading Test (SORT; Karlsen and Gardner, 1984) and the Word Study subtest of the Stanford Achievement Test (SAT; Gardner and colleagues, 1987), are designed for group administration. Even when administered to individuals, this feature allows clients to proceed through the items independently, if they can do so without frequent prompting and encouragement. Other subtests are designed to be administered individually. These include the Letter-Word Identification and Word Attack subtests from the WJPEB (Woodcock and Johnson, 1977) and the Word Attack subtests on both Form G and Form H of the WRMT-R (Woodcock, 1987). The administration of such instruments allows the clinician to control the pace of the evaluation. The WRAT-R (Jastak and Wilkenson, 1984) and the BDAE (Goodglass and Kaplan, 1983) also include subtests that require individuals to spell words to dictation.

If the person with TBI has difficulty maintaining attention, detecting and following sequences, or remembering directions, the examiner may choose to select the individually administered subtest to reduce the effects of these deficits on test performance. The increased structure imposed by individually administered tests helps to compensate for a person's cognitive deficits. It also eliminates the possibility of error as a result of skipping items inadvertently, marking responses incorrectly, or responding randomly to items without reading them, all of which are more common in individuals with involvement of right hemisphere processing deficits (Burns and colleagues, 1985). In addition, individual test administration allows the clinician to observe the client's use of spontaneous strategies. The result is a more precise understanding of the individual's word attack skills and the types and patterns of errors made.

Strategies that might be observed include sounding out individual letters, breaking longer words into syllables, using irregular as well as regular pronunciations for particular orthographic patterns, demonstrating differential skill for meaningful and nonsense words, and identifying prefixes, suffixes, and root words. Evidence of consistent errors on initial, medial, or final portions of words should be noted, as should reversal and inversion of letters, because such symptoms may signal the presence of visuoperceptual or visuomemory problems. Evidence of difficulty in decoding nonsense words in the presence of retained ability to pronounce real words suggests that the person has retained some holistic word level recognition skills accompanied by loss of (or lesser pretrauma ability in) phonemic decoding strategies.

The ability to spell is a complex neuropsychological process involving a number of visual, auditory, and motor skills. Because of its relationship to learning disabilities and other language-related disorders, spelling is receiving increased attention in the literature (Bookman, 1984; Horn and colleagues, 1988; Wallace and McLoughlin, 1988). Horn and colleagues (1988) studied spelling errors of learning disabled, TBI, and nondisabled young adults and showed that phonetically inaccurate spelling errors were significantly more prevalent among the learning disabled and TBI participants than among the nondisabled participants. They further demonstrated that phonetically inaccurate spelling patterns were associated with language disorder. Wallace and McLoughlin (1988) reported that spelling is a more sensitive indicator of language disabilities than reading is, probably because compensatory methods for spelling are fewer and less effective. That is, when the individual engages in the receptive language act of reading, contextual, structural, and configuration clues are all available to aid the process of constructing meaning, but when he or she engages in the productive act of spelling, such clues are typically not available to aid in reproducing words.

Wallace and McLoughlin (1988) commented that few published tests are available for assessing spelling skills and that informal techniques often provide information more useful than that obtained from formal tests anyway. Whether the clinician relies on formal or informal methods to gather samples of the spelling abilities of TBI individuals, particularly adults, it is important to determine the frequency and types of misspellings, such as errors involving additions and omissions of letters, letter order confusions and reversals, and letter substitutions. Word lists for testing should include both phonetically spelled and irregularly spelled words, as well as words that require the application of rules for combining prefixes and suffixes with root words. To assist in sorting out various elements of the integrative processes involved in spelling, it is also helpful for the clinician to distinguish between the examinee's ability to recognize spelling errors and to produce accurate spelling.

A test that can be used for differential diagnosis of interactive word analysis difficulties is the Boder Test of Reading-Spelling Patterns (Boder and Jarrico, 1982). This test includes procedures for identifying reading grade level based on the ability to read words aloud that alternate between those spelled either phonetically or nonphonetically. The reading test is followed by a spelling test constructed of known and unknown words from the reading test. This test is designed to identify dyslexia subtypes as *dysphonetic* (primary problems of integrating written symbols with their sounds), *dyseidetic* (primary problems of visual perception and memory for letters and whole-word configurations), and *mixed*. An interesting variation on tests of word attack and spelling is provided by the Comprehension of Oral Spelling subtest, which is part of the BDAE (Goodglass and Kaplan, 1983). The unique feature of this subtest is that the client is expected to be able to identify a word orally that has been spelled aloud.

Another spelling test that can be used with the TBI population, although not specifically designed for that purpose, is the Diagnostic Spelling Potential Test (DSPT; Arena, 1982). It consists of four subtests designed to assess spelling skills in the following areas: (1) writing words read aloud by the examiner, (2) word recognition through oral reading of isolated words, (3) visual recognition of correct spelling using a multiple choice format, and (4) auditory-visual recognition of correct spelling using a multiple choice format combined with oral presentation of the word list by the examiner. Alternate forms of the DSPT are available for pretesting and posttesting. Administration and scoring are reported to take about 25 to 40 minutes; however, experience has shown that administration time alone generally runs at least 30 minutes for TBI persons. The results of this test are useful for detecting patterns and types of spelling errors, distinguishing between production and recognition of correct spelling, and identifying performance differences, given visual or auditory input. Because the test takes a long time to administer, it is sometimes necessary to provide breaks between subtests. With TBI individuals, it is also important to observe their performance carefully during multiple choice subtests to ensure that directions are followed accurately.

Spelling subtests are often included within achievement test batteries. Although these subtests do not provide a comprehensive assessment of spelling skills, they may be more appropriate for use with TBI individuals than longer diagnostic spelling tests because of the problems of attention, concentration, memory, and direction following often associated with TBI. An example is the TOWL (Hammill and Larsen, 1983), which includes a 25-item spelling subtest for assessing the individual's ability to write words that have been read aloud by the examiner. The WRAT-R (Jastak and Wilkenson, 1984) also includes a subtest designed to measure word-level spelling to dictation. The WRAT-R is divided into two levels—one for use with children age 5 years 0 months to 11 years 11 months, and the other for use with persons ages 12 years 0 months to 74 years 11 months.

Vocabulary. Published tests and subtests of written vocabulary are designed to measure a person's knowledge of words and their meanings. Although vocabulary scores have often been considered to be the best single indicator of general intellectual ability, vocabulary abilities may be particularly vulnerable to TBI (Lezak, 1983). Lezak cautioned, therefore, that other verbal intelligence quotient (IQ) scores should be considered along with vocabulary scores when attempting to estimate a client's level of pretrauma verbal functioning.

Vocabulary measures differ from one another in the types of skills examined, method of administration, and format of presentation. Some measure simple word recognition, or sight vocabulary, as the person's ability to pronounce the word. Knowledge of word meaning is assumed for words that can be read aloud, rather than being assessed directly. Examples of this type of subtest include the Vocabulary subtest of the Gates-MacGinitie Reading Tests (Gates and MacGinitie, 1969), the Letter-Word Identification subtest of the WJPEB (Woodcock and Johnson, 1977), and the Word Identification subtest on Forms G and H of the WRMT-R (Woodcock, 1987).

The Blue Level of the SDRT (Karlsen and Gardner, 1984), which has a grade equivalent of 9 to 12, includes two subtests for measuring knowledge of word meaning. However, these subtests are timed, and test items are read and answered independently by the examinee. The abilities to maintain attention, to follow directions, and to comprehend printed material at the sentence level are all required of the individual. The Auditory Vocabulary subtest of the Brown Level of the SDRT, which has a grade equivalent of 5 to 8, and the Vocabulary subtest of the SAT (Gardner and colleagues, 1987) also measure knowledge of word meaning. However, for these subtests, both test items and answer choices are read aloud by the examiner. Although this reduces the possibility of some kinds of error on the examinee's part as a result of generalized cognitive and perceptual disabilities, it increases the possibility of others. Sentence-level auditory processing skills are required, because only the answer choices are printed on the examinee's response sheet.

The Word Comprehension subtest of the WRMT-R (Woodcock, 1987) uses an analogy format to assess knowledge of word meaning. Because TBI survivors often experience impaired reasoning ability, their performance is generally lower on this subtest than on other vocabulary measures.

To help sort out the specificity of written language and oral language problems, it may be helpful to administer the Peabody Picture Vocabulary Test-Revised (PPVT-R; Dunn and Dunn, 1981), because it does not require reading, writing, or verbal responding by the examinee. Lezak (1983) reported that the Age Equivalent Score (formerly the Mental Age Score) from the PPVT-R might provide the examiner with the best estimate of the individual's residual vocabulary and fund of information.

Most word-level tests of writing require individuals to write single words to dictation, as discussed in the previous section. A variation, which may provide greater opportunity to observe the ability to actually recall written words as vocabulary items, is the Written Confrontation Naming subtest of the BDAE (Goodglass and Kaplan, 1983). It requires individuals to write the names of pictured items they are shown.

Comprehension and Making Sense. Understanding printed material is the goal of reading. It is one that should not get lost in the search to identify mastery of various elements of reading subcomponents. In expression, the ability to convey meaning through writing is the ultimate goal.

Reading comprehension can be affected by many factors, including the length and complexity of passages, the reader's prior knowledge and experience with the topic, and the syntax and organizational patterns of the text. The clinician should consider all these factors when evaluating reading performance. This usually requires the administration of more than one assessment tool of reading comprehension.

When selecting reading comprehension assessment materials, several factors should be considered. If the individual's word reading skills are sufficiently intact, comprehension for sentences and short paragraphs can be assessed. Several published tests include passages of this length. The WJPEB (Woodcock and Johnson, 1977) and the WRMT-R (Woodcock, 1987) (Forms G and H) include passage comprehension subtests that use modified cloze techniques. Cloze techniques require readers to read passages silently and to tell examiners appropriate words to fill blanks that have been inserted in the passages. The level of difficulty for the passages in the WJPEB and WRMT-R ranges from first grade to college, but the length does not go beyond the level of a single short paragraph. Successful completion of these items calls for comprehension skills and the ability to use semantic and syntactic cues. Persons with word finding problems or other aphasic symptoms or speaking impairments associated with TBI may have difficulty responding in this format, and a multiple choice test may be more appropriate in such cases.

A number of standardized aphasia batteries include subtests for reading that evaluate comprehension of multiple sentence passages. However, caution is required when relying on these tests as comprehension measures because they may not provide valid estimates of ability to comprehend information from printed texts. As noted previously, the results of a study assessing the passage dependency of five aphasia batteries (Nicholas and colleagues, 1986) showed that more than half the test items for comprehension from these reading tests were answered correctly by a significantly greater than chance number of both aphasic and non-brain-damaged adults without reading the passages. In a later study, Nicholas and Brookshire (1987) found the Nelson Reading Skills Test (NRST; Hanna and colleagues, 1977) to be a more valid measure of paragraph-level written language comprehension than the five tests originally evaluated by Nicholas and colleagues (1986). Rand (1988) also found that the passage dependency of items on the Reading Comprehension Battery for Aphasia (LaPointe and Horner, 1979) was sufficient to test the written language comprehension of the individuals with TBI whom she studied.

Selections for evaluating should include multiple paragraph passages as well as single paragraphs. Persons with TBI who are able to comprehend sentences and short paragraphs frequently experience a significant decrease in comprehension when attempting to read longer passages. The Brown Level (grade equivalent 5 to 8) and Blue Level (grade equivalent 9 to 12) versions of the SDRT (Karlsen and Gardner, 1984) do include longer passages for measuring silent reading comprehension. These subtests are timed, and a written multiple choice format is used for responding. If the examiner has concerns about the examiner's ability to use an answer sheet accurately, the examinee can be instructed to mark responses directly in the test booklet. When tests such as this one or the *Gates-MacGinitie* (Gates and MacGinitie, 1969) are given, Lezak (1983) commented that, for individuals who process information slowly, time limits can be relaxed without much loss of reliability, because such individuals tend to fail items completed outside of established time limits anyway.

For information regarding comprehension of multiple pages of text, informal assessments can be constructed using short stories, such as those from *The Reader's Digest*. It is important to match the readability level of the selection to the client-performance level based on previous testing. As general guidelines, Chall (1983) indicated that by the end of sixth grade, normally developing children can read local newspapers, popular adult fiction, and popular magazines, such as *The Reader's Digest*, but that they still have difficulty with news magazines such as *Time* and *Newsweek*. By the end of 12th grade, most normally developing students have no difficulty comprehending various textbooks and reference works as well as more mature fiction, newspapers, and magazines (Chall, 1983). Another option for judging the readability of nonstandardized material is to use a readability formula, such as that proposed by Fry (1978) for using counts of syllables per 100 words to estimate grade level of the material. The problem with such formulas is that they measure only one limited aspect of text complexity.

When assessing reading comprehension for longer passages, a set of literal and inferential questions should be constructed about the material. Some examples of questions that can be asked about stories with a narrative structure are:

Who are the main characters in the story?
Where does the story mainly take place?
What problem occurs?
Why is it a problem?
What steps are taken to try to solve the problem?

How is the problem solved?
What kind of person is the main character? How can you tell?
What was the author's purpose (e.g., to entertain, to provide information, to persuade the reader)?

Passages that have expository structure (e.g., nonfiction selections, news magazines, science and social studies textbooks), rather than narrative structure, pose different kinds of challenges to the reader. Memory and organizational difficulties associated with TBI can interfere with the reader's ability to comprehend either narrative or expository texts. Such deficits reduce the ability to recall specific facts and details, to recall and describe a sequence of events, and to locate specific information in the passage.

Depending on the type of text, such difficulties may interfere in slightly different ways. For example, reasoning deficits affect the reader's ability to compare information and ideas, to draw conclusions, to evaluate information, and to integrate information with prior knowledge. Such skills might be tapped particularly when attempting to read a factual news magazine article and to answer questions about it. Short stories and novels also require the reader to keep information introduced at the beginning of the story alive as the story proceeds and to call on prior knowledge about the world and human motivations and emotions to interpret events in the story.

Throughout the reading comprehension assessment, the clinician should observe for signs of such difficulties and for any compensatory strategies the client might use, such as rereading, looking back for specific information to respond to questions, subvocalizing while reading, and taking notes or marking information in the text. To check for awareness of strategy use, the clinician should ask the client whether any special techniques or approaches were used to make understanding and remembering easier.

Prior knowledge and experience affect reading comprehension in a number of ways. Reading is usually easier when the reader has some familiarity with the topic, and this factor should be considered when selecting assessment materials. However, the clinician should bear in mind that individuals with TBI may respond to comprehension questions with information not stated or implied in the passage but related to the topic based on prior knowledge (Nicholas and colleagues, 1986; Rand, 1988) and may not recognize the distinction. In such cases, the results will not reflect the true severity of their reading difficulties. To check for possible effects of prior knowledge on passage comprehension, the clinician can ask clients which passage topics were familiar and compare accuracy of responses with questions regarding familiar and unfamiliar passages.

It is also important to assess individuals' abilities to *produce* written language texts that make sense and that follow the conventions of writing. The ability to write intelligibly draws on a number of skills that can be assessed with tasks at the word and sentence levels, but it is also important to assess how well an individual can perform when required to integrate complex skills on several levels simultaneously. The WJPEB (Woodcock and Johnson, 1977) includes two subtests that combine assessment in the areas of spelling, punctuation, capitalization, and usage. The Dictation subtest measures the examinee's ability to respond in writing to a variety of questions from these areas, such as, "Print the abbreviation for 'Avenue' " (item 16) and "Print the word that means more than one mouse; one mouse, two . . . what?" (item 17). The Proofing subtest requires the ability to identify and correct errors orally in one or two sentence passages. This subtest assumes that the individual has the ability to comprehend short written passages and to analyze for error detection. When administered to an individual with TBI, a low score on this subtest may be more indicative of underlying difficulties with reading comprehension and cognition than of lack of knowledge regarding rules for spelling, punctuation, capitalization, and usage.

If performance on tests of word-level spelling and writing mechanics indicates that the TBI client does have some writing ability at these levels, writing of connected texts should be evaluated. Unless a major goal is for the TBI individual to be able to engage competitively in academic or professional writing, it may be most appropriate for tasks in this area to relate to functional activities of daily living. For example, sample job applications or information questionnaires can be useful for eliciting rote information that is familiar to clients, such as their names and addresses. They can also be used to observe the client's ability to respond in short phrases and sentences to such written questions as, "What areas would you like to work on in therapy?"

The effects of language and cognitive disorders associated with TBI are frequently seen when individuals with TBI attempt to communicate long or complex ideas in writing. The effectiveness of written expression may be reduced by decreases in the person's ability to organize thoughts and ideas, as well as to recall words and how to spell them, accompanied by reduced ability to apply rules of punctuation, capitalization, syntax, and spacing. Some of the more common types of difficulties include insufficient classification and sequencing of ideas; incomplete or run-on sentence construction; distorted word order; incorrect usage of verbs, pronouns, and referents; and misuse or lack of punctuation. Clients who experience problems with hemispatial neglect or constructional difficulties will experience particular difficulty in organizing their writing on the page (Burns and colleagues, 1985).

Wallace and McLoughlin (1988) reported that the most effective and most widely used procedure for appraising written expression is evaluation of individuals' writing samples. Informal testing was also the most frequently mentioned tool for assessing writing in the Surges and Nelson (1988) study, being mentioned by 58 percent of the participants. The next most frequently mentioned tool, the BDAE; (Goodglass and Kaplan, 1983), was listed by only 34 percent of the participants. Although spontaneous writing samples offer the opportunity to observe the integration of multiple skills in tasks that may be designed to approximate functional written language tasks that occur naturally in the environment, factors related specifically to TBI must be considered when interpreting the results. For example, exaggerated difficulties with attention and organization may interfere with the TBI client's ability to convey meaning effectively while simultaneously applying rules related to the mechanics of writing. Because of the confounding of these factors, isolated direct assessment of the knowledge of discrete skills, such as the rules for punctuation, capitalization, and grammatical inflections ("word usage"), can be conducted apart from the application of writing skills within a connected writing sample. In this way, the clinician may be better able to analyze the separate effects of skill deficits and cognitive deficits on written expression.

One test that can assist in the process of differential diagnosis is the TOWL (Hammill and Larsen, 1983), which has been recently revised to become the TOWL-2 (Hammill and Larsen, 1988). The TOWL includes two subtests that measure skill in word usage and punctuation. The Word Usage subtest is a closure task of 25 sentence groups, each of which has a missing word the examinee is required to provide. Areas addressed include verb forms, auxiliary verbs, pronouns, plurals, and adjectives. The Style subtest also is made up of 25 items. In this case, sentences are written without capitalization or punctuation, and the examinee is expected to rewrite them using the rules for correct capitalization and punctuation. The Style subtest is useful for observing the individual's ability to copy words accurately.

Spontaneous writing of connected text can be observed with the TOWL as well. The Thematic Maturity subtest involves presentation of three related situation pictures printed on the response form. The examinee is instructed to write a complete story using all three pictures. The subtest is untimed, and the examinee is encouraged to take about 5 minutes to think about the story before beginning to write. The writing sample is evaluated against a set of criteria, and points are given for such aspects of content and organization as paragraphing, definite ending, naming of characters, inclusion of sequence or subplot, type of theme expressed, and attempted humor. TBI clients who have difficulty integrating, organizing, and expressing their thoughts are frequently observed to write three unrelated sentences in response to this task, one for each of the three stimulus pictures. The sentences may even be numbered. Although the use of writing conventions, such as those for punctuation, capitalization, usage, and spelling are not directly evaluated in the Thematic Maturity subtest, the clinician can check performance in these areas and compare the contextual performance with the performance on the isolated subtests designed specifically for these purposes.

The TOWL-2 includes some modifications in format and scoring from the original TOWL. For example, rather than a sequence of three pictures, one situation picture is used to elicit the story, reducing the likelihood that clients will write three unconnected sentences. Another change is that two forms are provided of the TOWL-2, making test-retest procedures more feasible with the revised instrument.

Oral Versus Silent Reading. Beyond assessing written language processing for differences according to levels of linguistic units, written language processing of TBI individuals should be assessed for unusually marked differences of processing in different modalities. Comprehension through silent reading is important to evaluate for several reasons. It is how most material is read by mature readers. Silent reading may also allow brain-injured persons to gain more immediate access to the meaning of written words if they have oral language production deficits that might impede that access. Johnson (1986), when discussing adult dyslexia, noted that readers with verbal expressive disorders read and comprehend better silently than orally. On the other hand, Johnson commented that readers with attention disorders often show improvement during oral reading because they must attend to all the words. In any case, analysis of oral reading as well as silent reading provides the clinician with additional information useful in pinpointing specific reading problems.

When assessing oral reading, passages of varied difficulty can be selected based on results from standardized assessments of paragraph level reading. The client should be tape recorded while reading the passages aloud to facilitate the clinician's ability to make observations while the client is reading and still obtain an accurate count of the number and types of oral reading errors. More or less formal observational methods can be used to guide the analysis process. For example, the clinician should look for such features as word-by-word reading, improper phrasing, inattention to punctuation, mispronunciations, omissions, repetitions, insertions, and substitutions.

It may aid the observational process to use the system of "reading miscue" analysis developed by Goodman (1976). Using this system, nothing the reader does is viewed as accidental. Rather, reading miscues provide evidence of the types of strategies the reader is using internally to read the text. It is particularly important to observe for reading miscues that result in words that maintain some visual or auditory similarity to the words printed on the page but violate the meaning of the text. Such miscues indicate reliance on phonemic decoding strategies, while ignoring semantic cues. This type of error is quite different from one in which the reader produces a word with associated meaning to the target word, but with little surface similarity, which may indicate inability to access graphophonemic decoding strategies. Both types of errors are serious if they happen so consistently that they indicate that the individual is using one approach to the exclusion of others. A normal mature reader should be able to demonstrate flexible switching among units of analysis and types of strategy as the task demands it. For the TBI individual, the rest of the comprehensive assessment, including pretrauma history and results of reading tasks using different types of words (real and nonsense, regularly and irregularly spelled) and passages, should help to sort out the relative effects of different factors on the reading process, and it should help to identify the person's access to flexible approaches.

Reading and Writing Rate. Assessment in the area of reading rate is concerned with how fast individuals can read while maintaining adequate levels of comprehension, along with how well they can scan or skim material for the purposes of previewing and locating specific information. Individuals who have experienced TBI are particularly at risk for demonstrating reduced reading rates as a result of visuoperceptual deficits, cognitive slowing, the implementation of time-consuming strategies to facilitate comprehension, and a lack of understanding of text organization and structure.

Not all reading batteries contain tests designed to measure reading rate. Both Brown (grades 5 to 8) and Blue (grades 9 to 12) Levels of the SDRT (Karlsen and Gardner, 1984) do contain Fast Reading subtests, which utilize a multiple-choice cloze format to measure an individual's ability to read easy material quickly and with comprehension. These tests are aimed for 2 minutes. The Blue Level also contains a timed subtest for Scanning and Skimming, which has two parts. In Part A, the examinee is presented with a page of questions and is asked to locate the answers in an accompanying article without reading it through. In Part B, the examinee is presented with an article to read, and, after 2 minutes, the article is removed and the examinee is asked to respond to 16 multiple-choice questions. Persons who have experienced TBI are likely to be frustrated by the scanning and skimming subtests, but such activities may be helpful in determining the ability of high-functioning individuals with TBI to return competitively to academic pursuits in secondary school or higher education. Such skills may or may not be important for a person seeking to return to work. The fast reading subtests are appropriate for most persons who have multiple sentence comprehension abilities. They should not be used for persons who are still at earlier levels of recovery.

No formal tests are available for assessing writing rate. However, clinicians can design informal measures for this ability when it is of concern. Tasks should differ depending on the source of concern. If the reason for concern about rate is one of linguistic recall and formulation, then spontaneous writing tasks of different types can be assigned, such as describing an event, listing words in a category, or writing a personal or business letter. Writing rates can be computed as numbers of syllables or words produced within a given time span. Writing rates for particular tasks can be compared as recovery progresses. It may also be helpful to record the length of processing pauses during the composition process so that they can be indicated, to be preserved for later comparison, on the written text.

If the reasons for concern about rate is more one of motor control, the other procedures can be used. In such cases, writing to dictation may be appropriate if reduction of auditory memory is not a problem, or copying of text may be used if visual tracking and perceptual skills are intact. Beukelman and colleagues (1985) and Dowden and Beukelman (1988) commented on the importance of measuring rate of output, along with accuracy and message flexibility, for individuals using augmentative and alternative communicative devices. Comparisons of pretraumatic and posttraumatic typing rates may be particularly helpful if such data are available.

ONGOING ASSESSMENT

The activities of the previous sections have been presented as those which might be an appropriate part of an initial assessment process. Because TBI persons may progress through a series of recovery levels, and they may transfer among rehabilitation programs during the process, they may be submitted to multiple initial assessments. The challenge to professionals in such cases is to judge the extent to which the new situation or changes within the individual justify a completely new set of evaluation activities. A balance must be achieved between the need to document progress and gather diagnostic information that is critical to program planning and the need to avoid the trap of continually reassessing and never getting to intervention. The information-gathering activities described earlier in this chapter can help reduce diagnostic redundancy.

On the other hand, frequent reassessments may be more critical for TBI survivors than they are for individuals with other types of disabilities. All children in schools who are labeled as handicapped and served under PL 94-142 must be provided with a comprehensive reevaluation at least once every 3 years. Such a schedule may not be frequent enough for children whose disabilities stem from TBI, because their status may change from month to month within the first several years aftertrauma.

One way to address the need for ongoing assessment without detracting too greatly from the time needed for intervention is to build strategies for ongoing assessment into the intervention process. This is often particularly easy to do when working with written language, because relatively permanent records are created. For example, written stories or letters can be duplicated, and features of them can be quantified as described previously. When working on writing using microcomputer word processing software programs, frequent printing of documents during stages of revision, with and without prompting, can demonstrate changes in clients' writing over time within a session and across sessions. Clinicians can also gather ongoing assessment records for their clients' oral reading skills by having them read aloud as the clinician simultaneously marks reading miscues (Goodman, 1976) on a duplicate transcript of the passage being read.

Systematic, ongoing assessment within the context of intervention is essential to successful rehabilitation for persons with TBI for several reasons. First, little research is available on the rehabilitation of reading and writing disorders following TBI, and the contribution of different brain areas and processes is not fully understood. Therefore, much intervention actually is based on educated clinical trial and error. This procedure involves applying what is known, observing for success or failure, and modifying intervention plans accordingly. A second reason is that it is difficult to predict the pattern and extent of recovery processes. The periods of spontaneous recovery and plateaus that occur after TBI affect the selection and relative success of various intervention methods. It has also been observed that improvement in one deficit area may reveal other areas of difficulty not apparent before intervention (Gouvier and colleagues, 1986). For all these reasons, the most effective clinical intervention program is likely to be one in which progress is monitored with activities of ongoing assessment.

INTERVENTION

Plans for intervention programs are made and modified based on all the assessment activities described previously. Intervention plans address deficit areas identified within the context of the individual's history and personal goals, taking into consideration the relative degree of impairment. Instructional sequences are defined, and relevant materials are selected. The appropriateness of strategy training is considered throughout the intervention period.

Levels of Impairment

Reading and writing abilities and disabilities vary considerably in different individuals after TBI. Those with the most severe disorders cannot read or write the letters of the alphabet, whereas those with less severe disorders may have functional reading and writing skills but experience difficulty with lengthy, complex passages requiring higher-order thought processes. Because of the considerable variation in severity and consequences of TBI, as well as the variation in history and goals of TBI survivors, clinicians may find it helpful to classify reading and writing disorders in terms of levels of impairment.

Webb (1987) presented operational definitions for three levels of impairment. These definitions provide general descriptions of impaired reading function for *severely impaired, moderately impaired,* and *mildly impaired* individuals. They also serve as a framework for understanding relative degrees of impairment, grouping intervention methods, and planning individualized instruction. In the following sections, Webb's (1987) original functional descriptions for levels of *reading impairment* are stated, and parallel functional descriptions for levels of *expressive writing impairment* are added. It should also be noted that the arrangement of neuropsychological processes is such that it is possible for a person to exhibit a more severe impairment in one area than the other (writing is usually more severely impaired, but not exclusively so).

Severely Impaired Persons. According to Webb (1987), who was writing about adults, the individual with a severe reading impairment is unable to read more than a few high-frequency or highly familiar words. Some evidence is available to suggest that children who acquire TBI during the preschool years are at even greater risk for having trouble acquiring skills they have not yet developed (Chadwick and colleagues, 1981a). A parallel severe *writing* impairment would involve the inability to write more than a few high-frequency words, such as the person's signature, often accompanied by inability to copy letters or geometric shapes.

TBI survivors who have severe impairments or whose pretrauma literacy functioning was low should have intervention goals to improve functional literacy skills for communication and to increase independence for daily living. Development of basic skills builds the foundation for successful performance of more complex tasks requiring these skills in later stages of recovery (Jacobs, 1988). However, a caveat is that exclusive focus on splinter skills may not result in transfer to functional literacy behaviors. A good general rule of intervention is to include activities using stimuli that approximate those of natural contexts and that are as intact as they can be without becoming too complex for the individual to be able to process them. With this caution in mind, the following tasks are suggested for use with severely impaired persons.

1. *Matching or copying shapes, letters, and words.* Symbols, letters, and words commonly found in the individual's environment provide functional stimulus materials for working on relearning reading and writing skills. Examples of such materials include circles or symbols with a diagonal line drawn through them to indicate "no" (smoking, eating, parking, etc.), abbreviations and acronyms, and directional signs. If visual processing limitations make reading impossible, the individual may still have auditory processing skills sufficient to enable them to benefit from such programs as Talking Books, which are available from the public library.

2. *Recognition and comprehension of single words.* Webb (1987) described a progression of intervention tasks designed to develop a core vocabulary of sight words and their meanings. Using nouns and verbs from lists of frequently occurring words in addition to lists of words with which the client should be familiar based on previous life experiences (e.g., the menu from a fast-food restaurant), the clinician can design tasks for matching words to pictures and selecting a target word from several alternatives. As the client progresses, contextual clues in phrases can be introduced to encourage the use of context to understand unfamiliar words.

3. *Written production of letters and single words.* Once the client is able to recognize letters and words, practice can be provided in writing letters or words spoken by the clinician. Again, the general rule of using stimuli in forms that are as intact as possible should be followed. The same word lists as those used for reading instruction can be used for writing instruction to encourage the establishment or recovery of associations among stimuli and types of processing. Stimuli for writing activities can also be drawn from functional living sources. For example, simple forms that require such personal identifying information as names and addresses can be used, if appropriate, and the individual can be encouraged to assist in such home management tasks as signing checks and writing items on shopping lists. Commercially available materials in this area include a program called *Fill in the Blanks* (Match, 1989) for practicing such skills, one called *Supermarket* (Tripp, 1976), in which problems related to such skills as grocery buying, making change, and check writing, and *Using the Telephone* (Cook, 1974), which contains exercises for common telephone usage, including using the telephone directory.

Moderately Impaired Persons. Webb (1987) described the individual with moderately impaired reading abilities as having comprehension of a good core vocabulary of single words and simple, short sentences or simple paragraphs presented at the factual level. Parallel impairments of writing abilities may be limited to expressing factual information in the format of short notes, fill-in-the-blank forms, or responding to direct, literal questions in phrases or simple sentences.

1. *Communication and independence.* TBI survivors with moderate impairments of literacy skills should have goals related to continued expansion of literacy skills for communication and increased independence in higher-order life skill areas. For adults, such areas include household business and housework, money management, community participation, caring for personal health and safety, and caring for children (Jacobs, 1988). Corcoran's (1985) *Reading for Survival* includes practice in reading newspaper articles, advertisements, regulations, package directions, time schedules, and warnings. In addition, recreational reading can be encouraged. *Reading Comprehension Materials* (Kilpatrick, 1982) can be used to provide stimuli from single words to complex stories on a fourth to tenth grade level. Some publishers (e.g., Fearon Education, A Division of Pittman Learning, Inc., Belmont, CA; Frank E. Richards Publishing Co., Inc., Phoenix, NY; Scholastic, Inc., Jefferson City, MO) specialize in providing high-interest–easy-reading materials for adolescents and adults, including materials aimed both at functional and recreational literacy skills.

2. *Special concerns for children and adolescents.* When children have moderate impairments, their goals can relate to the regular or special education curriculum if brain injury occurs during the elementary and middle school years. For such children, their needs can be addressed within academic settings, using the same kinds of stimulus materials and strategies that have been designed for working with individuals who have developmental reading disorders. However, the possibility that they might have retained some reading skills that were acquired pretraumatically should also be considered, as should the possible role of impairments related to generalized cognitive, attention, and memory deficits.

It is important that schools charged with providing free appropriate public educations for all handicapped children under PL 94-142 recognize some of the special concerns regarding children with TBI. They should not automatically place such children in programs for developmentally disabled children who are at a similar level of cognitive functioning. The cognitive profiles of children with TBI may vary considerably from those of children with developmental disorders. However, they often do need special education services, certainly when they are functioning at the level of moderate impairment.

When secondary level students sustain TBI, a more complex goal-setting process often must be conducted. In such cases, possible goals for postsecondary education may have to be reassessed as being unrealistic, but this should not occur too hastily, particularly if a college or university program is available that includes accommodations for persons with TBI. Functional reading and writing skills similar to those targeted for adults also should be addressed for moderately impaired secondary students.

3. *Computer-assisted instruction.* The individual with moderate impairment is a good candidate for computer-assisted reading instruction (Webb, 1987). Computer-assisted instruction is valuable for many reasons. It provides unlimited drill and practice opportunities; feedback is consistent and immediate; and authoring programs are available that allow clinicians to individualize intervention exercises. Program flexibility is particularly important because modifications in stimulus and response modes and timing variables often must be made to meet the individualized needs of a particular client with TBI. Data-collection provisions are also important. Examples of software programs (reviewed by Mills, 1987) that include some of these features are *Computerized Reading for Aphasics* (Major and Wilson, 1984), *Reading Recognition* (Mills and colleagues, 1986), *Cognitive Rehabilitation* (Smith, 1984), and *Language Stimulation Software* (Volin and Groher, 1985).

A software program that has been designed to be used with synthesized speech output to cue writers with words that they do not know how to spell (except for the initial letter) is *Cue-Write* (Beukelman and colleagues, 1988). This program can be set in two modes. In the "assist mode," the words in the person's individualized spelling vocabulary remain on the lower half of the screen as the person enters text into the top part of the screen. In the "tutor mode," the words disappear from the lower half of the screen after the second letter is entered. The *Cue-Write* program was useful in helping David, who was described in the first vignette at the beginning of this chapter, to recover enough spelling independence that he could write without assistance.

Because feedback on performance is immediate in computer-assisted intervention, and it is provided by the computer program, the clinician's role in using this approach is often one of facilitator, observing, modeling correct responses, and assisting the client with the mechanics of the task. These steps are particularly important when trying to establish rapport with an individual who is sensitive to feedback. However, Mills (1986, 1987), in discussing the use of microcomputer treatment for persons with aphasia and brain trauma, also cautioned that many clients should begin their computer-based treatment programs in a dependent mode and gradually move to clinic-based and home-based treatment modes. He pointed out that the clinician's presence is important in the early stages of intervention because clinicians are less rigid than the algorithms of computer programs and are able "to make repeated synergistic adjustments according to the behavior of the patient during a given therapy session" (Mills, 1986, p. 73). Such adjustments may be particularly important when addressing the problems exhibited by many persons with TBI in the areas of attention and initiation. This was the case with Chris, who was described in the second vignette at the beginning of this chapter.

A concern has been raised by some (e.g., Haarbauer-Krupa and colleagues, 1985) that uncritical overuse of computer-based cognitive retraining for TBI persons tends to address only splinter skills at basic levels, and little evidence is available to support its ability to improve "real-life performance of functional-integrative tasks" (Haarbauer-Krupa and colleagues, 1985, p. 335). However, if this limitation is kept in mind, even young children who were injured during prewriting or early-writing stages of their education can have their rehabilitation programs enhanced with the use of simple word processing programs. For example, Ylvisaker (1987), demonstrated how he has developed integrated programs for TBI children with marked attention and cognitive organization deficits. First, Ylvisaker interacted with a child using felt board characters and props to construct oral narratives about topics of interest to the child (e.g., a family camping trip). Then Ylvisaker reviewed and reinforced this activity by sitting at the computer with the child in his lap to direct the child's attention and to contain his activity level while jointly recalling elements from the "story" and dictating language for a written text, which the clinician typed as they worked. Ylvisaker reported that the child's ability to carry away a concrete product from his intervention session in the form of computer printout was a source of pride and a form of direct feedback to the family about what had occurred that day. It also facilitated parental reinforcement of the child's memory for the concepts discussed in a particular session.

4. *Comprehension and production of longer passages.* The focus of intervention for all moderately impaired persons is to increase the ability to comprehend and produce longer and more complex written language passages. Webb (1987) recommended having clients follow written directions as a means of improving comprehension of complex material at the sentence level. Simple directions can be used initially to introduce command verbs (e.g., *put, give, move*) and objects. Later, prepositional phrases (e.g., *under the*), independent

clauses (e.g., *before you*), and descriptive terms (e.g., *the blue book*) can be added to increase the length and complexity of tasks. *Practice in Survival Reading* (book series available from New Readers Press, Syracuse, NY) offers materials written at the third to sixth grade level that have interest levels appropriate for adult lifestyles.

Reading comprehension tasks for persons with moderate impairments should also include paragraph-length reading material. Developing the ability to identify main ideas and supporting details or event sequences facilitates comprehension and the development of basic support skills for comprehending longer passages. Materials for reading and writing intervention with adults and secondary students who exhibit moderate impairments are plentiful. For example, the Boning (1978, 1985) *Specific Skills Series* and *Supporting Reading Skills* series contain short story material followed by questions on main ideas, remembering details, and following directions. The *Reader's Digest Reading Skill Builders* and accompanying *Audio Lessons* (Readers Digest Services, Inc., Pleasantville, NY) include story material at varying reading grade levels, exercises, quizzes, and discussion questions following each story.

Newspaper and magazine articles are also useful for therapy tasks, provided that they are selected carefully with the client's background and vocabulary comprehension abilities in mind. *Using the Newspaper* (Parsky, 1989) is a set of materials that has been specifically designed for encouraging newspaper scanning and reading. *News for You* (New Readers Press) uses captioned pictures, headlines, and articles ranging from two to three related sentences up to approximately six paragraphs in a large print weekly newspaper at a fourth to sixth grade reading level. *Everyday Reading and Writing* (Laubach and colleagues, 1979) includes work not only in reading newspapers and magazines, but also in reading signs, labels, maps, instructions, reference books, and business and personal letters.

Interactive journal writing and letter writing are particularly useful activities for increasing the length and complexity of written expression. Social notes are also important spontaneous written language form for elementary school children. In such instances, individuals have the advantage of writing about familiar topics and may be motivated by focusing more on the communicativeness of the activities than on their correctness. Feedback about this kind of writing should consist of requests for clarification when the information is insufficient (as in interactive journals between the clinician and client) and avoid corrections based on errors of form. Other assignments can be given for encouraging the production of well-organized written texts.

Mildly Impaired Persons. Reading for individuals with mild impairments is slow, but comprehension is good if the person can tolerate the related rate of processing (Webb, 1987). Written expression may be relatively fluent (although slow) but ineffective in conveying intended meaning. The presentation of ideas and information may be disorganized, unclear, or ambiguous. If so, the person may benefit from the use of materials such as those provided by Brubaker (1978, 1983). Written expression may be too lengthy, too concrete, or lacking in sufficient detail, or it may diverge from the purpose or topic of the particular writing task. If so, exercises such as those provided by DeWitt (1984) may help the person regain or develop an ability to use figurative language.

1. *Increasing rate.* For the mildly impaired individual, the slow processing rate for comprehension of printed material is frustrating and often takes the pleasure out of what may have once been an enjoyable pasttime. Webb (1987) reported that some of the techniques for developing speed reading skills are useful when working with mildly impaired TBI individuals. For example, scanning the text for main ideas and general organization and adjusting reading rate to the nature of the task serve both to focus attention and to increase the rate of processing of written material.

   It is important to emphasize that acceleration of reading and writing rate should not be attempted until it has been determined that rate is the primary area of difficulty for the individual. As noted by Bawden and colleagues (1985), "the loss of the ability to formulate a plan of action is quite distinct from the ability to quickly execute the action" (p. 52). Accelerating rate when other reading or writing problems are evident may only worsen the situation by further reducing reading comprehension and the ability to construct meaning.

2. *Strategy development.* Mildly impaired individuals are often good candidates for strategy training. Their general cognitive levels and ability to maintain attention, coupled with their awareness of their deficits and need for compensation, increase the chance for success using such an approach. Compensatory strategy training facilitates optimal skill acquisition and reduces the impact of the functional limitations imposed by the cognitive deficits. It involves teaching the person with TBI to employ procedures and external aids deliberately for accomplishing difficult tasks (Ylvisaker and colleagues, 1987).

   Descriptions of strategies for improving reading and writing performance of mildly impaired persons can be found in the educational literature regarding students with learning disabilities. However, as Ylvisaker and colleagues (1987) pointed out, strategy choice and training with TBI survivors is a complicated process that must be carefully planned. For strategy intervention to be successful, the clinician must consider the person's needs and abilities, awareness of personal strengths and limitations, and issues related to generalization. Ylvisaker and colleagues (1987) provided an in-depth discussion of strategy intervention with persons who have experienced TBI that can be consulted for additional details regarding this type of approach.

3. *Types of strategies.* The goal of strategy instruction is to foster independent functioning in the learner. Many strategies are helpful in increasing reading comprehension and improving the effectiveness of written expression, including organizational strategies, self-monitoring strategies, and repair strategies.

Organizational strategies help the learner separate relevant from irrelevant information, focus attention on important points, and facilitate recall of information. Summarizing, highlighting, note taking, and outlining material during and after reading are examples of organizational strategies to improve reading comprehension. Organizational strategies for improving writing include outlines, clustering, and graphic organizers developed during the prewriting or planning stage of the writing process. Such strategies can be considered to be *metatextual* in that writers are encouraged to focus consciously on the way that texts are organized.

The encouragement of *self-monitoring strategies* can assist individuals during the reading and writing process by increasing their awareness of accuracy and facilitating detection of errors in the comprehension and expression of written language. Self-monitoring strategies for reading include self-questioning and paraphrasing during or immediately after reading. Self-monitoring also can lead the reader to adjust the rate of reading as necessary to ensure comprehension. Stimulus materials for individuals who demonstrate mild levels of impairment can be drawn primarily from functional materials important in the individual's environment, ranging from professional journals in the individual's vocational discipline to complex directions for building or sewing.

Writers can be assisted to self-monitor their work by referring to checklists, outlines, and other external sources while writing. Such strategies can be used to help the writer monitor accuracy in organization and expression of ideas, as well as the mechanics of writing. Prevo's (1986) *English That We Need* is a workbook designed to assist individuals in the mechanics of the English language and the practical aspects of its everyday usage.

Developing *repair strategies* enables individuals to correct errors once they are made. Repair strategies for reading comprehension include lookbacks, rereading, and checking outside resources such as dictionaries and other written references or knowledgable people. Proofreading (silently or aloud), editing, and referring to checklists and other outside sources are examples of repair strategies that can be used to improve written expression.

In some cases, individuals advance to the point that they can use *combined strategies*. One approach that requires an individual to use combined strategies has been presented in a number of forms since it was originally introduced as a method of improving the reading comprehension of soldiers in World War II. The "SQ3R" approach, as described by Robinson (1946), combines several organizational, self-monitoring, and repair strategies in a sequence. The title "SQ3R" serves as a mnemonic device for the five steps of the procedure: *survey* the material to be read; develop *questions* about the material using titles, subtitles, and headings; *read* to answer the questions; *recite* the answers in writing or aloud; and *review* by rereading the text to verify the answers. The SQ3R approach is useful when the goal for reading is new learning or comprehending lengthy passages, as it is in academic settings. It should be remembered that the approach is designed for reading expository and not fictional material and that each step must be taught directly and practiced under the clinician's supervision. A similar "multiple pass" approach has been presented in conjunction with techniques for modeling and reinforcement by Alley and Deshler (1979) and further discussed by Schumaker and colleagues (1982). Instructional objectives for this multipass procedure and other written language goals are provided by Nelson (1988).

Selecting Materials and Sequencing Instruction

When planning a sequence of instruction and selecting materials for use in intervention with TBI clients, the clinician must consider each person's current level of reading and writing abilities in conjunction with several factors that affect reading comprehension and effective written communication for such individuals. Such factors include those related to stimulus and response complexity, the degree of structure required for successful performance, the level of abstraction of materials, the client's familiarity with the content, and functional expectations.

Stimulus and Response Complexity. Webb and Love (1986) reported that the complexity of information in written material depends on the number of details found in it and on the semantic and syntactic levels of its linguistic expression. Materials and tasks selected for reading and writing intervention should be sequenced for presentation to the client according to level of complexity.

Reading tasks progress from letter matching and identification to comprehension of words and sentences, paragraphs, multiple paragraphs, and, finally, lengthier passages, such as book chapters and novels. Not only the complexity of the reading task itself, but also the complexity of responses required for demonstrating comprehension, should be analyzed and controlled. TBI survivors with expressive language difficulties may comprehend relatively complex printed material but may be unable to summarize the content due to difficulties with word retrieval or organization of ideas for expression. Multiple choice tasks are more appropriate for such individuals.

A progression of writing task complexity can also be used to guide intervention planning. Such a progression would extend from such tasks as (1) copying forms, letters, and words to (2) writing words and sentences to (3) dictation to (4) choosing or generating responses for performing sentence completion exercises to (5) writing lists and short notes and, finally, to (6) organizing ideas for writing such connected texts as paragraphs, letters, and stories.

Degree of Structure Required for Successful Performance. The clinician initially provides as much contextual structure as the client needs to complete a particular task successfully. Structure may include the provision of organized, straightforward stimulus materials that focus on one specific skill at a time; providing immediate, frequent feedback on task performance, providing cues as needed for recognition and correction of errors; establishing a predictable routine for therapy that may include frequent breaks to minimize the effects of fatigue and overload; minimizing environmental distractions; and facilitating on-task behavior.

Environmental restructuring is reduced as the individual learns organizational and self-monitoring strategies that increase independent performance. More functional, less predictable materials can be introduced as the client learns to implement organizational strategies to increase reading comprehension and written expression of complex ideas, to monitor the accuracy and consistency of responses through self-checking and reviewing strategies, to use external and internal strategies for maintaining attention to task in the presence of distractors, and to manage the effects of fatigue and overload.

Level of Abstraction of Materials. Lezak (1983) indicated that concrete thinking results from impaired conceptual functions that are sensitive to the effect of brain injury regardless of its site. She further reported that individuals who are unable to think abstractly have difficulty forming concepts, using categories, generalizing from a single instance, or applying procedural rules or principles. The clinician must therefore consider the level of abstraction of materials selected for use with TBI individuals.

Concrete activities for reading and writing intervention include those that require matching, concrete vocabulary selection, filling in blanks, recalling literal information, and identifying sequences. As a general rule, clients should not be expected to respond to inferential questions until at least 80 percent of literal information is understood and recalled (Webb, 1987). When individuals begin to recover or gain higher-order cognitive abilities, inferential comprehension skills can be introduced, along with writing tasks requiring abstract reasoning abilities.

Client Familiarity with Content. Written language that includes familiar content is more easily comprehended than written language that includes mostly new information. Similarly, it is easier to write about more familiar topics than to write about less familiar ones. For this reason, clinicians may choose to select reading material and writing activities related to clients' work and other interests. This provides opportunities for reading activities to focus primarily as confirmation of what is already known, using current knowledge to predict meaning. Similarly, writing efforts can be focused primarily on organized expression of existing, familiar knowledge and ideas.

As proficiency in reading and writing develops, less familiar material can be introduced. Instruction can then focus on reading for new meanings and integrating new information with that learned previously.

Functional Expectations. When establishing a plan for intervention, special consideration must be given to the client's needs for meeting functional environmental demands. The issue of environmental demands is described by Siedenberg (1988) as "the relationship between the setting in which the individual must function and his or her disability" (p. 58). Difficulty with generalization of newly learned skills and strategies to the everyday environment is a common procedure after TBI. Therefore, the individual who is successful with reading and writing activities in the clinic may be unable to perform similar types of activities in the home or workplace. Once outside the clinical setting, the client encounters factors that affect performance that may not have been directly addressed in formal intervention. Interferences may include auditory and visual distractions (including internal "noise"), interruptions, time constraints, and lack of internal structure or feedback necessary for monitoring performance levels. For example, a mother with young children who has experienced TBI may be able to read and summarize newspaper articles in the clinical setting but be unable to demonstrate this skill at home due to distractions in the environment. For such a client, it is not only important to remediate reading skills, but it is also essential to develop strategies for resuming reading after interruptions without sacrificing comprehension.

CONCLUSION

In conclusion, no single technique or set of materials is effective with all persons who have experienced TBI. The sequence of instruction and selection of materials should be flexible and adjusted according to the individual's current abilities and stage of recovery. Individuals who are severely impaired or who are in the earlier stages of recovery may benefit most from intervention activities that are highly structured, using predictable routines with simple, concrete materials, and frequent and immediate feedback on performance. Individuals who are less severely impaired, or who have progressed to moderate or mild levels of impairment during later stages of recovery, may benefit more from activities in which the complexity, length, and abstraction of stimuli have been increased and from the encouragement of self-monitoring and organizational strategies for increasing independent functioning.

It is also important for clinicians to remember that the complexity of intervention tasks that the client can handle interacts with the demands of the environmental context that the client can tolerate. Therefore, expanding such factors as the semantic complexity of reading material may necessitate a corresponding increase in the degree of structure provided by the clinician, at least until the client has become comfortable with the higher level of complexity and can handle it independently. If the intervention program includes ongoing assessment, intervention will have a better chance of being effective.

REFERENCES

Adamovich, B. B., Henderson, J. A., and Auerbach, S. (1985). *Cognitive rehabilitation of head injured patients: A dynamic approach.* San Diego, CA: College-Hill Press.

Alley, G. R., and Deshler, D. (1979). *Teaching the learning disabled adolescent: Strategies and methods.* Denver, CO: Love Publishing Co.

Arena, J. (1982). *Diagnostic spelling potential test* (DPST). Novato, CA: Academic Therapy Publications.

Bawden, H. N., Knights, R. M., and Winogron, H. W. (1985). Speeded performance following head injury in children. *Journal of Clinical and Experimental Neuropsychology, 7*, 39–54.

Becker, B. (1975). Intellectual changes after closed head injury. *Journal of Clinical Psychology, 31*, 307–309.

Bender, L. (1946). *Bender visual motor gestalt test.* Circle Pines, MN: American Guidance Service.

Benson, D. F. (1979). *Aphasia, alexia, and agraphia.* New York: Churchill Living-stone.

Benson, D. F. (1981). Alexia and the neuroanatomical basis of reading. In F. J. Pirozzolo and M. C. Wittrock (Eds.), *Neuropsychological and cognitive processes in reading* (pp. 69–92). New York: Academic Press.

Benton, A. L. (1977). Problems of test construction in the field of aphasia. *Cortex, 3,* 32–58.

Beukelman, D. R., Garrett, K., Lange, U., and Tice, R. (1988). *Cue-Write: Word processing with spelling assistance and practice* (Computer program). Tucson, AZ: Communication Skill Builders.

Beukelman, D. R., Yorkston, K. M., and Dowden, P. A. (1985). *Communication augmentation: A casebook of clinical management.* San Diego, CA: College-Hill Press.

Bever, T. G. (1975). Cerebral asymmetries in humans are due to the differentiation of two incompatible processes: Holistic and analytic. *Annals of the New York Academy of Sciences, 265,* 252–262.

Boder, E., and Jarrico, S. (1982). *The Boder test of reading-spelling patterns: A diagnostic screening test for subtypes of reading disability.* New York: Grune & Stratton.

Boning, R. (1978). *Specific skill series.* Baldwin, NY: Barnell Loft.

Boning, R. A. (1985). *Supporting reading skills.* Baldwin, NY: Barnell Loft.

Bookman, M. O. (1984). Spelling as a cognitive-developmental process. *Academic Therapy, 20,* 21–32.

Brink, J. D., Garrett, A. L., Hale, W. R., Woo-Sam, J., and Nickel, V. L. (1970). Recovery of motor and intellectual function in children sustaining severe head injuries. *Developmental Medicine and Child Neurology, 12,* 565–571.

Brooks, D. N. (1974). Recognition memory, and head injury. *Journal of Neurology, Neurosurgery, and Psychiatry, 37,* 794–801.

Brooks, D. N. (1976). Wechsler Memory Scale performance and its relationship to brain damage after severe closed head injury. *Journal of Neurology, Neurosurgery, and Psychiatry, 39,* 593–601.

Brooks, D. N., Aughton, M. E., Bond, M. R., Jones, P., and Rizvi, S. (1980). Cognitive sequelae in relationship to early indices of severity of brain damage after severe blunt head injury. *Journal of Neurology, Neurosurgery, and Psychiatry, 43,* 529–534.

Brown, G., Chadwick, O., Rutter, M., Shaffer, D., and Traub, M. (1981). A prospective study of children with head injuries. 111. Psychiatric sequelae. *Psychological Medicine, 11,* 63–78.

Brown, J., Nelson, M. J., and Denny, E. C. (1976). *The Nelson-Denny test.* Chicago, IL: Riverside.

Brubaker, S. (1978). *Workbook for aphasia: Exercises for the redevelopment of higher level language functioning.* Detroit, MI: Wayne State University Press.

Brubaker, S. (1983). *Workbook for reasoning skills: Exercises for cognitive facilitation.* Detroit, MI: Wayne State University Press.

Brown, V. L., Hammill, D. D., and Wiederholt, J. L. (1986). *Test of reading comprehension* (TORC). Austin, TX: Pro-Ed.

Burns, M., Halper, A., and Mogil, S. (1985). *Clinical management of right hemisphere dysfunction.* Rockville, MD: Aspen Publishers.

Chadwick, O., Rutter, M., Thompson, J., and Shaffer, D. (1981a). Intellectual performance and reading skills after localized head injury in childhood. *Journal of Child Psychology and Psychiatry, 22,* 117–139.

Chadwick, O., Rutter, M., Brown, G., Shaffer, D., and Traub, M. (1981b). A prospective study of children with head injuries. II. Cognitive sequelae. *Psychological Medicine, 11,* 49–61.

Chadwick, O., Rutter, M., Shaffer, D., and Shrout, P. E. (1981c). A prospective study of children with head injuries. IV. Specific cognitive deficits. *Journal of Clinical Neuropsychology, 3,* 101–120.

Chall, J. S. (1983). *Stages of reading development.* New York: McGraw-Hill.

Cook, C. (1974). *Using the telephone.* Syracuse, NY: New Readers Press.

Corcoran, E. L. (1985). *Reading for survival.* Phoenix, NY: Frank E. Richards Publishing Co.

DeWitt, J. (1984). *Means something else: Figures of speech, Writing book #1.* Marysville, MI: Pen-Dec Press.

Dowden, P., and Beukelman, D. R. (1988). Rate, accuracy, and message flexibility: Case studies in communication augmentation strategies. In L. Bernstein (Ed.), *The vocally impaired: Clinical practice and research* (pp. 295–311). Orlando, FL: Grune & Stratton.

Duffy, J. R., Goodglass, H., Holland, A. L., Horner, J., Kertersz, A., McNeil, M. R., and Porch, B. E. (1988, November). *Non-standard uses of standard aphasia tests: The authors speak.* Double miniseminar presented at the meeting of the American Speech-Language-Hearing Association, Boston, MA.

Dunn, L. M., and Dunn, L. M. (1981). *Peabody Picture Vocabulary Test-Revised* (PPVT-R). Circle Pines, MN: American Guidance Service.

Dunn, L. M., and Markwardt, F. G., Jr. (1988). *Peabody individual achievement test-Revised* (PIAT-R). Circle Pines, MN: American Guidance Service.

Durrell, D. D. (1955). *Durrell analysis of reading difficulty* (new ed.). New York: Harcourt Brace.

Frostig, M., and Horne, D. (1964). *The Frostig program for the development of visual perception.* Chicago: Follett.

Fry, E. B. (1978). *Fry readability scale.* Providence, RI: Jamestown Publishers.

Fuld, P. A., and Fisher, P. (1977). Recovery of intellectual ability after closed head-injury. *Developmental Medicine and Child Neurology, 19,* 495–502.

Gardner, B. F., Rudman, H. C., Karlsen, B., and Merwin, J. C. (1987). *Stanford achievement test* (SAT). San Antonio, TX: The Psychological Corporation, Harcourt Brace Jovanovich.

Gates, A. I., and MacGinitie, W. H. (1969). *Gates-MacGinitie Reading Tests.* NY: Teachers College Press, Columbia University.

Goodglass, H., and Kaplan, E. (1983). *The assessment of aphasia and related disorders* (ed. 2) (Manual for *The Boston diagnostic aphasia examination* (BDAE)). Philadelphia: Lea & Febiger.

Goodman, K. S. (1976). What we know about reading. In P. D. Allen and D. J. Watson (Eds.), *Findings in miscue analysis: Classroom implications* (pp. 57–70). Urbana, IL: National Council of Teachers of English.

Gouvier, W. D., Webster, J. S., and Blanton, P. D. (1986). Cognitive retraining with brain-damaged patients. In D. Wedding, A. M. Horton, and J. Webster (Eds.), *The neuropsychological handbook: Behavioral and clinical perspectives* (pp. 278–324). New York: Springer-Verlag Publishing Co.

Groher, M. (1977). Language and memory disorders following closed head trauma. *Journal of Speech and Hearing Research, 20,* 212–223.

Gronwall, D., and Wrightson, P. (1974). Delayed recovery of intellectual function after minor head injuries. *Lancet, 2,* 605–609.

Haarbauer-Krupa, J., Henry, K., Szekeres, S. F., and Ylvisaker, M. In M. Ylvisaker (Ed.). (1985). *Head injury rehabilitation: Children and adolescents* (pp. 311–343). San Diego, CA: College-Hill Press.

Hagen, C. (1981). Language disorders secondary to closed head injury: Diagnosis and treatment. *Topics in Language Disorders, 1*(4), 73–87.

Hammill, D. D., Brown, V., Larsen, S. C., and Wiederholt, J. L. (1987). *Test of adolescent language-2* (TOAL-2). Austin, TX: Pro-Ed.

Hammill, D. D., and Larsen, S. C. (1983). *Test of Written Language* (TOWL). Austin, TX: Pro-Ed.

Hammill, D. D., and Larsen, S. C. (1988). *Test of Written Language-2* (TOWL-2). Austin, TX: Pro-Ed.

Hanna, G., Schell, L. M., and Schreiner, R. (1977). *The Nelson reading skills test.* Chicago: Riverside.

Heilman, K. M., Safran, A., and Geschwind, N. (1971). Closed head trauma and aphasia. *Journal of Neurology, Neurosurgery, and Psychiatry, 34,* 265–269.

Heiskanen, O., and Kaste, M. (1974). Late prognosis of severe brain injury in children. *Developmental Medicine and Child Neurology, 16,* 11–14.

Herzog, J. (1988). Mutism as a sequel to closed head injury: A case history. *TEJAS (Texas Journal of Audiology and Speech Pathology), 14*(2), 15–17.

Horn, J. L., O'Donnell, J. P., and Leicht, D. J. (1988). Phonetically inaccurate spelling among learning-disabled, head-injured, and nondisabled young adults. *Brain and Language, 33,* 55–64.

Jacobs, H. E. (1988). The Los Angeles head injury survey: Procedures and initial findings. *Archives of Physical Medicine and Rehabilitation, 69,* 425–431.

Jastak, J. F., and Jastak, S. (1978). *Wide Range Achievement Test* (WRAT). Wilmington, DE: Jastak Associates.

Jastak, J. F., and Wilkenson, G. S. (1984). *Wide Range Achievement Test-Revised* (WRAT-R). Wilmington, DE: Jastak Associates.

Jennett, B., and Bond, M. (1975). Assessment of outcome after severe brain damage: A practical scale. *Lancet, 1,* 480–487.

Johnson, D. J. (1986). Remediation for dyslexic adults. In G. Th. Pavlidis and D. F. Fisher (Eds.), *Dyslexia: Its neuropsychology and treatment* (pp. 249–262). New York: Wiley.

Kaplan, E., and Goodglass, H. (1981). Aphasia-related disorders. In Sarno, M. T. (Ed.), *Acquired aphasia* (pp. 302–326). New York: Academic Press.

Karlsen, B., and Gardner, E. F. (1984). *Stanford diagnostic reading test* (SDRT) (ed. 3). San Antonio, TX: The Psychological Corporation, Harcourt Brace Jovanovich.

Kertesz, A. (1982). *Western aphasia battery* (WAB). New York: Grune & Stratton.

Kilpatrick, K. (1987). *Reading comprehension materials: Therapy guide for language and speech disorder* (Vol. 5). Akron, OH: Visiting Nurse Services, Inc.

Klonoff, H., Low, M. D., and Clark, C. (1977). Head injuries in children: A prospective five year follow-up. *Journal of Neurology, Neurosurgery, and Psychiatry, 40,* 1211–1219.

LaPointe, L., and Horner, J. (1979). *Reading comprehension battery for aphasia* (RCBA). Tigard, OR: CC Publications.

Laubach, F., Kirk, E., and Laubach, R. (1979). *Everyday reading and writing* (rev. ed.). Syracuse, NY: New Readers Press, Publishing Division of Laubach Literacy International.

Levin, H. S., and Eisenberg, H. M. (1979). Neuropsychological impairment after closed head injury in children and adolescents. *Journal of Pediatric Psychology, 4,* 389–402.

Levin, H. S., Eisenberg, H. M., Wigg, N. R., and Kobayashi, K. (1982). Memory and intellectual ability after head injury in children and adolescents. *Neurosurgery, 11,* 668–673.

Levin, H. S., Grossman, R. G., Rose, J. E., and Teasdale, G. (1979). Long-term neuropsychological outcome of closed head injury. *Journal of Neurosurgery, 50,* 412–422.

Lezak, M. D. (1983). *Neuropsychological assessment* (ed. 2). New York: Oxford University Press.

Major, B., and Wilson, K. (1984). *Computerized reading for aphasics* (Computer program). San Diego, CA: College-Hill Press.

Mandleberg, I. A., and Brooks, D. N. (1975). Cognitive recovery after severe head injury. I. Serial testing on the Weschler Adult Intelligence Scale. *Journal of Neurology, Neurosurgery, and Psychiatry, 38,* 1121–1126.

Match, S. D. (1989). *Fill in the blanks* (rev. ed.). Baltimore, MD: Media Materials.

Mills, R. H. (1986). Microcomputer applications in aphasia and head trauma. In J. L. Northern (Ed.), *The personal computer for speech, language, and hearing professionals* (pp. 85–99). Boston, MA: Little, Brown.

Mills, R. H. (1987). Dependent and independent use of microcomputers in aphasia rehabilitation. *Topics in Language Disorders, 8*(1), 72–85.

Mills, R. H., Burkhead, C., and Shappiro, M. (1986). *Reading recognition* (Computer program). Ann Arbor, MI: Brain-Link Software.

National Head Injury Foundation. (1988). *National Directory of Head Injury Rehabilitation.* Framingham, MA: author.

Neale, M. D. (1958). *Neale Analysis of Reading Ability (Manual).* London: Macmillan.

Nelson, N. W. (1988). *Planning individualized speech and language intervention programs* (rev. ed.). Tucson, AZ: Communication Skill Builders.

New Readers Press. (periodical, first issue, 1959). *News for you: A and B.* Syracuse, NY: Author, Publishing Division of Laubach Literacy International.

Nicholas, L. E., and Brookshire, R. H. (1987). Error analysis and passage dependency of test items from a standardized test of multiple-sentence reading comprehension for aphasic and non-brain damaged adults. *Journal of Speech and Hearing Disorders, 52,* 358–366.

Nicholas, L. E., MacLennan, D. L., and Brookshire, R. H. (1986). Validity of multiple-sentence in acquired dyslexia. *Journal of Speech and Hearing Disorders, 51,* 82–87.

Parsky, L. (1989). *Using the newspaper* (rev. ed.). Baltimore, MD: Media Materials.

Porch, B. E. (1967). *The Porch Index of Communicative Ability.* Palo Alto, CA: Consulting Psychologists Press.

Prevo, H. (1986). *English that we need.* Phoenix, NY: Frank E. Richards, Publishing Co., Inc.

Rand, M. B. (1988). *Reading assessment post head injury: How valid is it?* Unpublished master's thesis, The Ohio State University, Columbus, OH.

Readers Digest Reading Skill Builders (with accompanying *Audio Lessons*). Pleasantville, NY: Readers Digest Services, Inc.

Richardson, F. (1963). Some effects of severe head injury: A follow-up study of children and adolescents after protracted coma. *Developmental Medicine and Child Neurology, 5,* 471–482.

Rimel, R. W., and Jane, J. A. (1983). Characteristics of head-injured patients. In M. Rosenthal, E. Griffith, M. Bond, and J. D. Miller (Eds.), *Rehabilitation of the Head Injured Adult* (pp. 9–21). Philadelphia: Davis.

Robinson, F. P. (1946). *Effective study.* New York: Harper & Brothers.

Rosen, C. D., and Gerring, J. P. (1986). *Head trauma: Educational reintegration.* San Diego, CA: College-Hill Press.

Rutter, M. (1981). Psychological sequelae of brain damage in children. *The American Journal of Psychiatry, 138,* 1533–1544.

Sarno, M. T. (1980). The nature of verbal impairment after closed head injury. *The Journal of Nervous and Mental Disease, 168,* 685–692.

Schuell, H. (1965). *The Minnesota test for differential diagnosis of aphasia*. Minneapolis, MN: University of Minnesota Press.

Schumaker, J. B., Deshler, D., Alley, G. R., Warner, M. M., and Denton, P. H. (1982). Multipass: A learning strategy for improving reading comprehension. *Learning Disability Quarterly, 5,* 295–304.

Shaffer, D., Bijur, P., Chadwick, O. F. D., and Rutter, M. (1980). Head injury and later reading disability. *Journal of the American Academy of Child Psychiatry, 19,* 592–610.

Siedenberg, P. L. (1988). Cognitive and academic instructional intervention for learning-disabled adolescents. *Topics in Language Disorders, 8,* 56–71.

Singer, H., and Ruddell, R. B. (Eds.). (1985). *Theoretical models and processes of reading* (ed. 3). Newark, DE: International Reading Association.

Slosson, R. L. (1985). *Slosson intelligence test* (SIT). East Aurora, NY: Slosson Educational Publications, Inc.

Smith, E. (1974). Influence of site of impact on cognitive impairment persisting long after severe closed head injury. *Journal of Neurology, Neurosurgery, and Psychiatry, 37,* 719–726.

Smith, J. (1984). *Cognitive rehabilitation* (Computer program). Dimondale, MI: Hartley Courseware.

Spordone, R. J. (1987). A conceptual model of neuropsychologically-based cognitive rehabilitation. In J. M. Williams and C. J. Long (Eds.), *The rehabilitation of cognitive disabilities* (pp. 3–25). New York: Plenum Press.

Spreen, O., and Benton, A. L. (1969). *Manual for the Neurosensory Center comprehensive examination for aphasia*. Victoria, BC: University of Victoria, Neuropsychology Laboratory.

SPSS, Inc. (1988). *Statistical package for the social sciences (SPSS-X)*.

Surges, B., and Nelson, N. W. (1988). *Survey of management practices for written language abilties of persons with traumatic brain injuries*. Unpublished manuscript, Western Michigan University, Department of Speech Pathology and Audiology, Kalamazoo, MI.

Tripp, F. (1976). *Supermarket*. Dinuba, CA: Author. (Available from Fern Tripp, 2035 East Sierra Way, Dinuba, CA 93618).

Volin, R. A., and Groher, M. E. (1985). *Language stimulation software* (Computer program). Rockville, MD: Aspen Publishers.

Wallace, G., and McLoughlin, J. A. (1988). *Learning disabilities: Concepts and characteristics* (ed. 3). Columbus, OH: Merrill Publishing Company.

Webb, W. G. (1987). Treatment of acquired reading disorders. *Topics in Language Disorders. 8,* 51–60.

Webb, W. G., and Love, R. J. (1986). Therapy for retraining reading. In R. Chapey (Ed.), *Language intervention strategies in adult aphasia (2nd ed.)*. Baltimore, MD: Williams & Wilkins.

Wechsler, D. (1985). *Wechsler adult intelligence scale-Revised* (WAIS-R). New York: Psychological Corporation.

Wiederholt, J. L., and Bryant, B. R. (1986). *Gray oral reading tests—Revised* (GORT-R). Austin, TX: Pro-Ed.

Woodcock, R. W. (1987). *Woodcock Reading Mystery Tests-Revised* (WRMT-R; Forms G and H). Circle Pines, MN: American Guidance Service.

Woodcock, R. W., and Johnson, M. B. (1977). *Woodcock-Johnson Psycho-Educational Battery* (WJPEB). Allen, TX: DLM Teaching Resources.

Ylvisaker, M. (Ed.). (1985). *Head injury rehabilitation: Children and adolescents*. San Diego, CA: College-Hill Press.

Ylvisaker, M. (1987, October). *Language and cognitive rehabilitation following ac-*

quired brain injury in children. Videotape presented at the Van Riper Lecture Series, Kalamazoo, MI.

Ylvisaker, M., and Gobble, E. M. R. (Eds.). (1987). *Community re-entry for head injured adults.* Boston, MA: College-Hill Press.

Ylvisaker, M., Szekeres, S. F., Henry, K., Sullivan, D. M., and Wheeler, R. (1987). Topics in cognitive rehabilitation therapy. In M. Ylvisaker, and E. M. R. Gobble (Eds.), *Community re-entry for head injured adults* (pp. 137–220). Boston, MA: College-Hill Press.

PART   III

Motor Issues

CHAPTER 9

Motor Speech Disorders

KATHRYN M. YORKSTON
DAVID R. BEUKELMAN

At times, management of the communication needs of individuals with motor speech disorders as a result of traumatic brain injury (TBI) makes a speech-language pathologist feel like a character from a "Far Side" cartoon. A 1980 Gary Larson cartoon (Chronicle Features, Distributed by Universal Press Syndicate) depicts a scene in a doctor's office. The patient is sitting knee-to-knee with the examining physician. The patient's complaint seems obvious. A large bovine head is emerging from the top of his head, another from his back, another from his left elbow, and still another from his right knee. The doctor, looking the patient straight in the eye says, "I'm afraid you've got cows, Mr. Farnsworth." Patients with TBI, or perhaps their families, like Mr. Farnsworth, can already tell clinicians that there is a serious problem. What Mr. Farnsworth really wants to know are answers to more difficult questions. Will the cows go away by themselves? If not, how can I get rid of them? If they won't go away, how can I manage to live with them? Prediction of the extent and course of recovery, identification of the appropriate course of intervention, and long-term management of the handicap resulting from chronic disorders are issues that face the speech-language pathologist managing the communication needs of individuals following TBI. At times, because of clinicians' lack of information, they do little better than the doctor in the Gary Larson cartoon; they simply label the problem and stop there.

This chapter is an attempt to organize and report current management practices for motor speech disorders in the TBI population. It is an attempt to go beyond a labeling of the disorders and to review intervention approaches that clinical experience and research reports have identified as effective. Readers of this chapter will quickly realize that in some areas clinicians are well beyond the labeling stage and can outline some generally accepted intervention approaches. Unfortunately, in other areas, they have yet to settle even on the labels.

PERSPECTIVE ON MOTOR SPEECH DISORDERS

Motor speech disorders occur because of neurologic impairment that disrupts the planning or execution of the movements of speech production. The picture emerging from clinical experience with TBI is one of wide variability in type, pattern, and severity of motor speech disorders. These disorders following TBI may be temporary or persistent, mild or severe, compatible with other deficits or disproportionately severe, and they may or may not be accompanied by other language and cognitive disorders.

MODEL FOR CHRONIC DISORDERS

Motor speech disorders are usually associated with diseases and conditions that are chronic or long term, and TBI is certainly no exception. The authors have found the model of chronic disorders proposed by Bettinghaus (1980), Nagi (1965, 1969, 1976, 1977); and Wood (1980) to be helpful in developing a clinical perspective for the management of individuals with motor speech disorders. This model provides a framework for assessing performance and planning intervention as individuals with TBI make the transition from emergency care to acute rehabilitation to long-term rehabilitation and finally to community reentry. The authors have discussed this perspective in detail elsewhere (Yorkston and colleagues, 1988). According to this model, a disorder can be viewed as an *impairment* in that the motor speech disorder associated with TBI represents a "loss or abnormality of psychological, physiological or anatomical structure or function." Following TBI, there may be a loss of neuromotor control that is reflected in diminished motor planning or motor execution. A motor speech disorder can also be viewed as a *disability* in that it represents a restriction or lack (resulting from impairment) of the ability to perform an activity or function in the manner or within the range considered normal for a human being. While impairment reflects the lack of motor control, disability reflects the functional reduction in ability to produce rapid, intelligible, natural-sounding speech. Thus, the disability is a functional consequence of the impairment. Finally, a motor speech disorder can be viewed as a *handicap* in that the disabled individual experiences a disadvantage resulting from the impairment or the disability. This handicap limits or prevents the fulfillment of a role that is normal depending on age, gender, social, and cultural factors. An individual experiences a handicap resulting from a motor speech disorder if there is reduced ability to function in communication situations that require understandable, efficient, and natural-sounding speech. This disadvantage may be experienced as a lack of social, educational, and vocational opportunities.

PURPOSES OF INTERVENTION

The speech-language pathologist may intervene with a TBI individual for several different reasons, as outlined below. These reasons vary depending on the time after onset, level of severity of motor speech and other disorders, and overall rehabilitation goals.

Determining the Nature and Extent of the Impairment

As part of a transdisciplinary team that serves the individual with TBI, the speech-language pathologist is routinely expected to assess the impact of the injury on the motor speech capabilities of the individual. One aspect of this assessment is the effort to detect or confirm the presence of a motor speech impairment and to distinguish it from other cognitive and communication disorders. An experienced clinician usually uses perceptual approaches to make this determination in an effort to detect differences in performance from that expected for a nonimpaired person.

If the presence of an impairment in motor speech production is detected, an attempt is usually made to describe the nature of the impairment at several levels. The first is to determine a differential diagnosis of the type of motor speech disorder. In the case of TBI, this usually involves distinguishing among a variety of disorders including mutism, aphonia, apraxia of speech, and dysarthria. These disorders share the common characteristic of compromised speech production in the initiation, planning, or execution of motor speech production and are not solely attributable to cognitive or language impairments.

Determining the Nature and Extent of the Disability

In our work with persons with motor speech disorders, we have viewed three parameters as important indicators of the level of disability—speech intelligibility, speaking rate, and speech naturalness. Intelligibility refers to the understandability of speech. A measure of speech intelligibility is a useful index of the severity of the overall motor speech disorder. It is a comprehensive indicator of how well the speaker manages many of the components of speech production, including not only oral articulatory performance, but also respiratory, phonatory, and velopharyngeal function. We use the *Assessment of Intelligibility of Dysarthric Speech* (Yorkston and Beukelman, 1981a) or the *Computerized Assessment of Intelligibility of Dysarthric Speech* (Yorkston and colleagues, 1984) to assess sentence and single word intelligibility in a standard fashion. Changes in the impairment due to recovery, drug therapy, or other factors are frequently reflected in a change in intelligibility, the overall measure of severity. We also use speech intelligibility as a primary measure of disability because it is a concept that is quite easily understood by family members as well as by the TBI individual. Intelligibility measures can be understood without detailed knowledge of the physiology of speech production.

Speaking rate refers to the number of words or syllables per minute that a speaker produces. One characteristic of speakers with motor speech disorders is that their speaking rate is frequently reduced either as a result of the underlying impairment or as a compensation to achieve intelligible speech in the face of a motor control impairment. An example may be helpful to illustrate the role of speaking rate as a measure of disability. Suppose that a TBI dysarthric speaker is able to speak intelligibly at a rate of 60 words per minute (wpm). This individual is clearly more disabled than an individual who can speak with a similar level of intelligibility at a speaking rate of 120 wpm. It is equally clear that the individual who speaks intelligibly at 120 wpm is disabled compared with the nonimpaired individual who communicates effectively at 170 to 200 wpm. Thus, intelligibility alone can be an incomplete index of severity, and knowledge of speaking rate is a useful supplement to measures of intelligibility. There is commonly an interaction between speech intelligibility and speaking rate among persons with motor speech disorders. That is, some ataxic or hyperkinetic dysarthric speakers may be very unintelligible if they attempt to speak at rapid speaking rates. However, if their speaking rates are reduced, speech intelligibility may be improved (Yorkston and Beukelman, 1981b).

Speech naturalness is also an indicator of disability, especially for persons with a mild motor speech impairment. "Naturalness" is a complex phenomenon. Speech is natural if it conforms to the listener's standards of rate, rhythm, intonation, and stress patterning, and if it conforms to the syntactic structure of the utterance being produced. Although the range of speech that would be considered "natural" is limited, many features are necessary for speech to be considered natural. These features are extremely difficult to quantify objectively. If a precise definition of natural speech is difficult, then an adequate definition of the opposite of naturalness or bizarreness is nearly impossible to specify. Because natural speech is such a perceptually complex phenomenon, deviations from the norm or natural can take many different forms. Speech is considered unnatural or bizarre if it deviates from the expected or is unconventional in terms of the prosodic features of rate, rhythm, intonation, and stress patterning. Perhaps lack of speech naturalness is difficult to quantify or define because there are so many ways in which a speaker can be unnatural or bizarre. Unusual use of fundamental frequency, unusual rate or rhythm, and unusual breath grouping may all result in reduced naturalness. Individuals' speech is considered unnatural if their stress patterning is monotonous with no prominence assigned to any syllable or word within an utterance. Individuals' speech will also be considered unnatural if they signal excessive amounts of stress or signal stress in inappropriate locations.

Determining the Nature and Extent of the Handicap

The handicap resulting from a motor speech disorder involves the reduced ability to function in communication situations that require understandable, efficient, and natural-sounding speech, and it also involves the reactions of persons who affect the social, educational, and vocational opportunities and experiences of the disabled individual (Yorkston and colleagues, 1988a). The extent of handicap depends on a number of factors—the severity of the disability, the roles that the individual chooses to play, and societal attitudes. In some cases, individuals cannot fulfill roles because their speech intelligibility prevents them from being a public speaker or from interacting independently with the public in sales positions. However, in other cases, the attitudes of employers, fellow students, or even family members prevent or diminish a person's success in a certain role.

Assessing the Relationship Among Impairment, Disability and Handicap

The levels of the impairment, disability, and handicap may not be proportional to one another. Comparisons of severity across these dimensions of the disorder provides useful clinical management guidelines. For example, it is frequently the case early after onset that the level of disability is not proportional to the level of impairment. Perhaps as a result of cognitive deficits, the disability will be more severe than would have been expected from the documented level of impairment. Because acutely injured individuals may not monitor the adequacy of their speech production, they may fail to adequately compensate for the newly acquired motor control impairment. In this situation, one goal of intervention may be to achieve compatibility between the levels of disability and impairment. With proper self-monitoring, the levels of impairment and disability can be made consistent with one another.

In another clinically common example, the level of handicap cannot always be predicted solely on the basis of knowledge of the disability. In other words, two individuals with similar levels of disability may experience vastly different levels of handicap. Two individuals may both exhibit dysarthric speech that is intelligible but somewhat slow and unnatural. This level of disability may not be a handicap to the individual who must live in a sheltered environment because of cognitive, memory, and mobility problems. On the other hand, the young trial attorney seeking to return to a previous practice may be severely handicapped by anything less than superior speech production. Thus, the intervention process not only requires that the clinician describe motor speech production from the broadest of viewpoints, but it also requires that he or she must make a number of management decisions related to when, with whom, and how to intervene. These decisions are often based on a comparison of the level of impairment, disability, and handicap.

Reducing the Impairment, Disability, and Handicap

In addition to comparing and contrasting the relative severity and nature of various aspects of a motor speech disorder, another major purpose of intervention is to stabilize or reduce the severity of the disorder. The remainder of this chapter will focus on how the clinician can determine and then reduce motor speech disorders in TBI individuals. However, early efforts at communication intervention following TBI traditionally have focused on the impairment. Improvement in the level of motor control has been approached through preventing complications that hinder natural recovery; maximizing physiologic support through behavioral instruction; and using drug therapies. Improvement is commonly based on these efforts to reduce the extent of the impairment.

A second approach to intervention is to decrease the extent of the disability. At times, this can be accomplished by reducing the underlying motor impairment; however, at other times the individual is taught to compensate for a chronic, stable motor impairment to achieve more intelligible, natural-sound speech. An example of such a technique is rate control, in which individuals are taught to speak more slowly than normal to maximize intelligibility.

The third approach involves interventions that are designed to reduce the severity of the handicap. This phase of intervention occurs well into the recovery from TBI when it has become clear that the impairment is unlikely to be reduced in an important way. As was implied earlier, a reduction in the disability may reduce the handicap experienced by the individual. However, this is not always the case. For example, high school students with TBI may be placed at a considerable disadvantage by their peers even though their disability may be minimal. Generally, this aspect of handicap intervention must be managed through the education, regulation, or legislation of those interacting with the TBI individual. For example, a potential employer may need to be educated about the possibility that mildly dysarthric individuals are able to use the telephone effectively to communicate with other persons within the organization. The behavior of peer students may need to be regulated by school authorities so that a TBI student can participate comfortably in school activities. Finally, we are all aware of recent legislation that enables disabled persons to participate in public education and to have the opportunity for employment.

UNIQUE CHALLENGES IN MANAGING MOTOR SPEECH DISORDERS FOLLOWING TRAUMATIC BRAIN INJURY

A number of features make the management of motor speech disorders following TBI different from the management of motor speech disorders in other clinical populations. First, and perhaps the most obvious, is the fact that clinicians know so little about the management of TBI individuals. This is not particularly surprising when one compares the decades of study and interest in other motor speech disorders. For example, the effect of multiple sclerosis on motor speech has been studied for nearly a century. As discussed in Chapter 2, the relatively recent "silent epidemic" of TBI has provided clinicians with a new opportunity. Clinicians are thus faced with the dual challenges of a large TBI population and a relatively meager fund of past experience and expertise.

Second, the demographics of the TBI population are quite different from other populations with motor speech disorders. Traditionally, clinicians have dealt with the congenitally disabled population of cerebral palsied individuals or an elderly population of stroke patients with dysarthria or apraxia of speech. There is little experience dealing with a population typically in the young adult age range that may be somewhere less socially stable than the norm of the population. If an important motor speech disorder persists, these individuals can be expected to use the health care delivery system for many decades. Many of the dysarthrias traditionally of interest to speech-language pathology have been characterized by a degenerative course. Thus, speech-language pathologists became skilled in differential diagnosis, which requires that dysarthria be viewed as a symptom of an underlying neurologic process. Clinicians are somewhat less familiar with planning and implementing long-term interventions that have as their goal reducing the level of impairment, disability, and handicap.

Finally, TBI individuals with motor speech disorders are particularly challenging because their cognitive deficits interact with the motor speech–communication disorders in ways that are both complex and poorly understood. Bray and colleagues (1987) attempt to describe this interaction:

Communication functioning is dependent on both cognitive and motor recovery. Neuromuscular involvement of the speech mechanism (dysarthria) or inability to sequence oral movements for intelligible speech (apraxia) can result in the need to acquire another means of communication. Gross and fine motor problems as well as depressed cognitive functioning may severely restrict the domain of communicative options that are open. Perceptual and learning impairments may prevent the patient from acquiring a communicative system that is motorically feasible. Patients with limited self-awareness and impaired self-monitoring may not recognize the need to communicate more effectively. J. P., a head injured patient, who was unable to talk, illustrates several of these problems. She attempted to write as an alternative to speaking; however, her writing was illegible. Despite repeated demonstration that her writing could not be read, even by herself, she refused to try a keyboard (Bray and colleagues, 1987, p. 31).

Thus, TBI individuals may have difficulty adapting to the cognitive demands of augmentative communication systems. However, the sudden onset of less severe motor speech impairment may also necessitate the development of cognitively demanding compensatory strategies. Clinical experience suggests that some dysarthric speakers with TBI develop mal-adaptive behaviors that interfere with the adequacy of their speech production. These behaviors result in a level of disability more severe than would be predicted on the basis of their motor impairment. Other dysarthric individuals fail to compensate "automatically" for their suddenly disordered motor speech production mechanism. Thus, the diffuse cognitive deficits that permeate so many aspects of daily living in this population also have important consequences for motor speech production.

DISORDERS OF MOTOR INITIATION AND PLANNING

Mechanisms that control the voluntary production of speech have been a fruitful area of clinical and research investigation (Rosenbek, 1985; Rosenbek and colleagues, 1984; Wertz and colleagues, 1984). Any comprehensive model of speech production must have a means of accounting for how speakers are able to initiate and plan rapid, overlapping, and precise sequences of speech movement. Motor initiation and planning for speech are not well understood; however, it is reasonable to expect that severe diffuse neurologic damage may affect this complex process. A variety of speech disorders that appear to be related to motor initiation and planning have been described in the literature. Because the labels applied to these disorders have not always been consistent, the authors will attempt to describe the characteristics of various disorders and present whatever information related to prevalence and natural recovery pattern is available. They will also attempt to compare and contrast these motor disorders with other disorders of cognition and arousal.

MUTISM

Mutism refers to the inability or refusal to speak. It is not usually considered as a motor speech disorder, yet it will be discussed here briefly because if mutism is characterized by an underlying inability to initiate movement, it may rightfully be considered a motor speech disorder if the term *motor speech disorder* is viewed from the broadest possible perspective. Following severe traumatic TBI, an individual may be mute or unable to speak for several reasons. During coma, individuals are not expected to speak. Obviously, this failure to speak is not predictive of future ability to speak or future impairment of motor control. After arousal from coma, mutism persists in about 3 percent of individuals with TBI (Levin and colleagues, 1983).

Clinicians and researchers have observed differing patterns of mutism among individuals with TBI. Levin and colleagues studied 350 TBI individuals with mutism following arousal from coma. They suggest that

Two types of mutism may be distinguished after head injury. Interruption of speech following a left focal basal ganglia lesion is typically associated with more rapid recovery of consciousness and has a better prognosis for linguistic outcome, whereas mutism produced by severe diffuse TBI is more likely to lead to residual linguistic disorder (Levin and colleagues, 1983, p. 606).

Mutism should be distinguished from other forms of speechlessness that also occur in the TBI population. *Persistent vegetative state* (Jennet and Plum, 1972) refers to individuals who demonstrate no cognitive interaction with their environment. They do not follow commands and are totally unable to communicate. Their inability to speak is inseparable from their profound cognitive and arousal disorders. *Locked-in-syndrome* (Bauer and colleagues, 1979; Plum and Poser, 1980) is a term used to describe individuals with relatively preserved language comprehension who are unable to speak as a result of profound movement disorders. Many of these individuals may communicate by eye blinking or vertical eye movement; however, others are unable to achieve expressive communication.

Von Cramon (1981) studied 11 individuals who had suffered from acute traumatic midbrain syndrome. During the initial stage, mutism was characterized by the "complete loss of voluntary control of the laryngeal muscles." Although these individuals could cough or clear their throats reflexively, they were unable to do so voluntarily. During the second stage of their mutism, pain, disgust, or affirmation was signaled by nonverbal signals. In the final state of mutism, they produced verbalization in response to a stimulus, but not spontaneously. During this stage, speech was usually accompanied by a whisper or breathy phonation.

In a case study report of two TBI individuals with aphonia, Sapir and Aronson observed intact cough and swallowing abilities, and mildly impaired articulation, with an inability to phonate for speech. These authors argue against paralysis of the vocal folds and suggest that the aphonia may be due to a disturbance of the frontal lobe-limbic system. They write:

One explanation is that the aphonia was a consequence of an affective disorder secondary to damage or disturbance of the limbic system and its neocortical and subcortical, especially reticular and thalamic, connections. These neural systems allegedly do not participate in motor coordination nor in the execution of phonatory gestures, but seem to function as a drive-controlling mechanism that determines, by its activity, the readiness to phonate as well as the intensity of phonation (Sapir and Aronson, 1985, pp. 292–293).

Sapir and Aronson reported successful intervention with their two patients using approaches originally described for the treatment of hysterical aphonia (Aronson, 1980).

Clinical experience suggests that some individuals, as they emerge from coma, will experience a transient period in which they appear to be attempting to initiate phonation and are unable to do so even in response to verbal instructions. Their inability to produce phonation does not appear to be laryngeal paralysis or failure to follow simple directions. Oral articulation is often grossly intact. Often these persons "mouth words" in an attempt to communicate. Depending on their cognitive impairment, this may or may not be a successful communication strategy. These persons are able to protect their airway as they eat and to phonate when coughing or laughing, yet they cannot voluntarily initiate phonation on command or during speech. Some have required augmentative communication systems for a temporary period. At times, overlearned or automatic behaviors can be used to facilitate the initiation of phonation.* For example, an individual emerging from coma may be able to produce phonation when the telephone by their bedside rings and the receiver is handed to him or her with the comment, "Someone wants to talk to you." These same individuals may be unable to produce phonation in conversational speech or when instructed to do so. It has been the authors' experience that when voluntary phonation is achieved, these individuals become functional speakers in a brief period. We have been perplexed by these individuals and have been tempted to consider the possibility of apraxia of phonation. Although these individuals demonstrate a basic characteristic of apraxia, the impaired ability to perform voluntary movements in the presence of minimal or no impairment of reflexive movement, their rapid improvement is quite different from the rather systematic, gradual improvement of an individual with apraxia of speech.†

APRAXIA OF SPEECH

Prevalence and Characteristics

Apraxia of speech is an articulatory disorder resulting from impairment, as a result of brain damage, of the capacity to program the positioning of speech muscles and the sequencing of muscle movements for the volitional production of phonemes. No significant weakness, slowness, or incoordination of these muscles is observed in reflexive and automatic acts. Prosodic alternations may be associated with the articulatory prob-

---

*(Patricia Mitsuda, personal communication, March, 1989)
†(Jay Rosenbek, personal communication, August, 1988)

lem, perhaps in compensation for it (Darley, 1969, cited by Wertz 1985). A review of the apraxia of speech literature reveals that almost without exception the population being studied includes adults with left hemisphere cerebrovascular disorders. Apraxia of speech is rarely reported in published demographic studies of TBI; however, clinically it occurs frequently enough to be of concern to those managing the communication needs of individuals with TBI. The authors have observed TBI clients in their own clinical program who have demonstrated apraxic characteristics that range from very severe with no functional speech to mild with speech characteristics that are quite similar to the typical pattern of apraxia of speech associated with left hemisphere cerebrovascular disorders that has been so thoroughly reviewed by Rosenbek and colleagues (1984) and by Wertz and colleagues (1984). As literature descriptions suggest, the majority of apraxic patients exhibit concomitant language disorders. However, it is not highly unusual for mild apraxia of speech to persist after measurable language deficits have resolved. The following description of a 2-year, 6-month-old boy by Ewing-Cobbs (1986) and colleagues also reminds us that apraxia of speech is observed in the TBI population:

Language skills were evaluated 29 days post injury using the Sequenced Inventory of Communication Development (SICD) (Hedrick, Prather, and Tobin, 1975). The majority of receptive language tasks were performed at a 2 to 2 and one-half year level. The child was able to follow two-stage commands and demonstrated comprehension of certain function words. In contrast expressive language skills were consistent with a 4 to 12 months level. Meaningful single-word utterances were occasionally verbalized. Spontaneous speech considered largely of several vowels or consonant-vowel combinations. Although this child was able to imitate motor movements with the upper extremities, he was unable to imitate nonspeech sounds or oral movements. These findings were consistent with a severe nonfluent aphasia with moderate receptive language deficits. In addition, a severe oral-verbal apraxia was suspected (Levin and colleagues, 1983).

Severe Apraxia of Speech

Speech-language pathologists have observed numerous individuals who have been unable to speak because of failure to move their speech musculature to achieve the appropriate oral articulation or laryngeal gestures, yet these same individuals have demonstrated normal or minimally impaired movement during eating, coughing, and laughing. Clinicians have tended to describe these individuals as exhibiting apraxia of speech even though they realize that if that diagnosis is to be confirmed, other factors must be considered. Because of the severity of the overall motor disorder, it is difficult to document the influence of the accompanying dysarthria on speech production. It is common to observe that these severely involved individuals demonstrate dysarthric symptoms, weakness, slowness, and incoordination of movement in addition to a motor programming disorder. Yet, in the authors' opinion, the extent of their weakness does not explain their inability to execute the motor movements required for speech. Thus, with severe apraxia of speech, other motor control deficits may also be present.

Severe apraxia of speech may be confused with the failure to initiate movement that is present in some individuals with severe TBI. For example, some persons with severe frontal lobe injury experience difficulty in initiating voluntary as well as vegetative movements. We evaluated a young man with severe frontal lobe injury who would accept food into his mouth during assisted eating but had difficulty initiating a swallow at appropriate times. When the swallow was initiated, it appeared to be an efficient, functional act that cleared the oral cavity of food. He also demonstrated difficulty initiating movements of the speech mechanism for communication and limb movement for personal care. In cases such as this, the motor movement program appears to reflect a general inability to initiate activity rather than an apraxia of speech. When evaluating a severe impaired person with TBI, it is also necessary to confirm that the individual can cognitively comprehend the assessment task. At times, confused persons will fail to initiate movement or produce random or even groping movement patterns as they attempt to respond to instructions that they do not understand. These movement patterns may be confused with those associated with apraxia of speech. Thus, when assessing a TBI individual who is suspected of being severely apraxic, it is necessary to rule out other motor speech disorders, a generalized failure to initiate activity, and severe cognitive impairment as alternative explanations for an inability to voluntarily control the speech mechanism.

The authors have treated severely "apraxic" individuals due to TBI in much the same way that they treat severely dysarthric speakers. Generally, the individuals that they have served have been so severely impaired that they have been unable to speak functionally and require augmentative communication systems to communicate during the early phases of their recovery. As with severely dysarthric speakers, the authors have involved severely apraxic individuals in behavioral intervention activities to reestablish phonatory and oral articulatory control at minimal levels to support limited speech. As with the apraxia of speech that results from a cerebrovascular accident, a number of treatment principles are commonly applied. These include massed practice to reestablish the motor behavior, "deblocking" gestures to facilitate the natural flow of speech, and use of visual and auditory cues to improve the adequacy of speech production.

Moderate to Mild Apraxia of Speech

At this time, the authors are aware of no descriptions in the literature of moderately or mildly apraxia of speech due to TBI, nor have they collected data from a group of these speakers. Therefore, they have chosen to report a case study to document the presence of individuals with apraxia of speech due to TBI and recommend careful investigation of these individuals in the future.

Case Study. Our client was in his late twenties when he was involved in an automobile accident. He had graduated from college and was working in sales. At the time he became involved in our program, he was extremely agitated and was unable to communicate using natural speech. His lack of communicative success was frustrating to him and complicated by agitation. We provided him with a Canon Communicator and were surprised at the level of communicative ability. The messages he prepared on the Canon Communicator were grammatically well formed and correctly spelled; however, his cognitive confusions were apparent when he attempted to communicate his thoughts and concerns. Because his agitation was markedly reduced, he effectively communicated with a wide variety of family, friends, fellow patients, and rehabilitation staff.

Early in rehabilitation, his mobility and cognitive disorders, including severe memory deficits, were his primary concern. Although he participated in a speech intervention program, he was less concerned about spoken communication than his inability to move about independently and to remember his daily activities and routines. During a period of acute rehabilitation his mobility issues were resolved, strategies to compensate for his memory deficits were developed, and independent living and vocational activities became the major focus of intervention. It was during this outpatient program of reintegration into the community that he began to focus on restoration of natural-sounding speech. At approximately one year after onset, his speech was very similar to the pattern described in the literature for individuals with moderate apraxia of speech due to cerebrovascular accidents of the left hemisphere. He was largely an intelligible speaker, yet his articulatory efforts were inconsistent. His speaking rate was slow, and inconsistent articulatory errors were frequently noted. He was acutely aware of the errors, and he engaged in groping behavior as he attempted to achieve articulatory targets. Despite his awareness and acknowledgement of his motor speech disorder, he persisted in attempts to "speak like he used to." This meant that he would attempt to speak at what he perceived to be a "normal" rate. He did so only with unacceptable results. When he spoke at near normal rates, articulatory errors increased to the point where naive listeners could understand only approximately two thirds of his messages. In an effort to maintain "normal" rate, he reduced the number of pauses and breathed only when physiologically mandatory. This style of speech was not only very unnatural but also left the speaker exhausted after relatively brief periods. Although his speaking rate was 160 words per minute on a sentence production task as compared with a normal of approximately 190 words per minute, his articulation was much more accurate when he spoke at 130 words per minute.

In general our intervention program involved mass practice at appropriate speaking rates. We used the PACER computer program (Beukelman and colleagues, 1988) to help him control his speaking rate during treatment and during practice. The program paced his speaking rate by presenting the text of the passage on the computer screen and cued him to speak at a particular rate. We also taught him to "chunk" his production into appropriate breath group units based on the meaning of the utterance. In time he learned to enter his own passages into the PACER program. Routinely practicing every morning at what was judged to be an optimum rate assisted him to generalize this rate into his conversational speech.

This TBI man became a functional speaker who learned to speak as naturally as possible given the severity of his motor speech impairment. He is employed as a teaching assistant in a middle school setting, a position that requires considerable use of speech. Five years after his accident he continues to make apraxic-type articulatory errors. His mobility is not normal, but he has accepted that he walks well enough to get from "one place to another." He remains concerned about the residual cognitive limitations and his "less than perfect" speech. He continues to document words and word combinations that are difficult for him to say accurately and continues to practice the production of these words.

DYSARTHRIA

CHARACTERISTICS

Prevalence Following Traumatic Brain Injury

Dysarthria is a neurologic motor speech impairment characterized by slow, weak, imprecise, or uncoordinated movements of the speech musculature. The presence of dysarthria as a sequelae to TBI is commonly reported. Estimates of the prevalence of dysarthria in this population range from 8 to 100 percent depending on when measures were taken, what measures were used, and what population was studied (Dresser and colleagues, 1973; Groher, 1977, 1983; Sarno and colleagues, 1986; Rusk and colleagues, 1969). Rusk and colleagues (1969) reported that approximately one third of 96 patients with TBI exhibited dysarthria during the acute phase of their recovery. A followup study of 30 of the original dysarthric patients 5 to 15 years later revealed that half had improved and half had not changed. Thompsen (1983) reported that individuals with dysarthria secondary to TBI showed little or no improvement up to 15 years after injury. More recently, Sarno and colleagues (1986) examined 124 persons with closed head injury on a battery of communication tests. They reported that 34 percent of their subjects exhibited dysarthria ranging from mild articulatory imprecision to completely unintelligible speech. These authors reported that all dysarthric subjects also demonstrated "subclinical aphasia," which was defined as linguistic processing deficits in the absence of clinical manifestations of linguistic impairment (aphasia).

Thus, the information regarding the prevalence and natural course of dysarthria following TBI is somewhat confusing. Because this information is important to develop better evaluation and intervention approaches and to identify better prognostic indicators, this chapter will present the preliminary results of a clinical study carried out in the Department of Rehabilitation Medicine, University of Washington, and reported in detail elsewhere (Yorkston and colleagues, 1989). A total of 151 individuals with TBI were rated on six-point scales for presence and severity of (1) dysarthria, (2) swallowing disorders, and (3) level of cognitive function (Hagen and colleagues, 1979). Table 9-1 lists the speech and swallowing scales. Individuals were drawn from three different clinical populations—acute medicine, acute rehabilitation, and outpatient rehabilitation. Speech pathology services in the acute medical setting are primarily diagnostic, assessing the motor speech, swallowing, and cognitive-communication skills of acutely brain-injured patients. At this stage of hospitalization, short-term communication and swallowing management decisions are made, along with decisions regarding the need for further inpatient or outpatient rehabilitation. Patients drawn from the acute rehabilitation services have recovered sufficiently to allow them to participate in an intensive and comprehensive rehabilitation program. In the outpatient rehabilitation program special emphasis is placed on facilitating the patients' transition back to the community. Thus, the three populations surveyed represent generally different periods of time after onset.

Results of this survey are displayed in Figure 9-1 with mild to moderate indicating scaled scores of 4 or 5 and severe indicating scores of 1 to 3. Examination of the figure indicates that the highest prevalence of mild to moderate dysarthria (65 percent of the population) is found in the acute rehabilitation setting, followed by 42 percent in the acute medicine setting and 22 percent in the outpatient rehabilitation setting. The higher prevalence of mild to moderate dysarthria in the acute rehabilitation

Table 9-1. Rating scales for speech and swallowing disorders

SPEECH SCALE
1 No vocalization
2 Vocalizes as a signal or reflexively
3 Some functional speech, but it is judged to be less than 20 percent intelligible
4 Moderate dysarthria with speech intelligibility (between 20 and 85 percent)
5 Mild dysarthria with some slurring or sound production imprecision but intelligible speech
6 No dysarthria

SWALLOWING SCALE
1 Patient takes nothing by mouth secondary to risk of aspiration.
2 Patient takes nothing by mouth but is appropriate for swallowing treatment.
3 Patient is safe for oral intake with modified diet (e.g., pureed food with no thin liquids), and swallowing management precautions such as supervision of bite size and positioning are maintained. This patient is unable to meet nutritional needs orally.
4 Patient is safe for oral intake with modified diet and swallowing management precautions. With these modifications, the patient is able to meet nutritional needs orally.
5 Patient is safe for oral intake with either modified diet or swallowing management precautions.
6 Patient is safe for oral intake with premorbid diet and no precautions.

Source: Yorkston, K. M., Honsiger, M. J., Mitsuda, P. M., and Hammen, V. (1989c). The relationship between speech and swallowing disorders in head injured patients. J. Logemann (Ed.), *Journal of Head Trauma Rehabilitation*. 4(4): 1–16.

setting compared with the acute medicine setting may be explained by the fact the patients typically seen in acute medicine cross a broad range of severity levels, with many of the mildly involved individuals being discharged directly home rather than to the inpatient rehabilitation service. Severe dysarthria occurs most frequently in the acute medicine setting (24 percent), next in the acute rehabilitation setting (20 percent) and least frequently in the outpatient rehabilitation setting (10 percent).

The data presented thus far suggests that the prevalence and severity of dysarthria vary as a function of the treatment setting. Another important factor to consider when attempting to document the prevalence of dysarthria in the clinical population is the level of cognitive function. To explore the relationship between cognitive function and dysarthria, patients across treatment settings were grouped according to level of cognitive function. Results of this analysis appear in Figure 9-2 and suggest that prevalence and severity of dysarthria are greater for patients with more severe cognitive deficits. Note that 73 percent of the patients at level IV (Confused-Agitation) exhibited at least mild to moderate dysarthria. In contrast, only 5 percent of the TBI patients surveyed at cognitive level VIII (Purposeful and Appropriate) exhibited mild to moderate dysarthria.

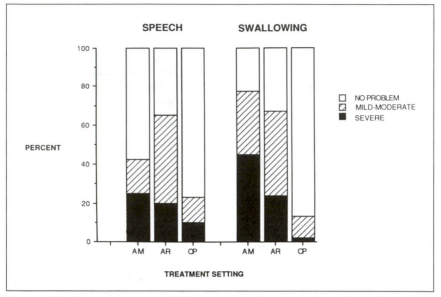

Figure 9-1. The proportion of TBI patients with no speech and swallowing problems, with mild-moderate problems, and with severe problems in the acute medicine (AM), acute rehabilitation (AR), and outpatient rehabilitation (OP) settings. From Yorkston, K.M., Honsinger, M.J., Mistuda, P.M., and Hammen, V. (1989c.) The relationship between speech and swallowing disorders in head injured patients. In J. Logemann (Ed.) *Journal of Head Trauma Rehabilitation* 4(4): 1–16.

Relationship Between Dysarthria and Swallowing Disorders

Although a detailed description of swallowing disorders following TBI can be found elsewhere in this text (see chap. 11), clinical experience suggests that speech and swallowing problems frequently co-occur in TBI. Speech and swallowing involve the same structures; however, Larson (1985) suggests that the behaviors are very different and the neural mechanisms that govern these behaviors may be quite different. Swallowing is generally reflexive except for the initial oral-preparatory stage, while speech is generally voluntary. Swallowing is thought to be controlled by a medullar swallowing center or central pattern generator that, once initiated, controls and coordinates the movement of swallowing in a stereotyped fashion. The center also precludes competing activity such as speech or respiration (Kennedy and Kent, 1985). Thus, once initiated, the complex motor activity of swallowing is completed without interruption. Speech, on the other hand, is an extremely complex move-

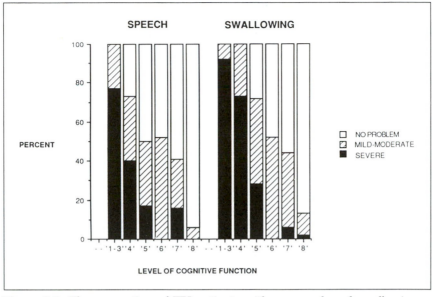

Figure 9-2. The proportion of TBI patients with no speech and swallowing problems, with mild-moderate problems, and with severe problems as a function of level of cognitive function Hagen, C., Malkmus, D., and Durham, P. [1979]. Levels of cognitive functioning. In *Rehabilitation of the head injured adult: Comprehensive physical management.* Downey, CA: Professional Staff Association of Rancho Los Amigos Hospital. Data are adapted from Yorkston, K.M., Honsinger, M.J., Mitsuda, P.M., and Hammen, V. (1989c). The relationship between speech and swallowing disorders in head injured patients. In J. Logemann (Ed.) *Journal of Head Trauma Rehabilitation* 4(4): 1–16.

ment governed by a number of cortical and subcortical regulatory mechanisms (see McClean, 1988).

The relationship between the severity of speech and swallowing disorders following TBI may be complicated by a number of factors, including time after onset and level of cognitive functioning. Table 9-2 contains data adapted from Yorkston and colleagues (in press). Both speech and swallowing functions were rated on six-point scales. Speech and swallowing functions were considered similar if they were within one scaled point of one another. Note that in the acute rehabilitation and outpatient rehabilitation settings, speech and swallowing functions were most often rated as similar. Only in the acute medical setting is swallowing considered more severely impaired than speech. These data suggest that the relationship between speech and swallowing is not a simple one. The relative severity of swallowing disorders early after onset may be a function of a combina-

Table 9-2. The relationship between severity of speech
and swallowing disorders as a function of treatment
setting in the traumatically brain-injured population

	Acute medicine (%)	*Acute rehabilitation (%)*	*Outpatient rehabilitation (%)*
Swallow worse than speech	45	15	0
Swallow similar to speech	52	83	100
Swallow better than speech	2	2	0

Source: Yorkston, K. M., Honsinger, M. J., Mitsuda, P. M., and Hammen, V. (In press). The relationship between speech and swallowing disorders in head injured patients. J. Logemann (Ed.), *Journal of Head Trauma Rehabilitation* 4(4): 1–16.

tion of the cognitive impairment and failure to develop the strategies to compensate for the newly acquired impairment.

Types of Dysarthria

There appear to be no research studies that focus primarily on describing the dysarthric characteristics of the TBI population. However, there is growing evidence, from a series of intervention studies, of the diversity of characteristics that depend on the locus and severity of the TBI. Predominantly ataxic dysarthria was observed in the TBI patients studied by Simmons (1983), Yorkston and Beukelman (1981a), and Yorkston and colleagues (1984). Predominantly flaccid dysarthria was reported for a single patient by Netsell and Daniel (1979). Yorkston and Beukelman (1981b) described TBI individuals with mixed flaccid-spastic dysarthria and mixed spastic-ataxia dysarthria. Because of the diffuse nature of most brain injuries, the dysarthria type is usually mixed to some extent. To date there have been no studies reporting the prevalence of the various types of dysarthria in this population.

ESTABLISHING COMMUNICATION

Selection of Augumentative Approaches

Following TBI, the initial goal of an intervention program usually is to develop an early, effective approach to communication. In Chapter 10 DeRuyter and Kennedy describe in detail the augmentative and alternative communication (AAC) strategies and systems used with TBI persons, so a discussion of early communication approaches will not be presented here.

Speech in Conjunction with Augmentative and Alternative Communication (AAC) Approaches

After an AAC system is in place for a severely communicative disordered individual with TBI, an aggressive attempt to reestablish natural speech should be initiated. Intelligible natural speech is obviously far superior to any current AAC-based communication in terms of rate, efficiency, and flexibility. However, natural speech need not be completely intelligible to facilitate communication. In communication settings in which the context is quite specific, such as greetings, answers to yes and no and multiple choice questions, even highly distorted speech can be effective. In many rehabilitation settings, context provides powerful assistance in making severely distorted natural speech functional. Thus, natural speech is frequently an important component of an overall AAC approach and may be used in predictable situations. Other AAC approaches may be used to introduce new topics, share novel information, or resolve communication breakdowns.

Many individuals with TBI require specific and extended instruction to learn when to use their AAC systems and when to use natural speech. Instruction is probably necessary in this complex decision for several reasons. First, persons with acquired severe communication disorders due to TBI have had no previous experience integrating the use of AAC systems and natural speech; therefore, they bring no "old knowledge" to this task. Second, one must monitor the type of interaction to decide if the context is apparent enough to the listener to allow for the use of natural speech. Third, one must decide whether the listener has successfully understood a message and whether communication breakdown resolution is necessary. Finally, one must determine the listener's capability. For example, listeners who are familiar with severe communicatively impaired persons often are able to understand natural speech more easily than are others, since these familiar listeners often possess enough shared information to enhance their effectiveness as listeners.

Instruction to assist the severely dysarthric individual in knowing when to use natural speech and when to use an AAC approach involves the system user as well as the most frequent listeners. Initially, it is often helpful to have the listeners "coach" the individual regarding when to attempt speech and when to use the AAC system. In this way, the TBI individual who is using an AAC system can be taught by listeners in natural context.

Supplemented Speech

The current authors (Beukelman and Yorkston, 1977) reported the use of an alphabet supplementation approach, in which the dysarthria speaker pointed to the first word on an alphabet board as the word was spoken. They reported on the impact of the alphabet board supplementing approach on the speech intelligibility and speaking rate of a 17-year-old high school student who suffered a brainstem injury in a motor vehicle accident. The supplementation approach reduced this individual's speaking rate from 86 wpm (habitual) to 28 wpm (supplemented). Speech intelligibility increased from 32 percent (habitual) to 75 percent (supplemented).

Several reasons may be considered for the increase in speech intelligibility during the supplemented speech condition. First, additional information is provided to the listener when that individual is able to see the letters that the user identifies. However, there is some evidence that for some speakers, the change in speech rate or other aspects of speech production may also contribute to improved intelligibility. The high school student with TBI described earlier achieved a speech intelligibility percentage of 58 percent when he pointed to the first letter of the word as he spoke but without the listener's seeing the alphabet board. Thus, considering that his habitual intelligibility score was 32 percent, he achieved a 26 percent increase in intelligibility just from the change in speech production. An additional 22 percent intelligibility increase occurred when the first letters of words could also be viewed. The impact of alphabet supplementation has also been studied by Crow and Enderby (1989), who measured the single word and sentence intelligibility of six dysarthric individuals using this approach. In this study, judges listened to audio tapes and thus were not provided with information about the identity of the initial letter of the word. Despite this judging format, intelligibility of both single word and sentence productions improved. The slowing of speaking rate necessitated by the pointing task may have contributed to improved sentence production. Improvement in single word production is more difficult to explain. One possible explanation is an increase in articulatory precision.

Obviously, not all dysarthric speakers achieve an increase in speech intelligibility when they use supplemented speech. However, the potential for an important improvement in speech intelligibility associated with this simple technique warrants its consideration when managing the resolving motor speech disorders in the TBI population. Generally, candidates for the alphabet supplementation approach are severely dysarthric individuals who are using an alphabet approach as an AAC technique. These individuals have some speech, but reduced intelligibility limits its usefulness. Minimal speech production requirements are needed for successful use of the alphabet board supplementation approach. Individuals using this approach must be able to achieve consistent, voluntary phonation or at least an audible whisper. Because the first letter of each word is identified for the listener, often treatment initially focuses on vowel differentiation and later on the inclusion of final consonants.

Most often, individuals using this approach point to the letters on the alphabet board with their hands. In cases where individuals are unable to indicate the letters by pointing, other options, such as a headlight pointer, should be attempted. Individuals using the alphabet supplementation approach must have sufficient spelling skills to identify initial letters of words correctly. Our experience has shown that this is not a demanding task since spelling skills are often retained by persons with TBI (see Chaps. 7 and 8).

As discussed earlier, the alphabet supplementation approach is not a cognitively demanding task. However, TBI individuals with severe cognitive deficits may need more training in the use of this approach than other dysarthric speakers with intact cognition. Dysarthric individuals who use spelling-based devices or alphabet boards must make a number of changes in their communication style as they make the transition to the speech supplementation approach. They often prefer to use the alphabet board supplementation approach because it is much more rapid than letter-by-letter AAC approaches. Because of the severity of dysarthria among speakers who use the supplementation approach, at times communication breakdown will occur. Many individuals choose to resolve communication breakdowns by spelling the word on a letter-by-letter basis and then proceeding on a supplemented basis. For some persons with severe cognitive limitations who use the supplemented approach, using the alphabet board both in the supplemented (first letter) fashion and in the letter by letter fashion is confusing. The authors have found it necessary to use two different alphabet boards with some of these individuals. One board is used for the supplemented approach, and the other is used to resolve communication breakdowns. Ideally, the alphabet boards should differ sufficiently so that they can be easily distinguished by the listener and the user. The authors have successfully distinguished alphabet boards with white letters on a black background for one purpose and black letters on a white background for the other.

In summary, the alphabet supplementation approach has many advantages for the TBI population. First, it is not cognitively demanding and relies on usually preserved spelling skills. Second, it is an effective means of reducing the speaking rate, often at a time in recovery when other behavior rate reduction techniques are ineffective. Third, because the alphabet board is continually present, severely dysarthric individuals always have a ready means of breakdown repair available to them. The final benefit of the system may be the most important one. The alphabet supplementation approach allows for extensive practice of motor speech production before natural speech alone would support successful communication. This continual practice may facilitate and enhance the natural recovery of motor speech production.

Despite these advantages, a word of caution is warranted regarding the use of alphabet supplementation with TBI individuals. Use of the approach with severely dysarthric speakers usually necessitated a one-word-at-a-time speech pattern. This pattern is often consistent with the poor respiratory support exhibited by these individuals. Transition from use of alphabet supplementation to independent use of natural speech should be encouraged when physiologic support warrants it. Some speakers, when making the transition from the alphabet board to independent use of natural speech, will need some training to eliminate the one-word-at-a-time breath patterning habit.

ESTABLISHING RESPIRATORY SUPPORT FOR SPEECH

Normal Respiratory Function During Speech

The respiratory system is the source of aerodynamic energy for speech. Generally, the respiratory goal of a speaker is to generate a relatively steady level of subglottal air pressure for the duration of a breath group, with slight variations to support stress patterning. In normal speech, adequate loudness levels are maintained throughout an utterance. Normal speech is characterized by a rapid inhalation and a prolonged exhalation. Typically, the normal speaker inhales to a point slightly more than 60 percent of lung volume level and then, depending on the length of the utterance, continues to speak until reaching a point about 35 percent of lung volume level. The speaker then inhales again and continues to speak. Usually, the speaker inhales to a greater lung volume level before long utterances and to a lesser lung volume level before short utterances. For normal speakers, respiratory patterning for speech is tied to the meaning of the utterance. Thus, breath group length is controlled by the form of the message that is produced, with speakers more likely to terminate a breath group at the conclusion of a sentence or a phrase than in response to physiologic demand. A description of this complex motor control process is beyond the scope of this chapter; however, the interested reader is referred to Hixon (1973, 1987), Hixon, and colleagues (1976), Folkins and Kuehn (1982), and Weismer (1985) for excellent discussions of normal respiration during speech.

Respiratory Impairment in Traumatic Brain Injury

The restoration of intelligible speech does not always occur in TBI persons who are unable to speak because of severe dysarthria. However, several authors have reported the restoration of intelligible natural speech following a long period of AAC system use—13 years (Workinger and Netsell, 1988) and 3 years (Light and colleagues, 1988). Each of the individuals described had used AAC systems to support communication and had been involved in long-term programs to establish the physiologic control necessary for intelligible speech. It has been the authors' clinical experience that failure to establish respiratory-phonatory support for speech is an important factor necessitating the long-term use of AAC approaches.

The authors' speech intervention approach for severely dysarthric, TBI speakers is somewhat different than the one used with less severely impaired speakers. When working with moderately severe dysarthric speakers, who are capable of achieving at least some intelligible speech, they attempt to work on speech as an integrated activity. In doing so, they usually do not focus on intervention activities or drills that focus on a single component (phonation, respiration, etc.) of the speech mechanism. For example, the authors would not require a client to sustain phonation until they achieve normal levels of performance. Especially with TBI individuals, the authors attempt to work in the context of natural speech as much as possible, so that extensive generalization instruction is not required. However, for the very severely dysarthric speaker who is unable to produce speech, the authors are often forced to develop the physiologic support for speech before proceeding to a more integrated intervention approach.

In some ways, this early phase of intervention is analogous to creating the physiologic building blocks of speech. These building blocks can be considered the minimal physiologic requirements to support intelligible speech. If the building blocks or minimal requirements already exist (as is the case with most moderate or mildly involved speakers), then one simply proceeds to create the structure. If they are not present (as is the case with most severely involved speakers making the transition from use of an AAC system to natural speech), then one must work to develop the building blocks or the components of speech production. For a detailed description of the authors' efforts to develop the physiologic support for speech, the interested reader is referred to Yorkston and colleagues (1988a). Their approach is presented in abbreviated form in the following sections.

The impact of respiratory impairment on the performance of a dysarthric speaker is a complex phenomenon. Some individuals with severely impaired respiratory function perform remarkably well during speech, while others with apparently much less involvement of the respiratory system use unusual and maladaptive respiratory patterns. Some speakers modify their respiratory function very well in response to behavioral instruction; however, others remain rigid in their respiratory patterning. Unfortunately, the research literature contains no group studies that explore the performance of dysarthric speakers due to TBI. However, through the years, the authors have had extensive experience with TBI persons and have intervened to modify their respiratory patterns to achieve more functional speech. An understanding of the respiratory aspects of speech is critical to clinical management of all types of dysarthria. This is particularly true in TBI individuals, since the respiratory impairment in this population ranges from the inability to modify rest breathing patterns to extensively maladaptive respiratory patterns to essentially normal respiratory patterns for speech.

Assessment

The speech-language pathologist attempting to understand the physiologic capabilities of a dysarthric speaker is faced with what seems to be an almost endless number of aspects of speech production that can be measured. However, the pressing demands of clinical time available for assessment and patients' tolerance for protracted testing necessitate a focused assessment process. Experience teaches clincans to do what is necessary to make intervention decisions. The authors' clinical assessment approaches usually involve two phases. In the first phase, perceptual judgments are made about the adequacy of various aspects of speech production. Perceptual judgments allow the clinician to generate hypotheses about the various contributors to the speech disorder. The second phase of clinical assessment usually involves instrumental measures of various aspects of speech production. These "objective" measures allow the clinician to affirm or refute the perceptually derived hypotheses that are necessary to develop an appropriate and specific intervention plan.

Perceptual Indicators of Respiratory Impairment. If respiratory performance is severely impaired, adequate speech may be impossible. Diminished respiratory capability can be identified perceptually. The inability to sustain an adequate level of subglottal air pressure during speech can affect speech performance in several ways. Because the level of voice loudness is very closely related to the level of subglottal air pressure, if air pressure cannot be sustained within the normal range, reduction in vocal intensity is commonly observed. A second characteristic is the modification of breath group length and patterning of respiratory movements during speech. During the initial perceptual aspect of the respiratory evaluation, the clinician should listen for abnormal patterns of timing of inhalation and exhalation. With inadequate respiratory support for speech, the length of the breath group is more commonly determined by the level of physiologic support rather than the form of the message. Therefore, speakers may terminate breath groups when they need to take a breath rather than at syntactically appropriate junctions.

Although voice loudness and breath patterning abnormalities are the perceptual features most closely associated with respiratory adequacy, impairment in respiratory support may also complicate other aspects of speech production. Inadequate subglottal air pressure is usually associated with the inability to generate intraoral air pressure. If adequate air pressure cannot be impounded in the oral cavity, oral articulation will become imprecise, especially for those sounds that require a buildup of intraoral air pressure, such as plosives and fricatives. Inadequate respiratory support also severely limits the prosodic variations such as intonation and stress patterning that are necessary for natural-sounding speech.

The first phase of the respiratory assessment involves listening to a sample of connected speech and attempting to identify perceptual indica-

Table 9-3. Perceptual indicators of respiratory inadequacy.

INITIATION OF PHONATION
Can the speaker voluntarily initiate phonation on a nonspeech task such as sustained phonation?
Are speech attempts associated with phonation?
LOUDNESS ALTERATIONS
Is the overall loudness level too low or too high?
Is the loudness level consistent?
Are sudden uncontrolled alterations in loudness present?
Does loudness diminish over the course of a single breath group unit?
Does loudness diminish over the course of extended speech?
Can the speaker increase loudness (shout)?
Can the speaker produce quiet phonation?
Does the speaker complain of fatigue when speaking for extended periods at conversational loudness levels?
BREATH PATTERNING ABNORMALITIES
Is the respiratory pattern different from the normal pattern of a quick inhalation phase followed by a prolonged exhalation phase?
Does the speaker inhale to an appropriate lung volume level?
At what point in the respiratory cycle does the speaker initiate an utterance?
Is there a quick preparatory inhalation before the initiation of an utterance?
Does the speaker use pauses for emphasis, or do all pauses contain an inhalation?
Do exaggerated respiratory maneuvers, such as excessive elevation of the shoulders during inhalation, appear during speech?
Does the speaker appear to run out of breath before inhaling?
CONSONANT PRODUCTION
Is the speaker able to produce pressure consonants?
Does the ability to produce pressure consonants vary within a breath group unit?

tors of respiratory inadequacy. Table 9-3 contains a list of questions that may be used to structure this perceptual assessment. Note that some of the questions relate to initiation of phonation, others to the voice loudness and breath patterning, and still others to production of pressure consonants. If the perceptual assessment leads one to suspect respiratory inadequacy, then an in-depth examination of respiratory impairment is warranted.

In-Depth Examination of Respiratory Impairment. Once the presence of inadequate respiratory support has been confirmed through perceptual evaluation, an attempt is usually made to describe the respiratory function in depth. The two major areas of focus in this phase of the assessment are the adequacy of respiratory support (the speaker's ability to sustain adequate levels of subglottal air pressure) and the pattern of respiratory movements.

1. *Adequacy of respiratory support.* The clinician should begin the detailed respiratory assessment by examining the energy source for speech as it is reflected in a measure of subglottal air pressure. In persons with tracheostomies, subglottal air pressure can be sensed through the tracheostomy tube or tracheostomy button. However, in patients without tracheostomy, direct measures of subglottal air pressure are difficult. Rather, subglottal air pressure levels are estimated by measuring the amount of intraoral air pressure during the stop phase of a voiceless stop consonant and estimating the corresponding level of subglottal air pressure. Selection of the stop phase of voiceless stop consonants fulfills several requirements. First, the glottis is open during the stop phase of a voiceless plosive sound /p/. The oral cavity is a sealed system because the velopharyngeal port is closed and the lips are closed. Because the vocal folds are separated and the remaining system is sealed, the oral and subglottal cavities can be considered to function as a single cavity from an aerodynamic point of view (Netsell, 1969; Smitheran and Hixon, 1981). By measuring oral air pressure during the stop phase of the voiceless plosive sound, the clinician can estimate the amount of subglottal air pressure a speaker is using. During conversational speech by the normal adult, subglottal air pressure usually averages between 7 and 10 cm H_2O. If a TBI individual is generating only 1 or 2 cm H_2O, this is a good indication that the respiratory support for functional speech is not adequate.

When instrumentation to quantify accurately the intraoral air pressure generated during an utterance is unavailable, respiratory adequacy can also be estimated using a simple U-tube manometer or even simpler "homemade" apparatus depicted in Figure 9-3. The apparatus consists of a clear water glass with a tape marked in centimeter units attached to

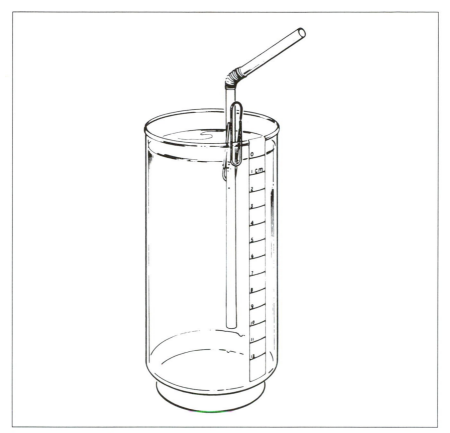

Figure 9-3. A drinking glass with a straw inserted to a depth of 10 cm. This device can be used to indicate respiratory support in dysarthria. From Hixon, T., Hawley, J., and Wilson, J. (1982). An around-the-house device for the clinical determination of respiratory driving pressure: A note on making simple even simpler. *Journal of Speech and Hearing Disorders, 47,* 413.

the side. The glass is filled with water to the "zero" mark, and a straw is inserted into the water to the desired depth, which is the 10-cm level in Figure 9-3. By asking the dysarthric speaker to blow into the straw and sustain a stream of bubbles for as long as possible, one is able to estimate respiratory support. Clinically, the authors have found Netsell and Hixon's (1978) "five-for-five" rule to be very helpful. This rule suggests that if an individual is able to sustain 5 cm of water pressure with a bleed in the system for 5 seconds, then respiratory support should be adequate for speech. Some individuals are unable to achieve the target of 5 cm H_2O for any time. Others, especially those with an ataxic component to their movement disorder, will be able to generate adequate levels but will have difficulty controlling their output at the steady level associated with adequate speech production.

Respiratory support for speech can also be estimated by assessing the speaker's ability to produce sustained phonation. Most normal individuals can sustain phonation for a minimum of 15 seconds for adult males and 14.3 seconds for females (Hirano and colleagues, 1968). The respiratory capabilities for normal individuals are far greater than the respiratory demands for conversational speech. The authors' approach clinically is not to require maximum phonation but rather request that the speaker produce phonation for a relatively brief time—8 to 10 seconds. In this way the task more closely reflects the respiratory demands of speech. Production of sustained phonation obviously reflects both respiratory and laryngeal function. Sustained phonation time may be greatly reduced with laryngeal paralysis or with spastic vocal fold function.

2. *Respiratory movements.* The respiratory movements of a dysarthric speaker may suggest a variety of impairments. Some individuals exhibit excessive movements during speech, such as excessive elevation of the shoulders. An expansion of the thorax may indicate compensation for poor abdominal control. In other cases, observations of changes in respiratory shape may reveal paradoxic movements of the thorax and the abdomen. Paradoxing is a maneuver in which the circumference of the thorax is increased during inhalation while the circumference of the abdomen is decreased, or vice versa. Because the two movements are, in effect, working at cross-purposes, inadequate respiratory control for speech may result.

Changes in respiratory shape (thorax and abdomen) can be observed perceptually by placing one hand over the diaphragm and the other on the rib cage. It is obvious that these perceptual observations are extremely informal and do not yield precise or objective measures of the shape, timing, or respiratory volume. Currently, the most popular devices for objective measurement of respiratory shape are the magnetometer system used by Putnam and Hixon (1984) and the Respitrace described by Hunker and colleagues (1981).

Disorders of respiratory movement may be reflected by a reduced vital capacity, which makes it difficult for some speakers to generate adequate subglottal air pressure amplitudes and durations for speech when utterances are initiated at 60 percent of a reduced vital capacity. These individuals may routinely need to initiate utterances at levels greater than 60 percent of their reduced vital capacity.

Some speakers initiate utterances at their prevailing lung volume level without taking a preparatory inhalation before speech. This pattern is sometimes seen in individuals with TBI. In this situation, the individual frequently initiates speech at improper lung volume levels and, over the course of sustained speech, may initiate talking at a series of inconsistent lung volume levels. This demands that the individual make extensive adjustment in utterance length and in the performance of upper airway structures to compensate for this inconsistency.

Some individuals speak at a reduced lung volume level because they are unable to modify their breathing pattern at rest. In severe TBI, the inability to modify the breathing pattern at rest voluntarily is not uncommon. These individuals find it difficult to inhale to a greater lung volume level in preparation for a lengthy utterance. They also experience difficulty sustaining the respiratory support for a long utterance in that they are used to managing their respiratory system consistent with the pattern that they habitually used for rest breathing with essentially equal durations of inhalation and exhalation.

Finally, some individuals with TBI will use excessive lung volume levels. In an effort to compensate for phonatory, velopharyngeal, and articulatory function, some dysarthric speakers inhale to excessive lung volume levels before they initiate speech. The resulting high level of subglottal air pressure is often associated with excessively loud speech for those who are able to initiate phonation at such high lung volume levels. For those who are unable to initiate phonation at the high lung volume levels, there may be excessive air wastage. In TBI, the use of excessive lung volume levels may be a maladaptive respiratory behavior that has not been modified in the presence of a changing physiologic capability. Early in their recovery, some individuals are required to generate excessive subglottal air pressure levels to initiate phonation. As their phonatory control improves, some of them do not modify this pattern.

Treatment

The overall treatment goal for patients with respiratory impairments in motor speech disorders is to achieve a consistent subglottal air pressure level during speech that is produced with minimal fatigue and appropriate breath group lengths. This is generally accomplished by one of a number of general approaches. First, the speaker is taught to compensate for the neuromotor impairment by maximally using his or her potential respiratory support. Second, the speaker may be involved in an intervention program designed to decrease the extent of neuromotor involvement through pharmacologic therapy or neuromotor training. Third, a prosthetic approach may be used to increase the adequacy of respiratory support for speech. Finally, the level of the respiratory impairment may be minimized by increasing the efficiency of the laryngeal, velopharyngeal, or oral articulatory valves. The following discussion will be organized in a manner that reflects a sequential approach to respiratory problems observed in the dysarthric population.

Establishing Respiratory Support. In an effort to develop a consistent subglottal air pressure, Netsell and Daniel (1979) suggested a biofeedback approach to train a flaccid dysarthric client to sustain air pressures within the range used for speech (5 to 10 cm H_2O). At the beginning of treatment their client generated only 1 or 2 cm H_2O for less than 3 seconds. They instructed him to blow into a pressure sensor as a "leak tube" allowed air to escape at a rate associated with normal phonation (75 to 125 cm/sec). These authors report that their client was able to learn to generate 10 cm H_2O for 10 seconds by the end of eight 20-minute training sessions.

The authors have modified the simple device described by Hixon and colleagues (1982) by using slightly different materials. They use a plastic bottle with a hole in the cover. A tube is then inserted through the hole and into the water. In this way, risk of breakage and water spillage is reduced and the apparatus can be sent home with the patient with a recommendation for daily practice. The authors have found that families and personal care attendants can have severely dysarthric speakers practice this procedure as a beginning effort to establish consistent control of the respiratory system. As in the assessment phase, 5 cm is used for a 5-second target level. Once a patient has achieved this level of function, the next step is typically speech production tasks. Setting higher target levels often is associated with undesirable features. In attempting to "overdrive" the respiratory-phonatory system, the speaker often begins to produce a harsh, strained, strangled voice quality.

In addition to the blowing techniques, another approach to train consistent air-pressure generation is to have a client sustain vowel sounds. The intensity level of the vowel can be monitored on a voltage meter or with an intensity measurement device such as a Visipitch. This task can be used successfully if pharyngeal control is adequate. Once respiratory support for phonation can be controlled, the client can participate in more speechlike tasks, such as the repetition of syllables.

Postural Adjustments. Some persons with severe motor impairment are unable to generate consistent air pressure values in the seated position. In these cases, postural adjustments or prosthetic assistance may be necessary. For example, a number of TBI individuals are unable to initiate phonation in the upright position but can achieve phonatory and respiratory control to initiate phonation when supine. For speakers who benefit from postural adjustment, appropriate positioning can be accomplished by placing the individual in a wheelchair or a lawn chair with an adjustable back (Collins and colleagues, 1982). Proper wheelchair positioning, that is, with adequate trunk support, is associated with optimum respiratory-phonatory control.

Respiratory Prosthesis. Two types of respiratory prostheses have been used to supplement expiratory forces during speech. A corset (abdominal binder) has been used routinely with persons with spinal cord injuries who have intact diaphragmatic innervation but minimal or no innervation of the expiratory muscles. For some persons with head injury, the abdominal binder provides improved respiratory support for speech. For the speaker with inspiratory weakness, the binder may be effective but potentially dangerous; its use in treatment must involve medical approval and supervision.

The second type of abdominal prosthesis is the expiratory "board" or "paddle" described by Rosenbek and LaPointe (1985). This board is attached to a wheelchair so that it can be swung into position just anterior to the abdomen. As the individual prepares to speak, he or she leans forward into the board, thus increasing expiratory forces. Because the individual can lean back away from the board, this approach does not interfere with inhalation. The efficient use of the board requires some trunk strength and the balance to lean forward and back at appropriate times. Although the authors have found the expiratory board to be useful occasionally, usually the speakers who need it most do not have the trunk balance or strength to use it effectively.

Stabilizing the Respiratory Pattern. Even after individuals can generate the subglottal air pressures necessary for speech, it is still necessary to teach some of them to stabilize the respiratory pattern that they use. The first step to stabilize the pattern of severe and moderately dysarthric individuals is to identify a functional lung volume range for them to use during speech. As mentioned previously, normal speakers generally inhale to approximately 60 percent of lung volume level before initiating speech. Persons with motor impairment may need to inhale to a slightly higher level to generate the subglottal air pressure levels that they require for speech. Once an effective lung volume level range has been selected, many TBI individuals require instruction to inhale consistently to that lung volume level before initiating speech rather than to begin to speak at whatever lung volume level they happen to be at the moment.

Chest Wall Shape. According to Hardy (1983), there is no "best" respiratory shape for a dysarthric speaker. However, some speakers have adopted chest wall shape patterns that are extremely fatiguing or maladaptive. These patients should be taught a more effective respiratory pattern. The most common of these maladaptive patterns is for an individual to elevate the shoulders excessively during each inhalation. In this situation the individual should learn to use a coordinated pattern of thoracic and abdominal breathing.

Elimination of Abnormal Respiratory Behaviors. Although the research documenting the use of abnormal respiratory behaviors by TBI individuals is extremely limited, anecdotal reports of maladaptive behaviors are common. It is not unusual for a TBI individual to retain a maladaptive respiratory pattern that was necessary early in recovery and continue to use this pattern long after more normal respiratory control is possible. For example, the authors treated a young woman who inhaled after the first syllable of each utterance. Once she had taken the initial inhalation, it was not uncommon for her to speak several syllables before she inhaled again. We were unable to change this maladaptive respiratory behavior. Perhaps she had developed this pattern when she began to speak again and when her respiratory support was inadequate to produce more than one syllable per breath group.

Increasing Respiratory Flexibility. The authors attempt to increase the consistency with which severe dysarthric individuals manage their respiratory system and to increase flexibility in mildly dysarthric speakers. Candidates for this phase of intervention may include (1) speakers who produce utterances with stereotype breath group lengths, (2) speakers who never pause without inhaling, and (3) speakers who are unable to manage the "quick" inhalation needed to support the short breath group utterance. Once again, it is quite common to find dysarthric individuals with TBI who retain a respiratory pattern that they learned early in their recovery. For example, Bellaire and colleagues (1986) report on a young man with TBI who spoke with a habitual breath group of five to six syllables, yet he was able to produce utterances of over 20 syllables on instruction. In this case, he required an intervention program to encourage the flexible use of his respiratory system during speech to accommodate utterances of various lengths and of various prosodic patterns.

LARYNGEAL FUNCTION

Some level of phonatory dysfunction is present in a very large percentage of dysarthric speakers with TBI. This dysfunction may range in severity from mild impairment with no associated disability to an impairment that is so severe that it is the primary factor limiting communication. Because respiratory support and phonatory ability are so closely related, especially in early recovery for motor speech disorders related to TBI, many of the assessment and intervention approaches just described for respiration also apply to phonatory function. For example, when the clinician attempts to understand a severe phonatory impairment and to establish voluntary phonation, one component of the assessment would be to describe the respiratory support; an intervention program might include efforts to maximize respiratory support and explore the potential benefits of postural adjustments. Thus, although it is impossible to separate respiratory from phonatory function, the following discussion outlines assessment and intervention strategies for laryngeal impairment in TBI.

Assessment

Generally, assessment proceeds along the same lines as the clinical assessment of other components. The first phase involves documentation of the presence of phonatory impairment and a perceptual description of its characteristics and severity. This stage usually serves as a screening process. The second phase of the assessment involves an in-depth analysis of phonatory function. In the second phase a series of questions are posed that are related to the mechanisms underlying the perceptual features of phonation. A plan for intervention is then developed from this in-depth assessment.

Perceptual Assessment. When discussing assessment of voice disorders, Aronson (1980) writes that "the trained ear and mind are, at present, the most useful instrument" (p. 182). Much of the current clinical assessment of phonatory dysfunction of dysarthric speakers is made using perceptual judgments. However, the specific phonatory functions are gradually being assessed more often using instrumental measurement techniques, such as acoustic analysis or aerodynamic resistance. The perceptual assessment of phonatory impairment is usually quantified using a scaling procedure, perhaps somewhat similar to the equal-appearing interval scale reported by Darley and colleagues (1969). Table 9-4 contains a listing of the perceptual indicators of phonatory impairment. Note that a number of these features may be associated with other components of the speech production in addition to phonation. For example, the perceptual indicator, "short phrases," may reflect the combined reduction of respiratory support and inefficient valving at the laryngeal, velopharyngeal, or oral articulatory levels.

In-depth Assessment of Laryngeal Dysfunction. Because dysarthria is typically characterized by impairment in multiple speech components, it is necessary to examine the relationship of phonatory impairment with other aspects of phonation. It is possible that what appears to be an impairment in phonation may instead reflect an impairment in respiratory or velopharyngeal performance. For example, poor respiratory sup-

Table 9-4. Perceptual indicators of phonatory impairment

Inability to produce phonation
Abnormal pitch level
Pitch breaks
Monotone pitch
Voice tremor
Monotone loudness
Excessive loudness variation
Loudness decay
Alternating loudness
Harsh voice
Hoarse voice
Breathy voice
Strained-strangled voice
Short phrases
Ability to distinguish voiced versus voiceless cognate pairs

port may result in deviations of voice loudness and length of phrase. Answers to the following questions are needed to interpret the data derived from the assessment of phonatory performance (Yorkston and colleagues, 1988a):

Is the level of subglottal air pressure adequate to support phonatory function?
Does the speaker "overdrive" the respiratory system when attempting to produce phonation?
How flexible is the respiratory system?
Can the respiratory system be controlled in a coordinated fashion?
How efficient is the velopharyngeal valve?
Is the speaker able to achieve complete velopharyngeal closure?
Is the closure timed in relationship to other aspects of speech production?

The assessment of the laryngeal function usually involves some measure of laryngeal efficiency in terms of how well the expiratory air stream is valved at the level of the vocal folds. This can be assessed through one's perceptual characteristics of the client's voice. Several perceptual features may signal the laryngeal insufficiency. A breathy voice may indicate air wastage and thus signal inadequate laryngeal closure. On the other hand, a voice with strained-strangled quality may reflect excessive adduction of the vocal folds. The efficiency of glottal closure may also be assessed by listening to the quality of the cough, a throat-clearing maneuver, or a hard glottal attack. A weak or "mushy" cough may indicate vocal fold weakness.

The duration of sustained phonation time has also been taken as a measure of laryngeal efficiency. Prator and Swift (1984) used the following formulas that include measures of vital capacity to predict maximum phonation time for adults:

For males: VC divided by 110 × 0.67 = maximum phonation time
For females: VC divided by 100 × 0.59 = maximum phonation time

Obviously, a performance on this task depends not only on the efficiency of glottal closure but also on the level of respiratory support.

Measures and estimates of air flow during phonation have also been used to measure laryngeal efficiency. Mean air flow rates are computed by dividing volume exhalation during phonation by time. For males, mean flow rates average 115 ml/per second; for females, they average 100 ml/per second (Yanagihara and colleagues, 1966). Because of possible inconsistent laryngeal control by dysarthric speakers, average levels of air flow may not reflect the status of the actual function (Netsell and colleagues, 1984).

Estimates of laryngeal resistance have been used to estimate the opposition to air flow imposed by the larynx. Although this measure cannot be taken directly, Smitheran and Hixon (1981) describe an approach to estimate the aerodynamic impedance of the laryngeal structures. For a detailed description of aerodynamic and fiberoptic laryngeal assessment, see Netsell and colleagues (1989). One limitation of this procedure with dysarthric speakers is that the measure does not necessarily reflect the stiffness of the vocal fold. For example, in a severely spastic individual, the vocal folds may be very stiff yet, because of the vocal fold position, produce a breathy voice quality.

Finally, laryngeal efficiency may be estimated by observing the movement of the vocal fold through laryngoscopy. This technique is useful when evaluating vocal fold paralysis. However, the rapid movement of the vocal fold does not permit cycle-by-cycle evaluation of the vocal folds using this technique. During recent years, the use of the fiberscope, a stoboscopic light source, and video recording has shown promise for visualizing and measuring vocal fold movement in dysarthric speakers.

Vocal flexibility refers to variations of pitch and loudness that aid in the expression of meaning. This aspect of voice can be assessed perceptually by judging the parameters of pitch variation, loudness, and quality. Generally these measures are made clinically through perceptual means. However, vocal flexibility can be measured acoustically with parameters related to fundamental frequency, such as range of fundamental frequency within an utterance, range of peak fundamental frequencies of each syllable within an utterance, slope of fundamental frequency contour, and so on.

Treatment of Laryngeal Dysfunction

Establishing Voluntary Phonation. This discussion of treatment will be organized according to severity. The first step in treating an aphonic individual is to evaluate "reflexive" phonation. Some severely dysarthric individuals who are unable to voluntarily produce phonation are able to produce phonation in conjunction with reflexive activities. These non-speech reflex patterns would include laughing, coughing, sighing, and expressions of pain and discomfort. When phonation occurs, note should be taken not only of the type of activity (laughing) but also of the speaker's position (supine, prone, or sitting). When respiratory drive is weak, the speaker's efforts might be supplemented with abdominal pressing to increase the subglottal air pressure being generated. Family members and attendant staff are encouraged to keep a diary of the times when phonation occurs (Yorkston and colleagues, 1988a). The following instructions may be given for such monitoring:

Remember to include information about date, voicing behavior, consistency, position when voicing occurs, and stimulus and whether or not the speaker could continue to produce voicing. Make an entry at least once a week. Pick a particular day each week if that will help you be consistent. (Yorkston and colleagues, 1988a)

The information obtained from such a diary can be used in planning treatment. The authors have used the diary approach extensively with slow-to-recover TBI individuals. Frequently when severe dysarthric patients are evaluated through the outpatient clinic, they will be unable to produce voluntary phonation regardless of positioning, physical assistance, or behavioral instruction. However, the families may indicate that they have heard voicing on occasion. When this is the case, families are asked to complete a diary. By completing the diary for 1 month, one can see if voicing is occurring with increasing frequency. If it is increasing, one can see which factors appear in association with it. For example, in one case, voicing was noted most often in the time just following meals. Once this pattern was established, a postmealtime practice routine for facilitation of voluntary phonation was developed.

To develop voluntary phonation, often there is a transition from the reflexive phonatory behaviors reported above. For some, this transition is almost immediate; however, for others, the transition may take months or even years. The authors commonly ask individuals to attempt to produce reflexive behavior on a repetitive basis and next to produce phonation voluntarily. Typically, these speakers are simultaneously participating in a program designed to increase their ability to generate subglottal air pressure. During the phonatory practice sessions, the patient is usually positioned for maximal generation of subglottal air pressure when attempting phonation. Thus, many patients are positioned supine with an abdominal press to increase subglottal air pressure. Rarely is early phonation most effectively initiated in the upright or seated position. Because the goal of this early phase of intervention is more forcible, vocal fold adduction, traditional pushing or pulling exercises such as those described by Prator and Swift (1984) may be used. Workinger and Netsell (1988) report a case study in which a man with TBI was instructed to pull on a hand grip to initiate phonation during practice activities as well as during speech. Once severely dysarthric speakers are consistently able to initiate phonation, they are asked to attempt to shape the oral cavity to produce a number of different glottal sounds and to initiate phonation while assuming these articulatory positions.

Increasing Loudness. Reduced voice loudness is a relatively common dysfunction among dysarthric individuals. Behaviorally, training to increase vocal loudness may involve instructing the speaker to generate greater levels of subglottal air pressure. These and other techniques are discussed earlier in the chapter. When speakers are unable to change their respiratory pattern, loudness may be enhanced by a portable amplification system. Amplification systems should be small enough to be carried in a pocket or purse with a boom microphone small enough to be mounted on eye glasses or behind the ear. Such amplifiers are useful because they do not need to be held and tend to minimize environmental sounds.

Improving Vocal Quality. Depending on the neurologic impairment, a variety of vocal quality characteristics may mark the speech of dysarthric individuals with TBI. Rough, hoarse, harsh, or breathy voices are common. When these symptoms are not handicapping, often they are left untreated. For severely involved dysarthric speakers, other aspects of speech production may be more critical to the improvement of speech intelligibility and reduction of communication disability than a change in voice quality. When voice quality impairment is present and is felt to contribute to overall disability and handicap, intervention may be warranted.

When voice quality disorders are associated with hyperadduction of vocal folds, a traditional voice therapy technique designed to reduce laryngeal hyperadduction and increase airflow through the glottis may be appropriate (see Prator and Swift, 1984). At times, vocal quality disorders may occur because of excessive respiratory drive in the presence of diminished phonatory control. The rough, hoarse, or harsh voice that accompanies such a pattern may be diminished by having the speaker adopt a level of subglottal air pressure that is appropriate for the particular function of communication and is also consistent with the level of laryngeal control that he or she can achieve. Some TBI clients with cognitive difficulties seem to have difficulty making judgments about appropriate loudness levels. At times, specific instruction is required to maximize respiratory-phonatory coordination. Portable amplification may be used in an attempt to reduce "respiratory overdrive" common in severely dysarthric individuals. Amplification assists them to learn to "not work so hard" when attempting to speak.

VELOPHARYNGEAL FUNCTION

Velopharyngeal dysfunction of dysarthric speakers with TBI is of critical interest to the speech-language pathologist for a number of reasons. First velopharyngeal impairment occurs frequently in this population. Second, velopharyngeal impairment is extremely important clinically because it tends to exaggerate the impairment of other aspects of the speech mechanism. For example, if an individual has reduced respiratory support for speech, the reduced level of air pressure that can be produced by the individual may be further diminished because of the escape of air through the velopharyngeal port. Velopharyngeal dysfunction distorts the production of vowel and consonant sounds even though they may be produced with an accurate, oral articulatory gesture. In the presence of velopharyngeal dysfunctions, vowels are perceived as hypernasal and many consonants may be perceived as imprecise. Finally velopharyngeal impairment is of concern clinically because frequently clinicians can intervene successfully to compensate for this impairment. For example, there exists a growing number of literature reports of successful management of velopharyngeal incompetence using palatal lifts (see Yorkston and colleagues [1988a] for a more detailed discussion in this area).

Normal Velopharyngeal Function

The role of the velopharyngeal mechanism during normal speech varies depending on the task. During the production of nonnasal consonant sounds, the velopharyngeal mechanism can be viewed as an aerodynamic valve that it is completely sealed to prevent the escape of air flow from the oral cavity through the nasal cavity. For most speakers, the velopharyngeal seal is complete during some aspect of "pressure consonant" production; however, the pattern and duration of closure varies from speaker to speaker. A small number of "normal" speakers demonstrate very small velopharyngeal openings during the production of some nonnasal sounds. During the production of nasal consonants, the velopharyngeal mechanism is opened to allow the coupling of the oropharyngeal and the nasal cavities. This allows a resonance pattern associated with a normal degree of nasality. During vowel production, the status of the velopharyngeal mechanism is influenced by the requirements of the adjacent consonants. Some nasalization is common. In fact, the complete closure of the velopharyngeal mechanism results in a denasal quality that is judged to be abnormal.

Characteristics in Dysarthric Speakers

Although velopharyngeal function in dysarthric speakers has not been studied as thoroughly as it has for normal and cleft palate speakers, increased reports of dysarthric speakers suggest different patterns and severity of velopharyngeal dysfunction. Table 9-5 contains a rating scale for estimating the level of severity of velopharyngeal dysfunction developed by Netsell and colleagues (1989). Note that the narrative statements reflect such aspects of velopharyngeal function as timing of movements related to other articulators, extent of velopharyngeal contact, and consistency of movement. The rating scale is based on examiner's viewing of midsagital videofluoroscopy.

The relationship between severity of velopharyngeal dysfunction to overall articulatory adequacy in TBI speakers has received some recent

Table 9-5. Estimated level of severity of velopharyngeal
dysfunction and corresponding narrative statements
based on examiner's viewing of midsagital videofluoroscopy

Level of severity	Narrative statements
WLN	Within normal limits; closure when expected and opening occurs at proper times for nasal consonant environment
1	Near normal function; VP movements well timed with other articulators; velar height and extent of pharyngeal contact somewhat less than normal
2	Performance is somewhere between levels 1 and 3
3	Closure achieved on approximately 50% of oral consonants, or opening seen on oral consonants adjacent to nasal consonants, or both
4	Consistent VP opening (1–2 mm gap) for oral consonants
5	Performance is somewhere between levels 4 and 6
6	Closure never achieved; velar movements never close more than 50% of the VP space
7	Minimal (1–2 mm) or no velar movement; closure never achieved

WNL = within normal limits. VP = velopharyngeal Source: Netsell, R., Lotz, W., and Barlow, S. (1989). A speech physiology examination for individuals with dysarthria. In K. M. Yorkston and D. R. Beukelman (Eds.), *Recent advances in dysarthria*. Boston: College-Hill Press.

attention (Yorkston and colleagues, 1989). A group of 24 dysarthric adults (21 of whom were recovering from TBI) were placed into one of two groups based on aerodynamic measure of velopharyngeal status. All had perceptual characteristics suggestive of velopharyngeal dysfunction, including hypernasality. Group I contained 13 individuals who were velopharyngeally incompetent in that nasal air flow was always noted during the stop phase of voiceless plosive sounds (see the section on assessment below for a detailed description of the measurement task). These individuals would probably have been rated as 7 on the Netsell and colleagues (1989) scale. Group II contained 11 individuals who at times were achieving complete velopharyngeal closure. Articulatory adequacy was measured using a phoneme identification task (Yorkston and colleagues, 1988b), a computer-generated articulatory inventory. Results indicated that not only did overall articulatory adequacy vary as a function of the severity of velopharyngeal dysfunction, but the pattern of articulatory errors distinguished those speakers who were completely incompetent from those with more moderate levels of velopharyngeal dysfunction. Specifically, the more severely involved speakers exhibited disproportionately greater problems in producing pressure consonants. Those who at times were achieving velopharyngeal closure did not exhibit a marked difference between the production of pressure consonants and the category of nasals and glides. Thus, severe velopharyngeal involvement has an impact not only on resonance characteristics but also may affect more general aspects of articulatory function.

Assessment

During the assessment of a dysarthric speaker, the clinician usually attempts to address several questions regarding velopharyngeal function (Yorkston and colleagues, 1988a):

Is there evidence of velopharyngeal dysfunction in the speaker?
What is the extent and pattern of dysfunction?
Does the velopharyngeal dysfunction influence other aspects of speech performance?
What options are available to improve velopharyngeal function in the speaker?

The initial assessment of velopharyngeal dysfunction is usually a perceptual assessment. There are three perceptual indicators of velopharyngeal dysfunction—hypernasality, occurrence of nasal emission, and a disproportionate inability to produce pressure consonants. If any of these perceptual features is present, then a more in-depth assessment of velopharyngeal dysfunction is warranted.

Once the presence of a velopharyngeal dysfunction is confirmed, additional measures may be necessary to describe the exact nature of the dysfunction. Aerodynamic measures of oral air pressure and volume velocity of air flow across the velopharyngeal port are indicators of velopharyngeal function. These techniques do not provide a direct measure of velopharyngeal movement but are used to make estimates of velopharyngeal resistance. The equipment and procedures used in these measures are described in Kuehn (1982), Netsell (1969), Warren (1975), and most recently in Netsell and colleagues (1989). These aerodynamic measures allow the clinician to make precise inferences about the extent and timing of velopharyngeal closure. However, they have some limitations. The shape of the velopharyngeal port during speech is not described.

Radiographic techniques are also used to measure velopharyngeal function. These techniques have been used extensively with cleft palate speakers but may also prove useful with dysarthric speakers. Rather than rely on inference about the movement from a perceptual observation, these techniques allow for the examination of movements from structures typically hidden from view. In the dysarthria field, radiographic procedures have been used somewhat more sparingly than in cleft palate. Although the authors do not use radiographic procedures as a routine part of our examination of persons with dysarthria, they are frequently employed by some in the palatal lift fitting process.

Direct visualization of the velopharyngeal mechanism can be achieved using fiberoptic equipment. The flexible shaft of the fiberscope is inserted through the nares and the nasal cavity until the soft palate in the pharyngeal walls can be observed. This technique allows the observation of the movements of the structures. Several features of the fiberoptic equipment have limited its use with dysarthric speakers secondary to TBI (1) many individuals are unable to tolerate the presence of the fiberscope in the nasal cavity, (2) the fiberscope does not provide a written record of velopharyngeal function that can be compared with performance at another time, and (3) the size estimates of a structure are difficult because the size of the image depends on the distance between the object being viewed and the lens of the scope.

The final phase of the assessment of velopharyngeal function is to estimate the impact of intervention. A number of techniques have been employed to modify velopharyngeal function (Yorkston and colleagues, 1988a). The nares may be occluded to eliminate the escape of air through the nasal cavity. Speech loudness and articulatory precision are then assessed with and without the nares included. Of course, valving the speech mechanism in this way does not precisely mimic adequate velopharyngeal function, but it does provide a gross estimation of improved function if one selectively observes such features as adequacy of pressure consonant production. The flaccid dysarthric speaker may experience improved velopharyngeal function in the supine position with gravity assisting the soft palate to approximate the posterior pharyngeal wall.

Treatment

Behavioral Treatment of Velopharyngeal Dysfunction. The three general categories of treatment approaches with persons with velopharyngeal dysfunction are behavioral, prosthetic, and surgical. Behavioral approaches for the management of velopharyngeal dysfunction in dysarthric speakers with TBI have received scant attention in the literature. Generally, behavioral approaches are only considered with persons who have mild or moderate velopharyngeal dysfunction. In other words, those individuals are able to achieve adequate closure if they are speaking at appropriate rates and are adequately monitoring their general articulatory precision. It is most common to treat velopharyngeal dysfunction in this portion of the population simply as an articulation problem. The control of speaking rate has been reported to have a positive impact on velopharyngeal performance in selected individuals with ataxic dysarthria (Yorkston and Beukelman, 1981b). As the speaking rate of these individuals was reduced, they became increasingly successful at achieving articulatory targets including accuracy of velopharyngeal closure. Despite the appropriateness of behavioral intervention for some dysarthric speakers with TBI, there is no indication that a reduction in speaking rate will improve the velopharyngeal function of more severely involved dysarthric speakers. Froeschels (1943) and Froeschels and colleagues (1955) have suggested a pushing technique for speakers with velopharyngeal paralysis. Their rationale is that voluntary contraction of one group of muscles will overflow into other muscles.

Prosthetic Treatment of Velopharyngeal Dysfunction. The most common prosthetic method of treating velopharyngeal dysfunction in dysarthric speakers involves fitting of a palatal lift. A lift consists of a retentive portion that covers the hard palate and fastens to the maxillary teeth by wires and a lift portion that extends along the oral surface of the soft palate. At times, orthodontic bands or acrylic ridges are added to selected teeth to improve the lift's retention capability.

Rather than presenting a complete review of palatal lift fitting, the guidelines for *candidacy* for palatal lift in the TBI population will be presented here. The requirements for palatal lift candidacy appear to differ from center to center. The following guidelines tend to cover the major considerations (Gonzales and Aronson, 1970; Netsell and Rosenbek, 1985; Rosenbek and LaPointe, 1985):

1. *Severity of dysfunction.* A palatal lift should be considered for speakers who demonstrate consistent inability to achieve velopharyngeal closure. For such individuals, behavioral intervention, in the absence of spontaneous recovery, is usually ineffective. For individuals who are able to achieve closure during some, but not all, speech attempts, palatal lift intervention is less clear cut. If the disorder is mild, behavioral intervention may be useful. Typically, a brief trial intervention can indicate whether the behavioral approach will be likely to succeed.

2. *Impairment of other speech components.* Palatal lifts are most likely to succeed immediately with those individuals who exhibit a relatively isolated velopharyngeal impairment. Unfortunately, for most dysarthric speakers with TBI, velopharyngeal dysfunction is most frequently accompanied by respiratory, phonatory, or oral articulatory impairment. Although speakers with severe articulatory or respiratory disorders may be considered for palatal lift fitting, clinicians should not expect more from the lift than the speaker's symptom complex will allow (Rosenbek and LaPointe, 1985). When multiple speech components are involved, palatal lift fittings should be followed by a traditional program of respiratory or articulatory training. For the severely involved speaker, managing the velopharyngeal mechanism may serve to improve the efficiency of the respiratory system and to allow for progress in the modification of oral articulation.

3. *Cooperation.* Lack of motivation and failure to cooperate are frequently cited as counterindications for palatal lift fitting (Gonzales and Aronson, 1970; Dworkin and Johns, 1980). The authors do not consider palatal lifts for speakers with severe TBI who are still easily agitated, unable to tolerate minimal amounts of discomfort, or unable to understand the purpose of the intervention.

4. *Palatal spasticity.* Speakers with extremely spastic palates may be difficult to fit with a palatal lift. The result of spasticity is a stiff soft palate that may not tolerate elevation and may make retention more difficult.

4. *Swallowing difficulties.* If a speaker has difficulty swallowing secretions without aspiration or difficulty initiating the swallowing reflex, the presence of the palatal lift will probably reduce swallowing efficiency to some extent. Typically, the flow of saliva is increased during the phase in which the speaker is accommodating to the lift. This period is typically a brief one.

6. *Dentition.* Because retention of the palatal life depends on adequate dentition, dental care and maintenance of good oral hygiene are particularly important for severely dysarthric individuals who are candidates for palatal lift fitting. Edentulous persons are consid-

ered difficult to fit with palatal lifts by some centers, whereas other centers report considerable success with this group of speakers. Ill-fitting dentures are particularly problematic when combined with a spastic soft palate.

7. *Hypersensitivity.* At times, hypersensitivity can be managed behaviorally. Daniel (1982) suggested that there are individuals who have difficulty adjusting to a palatal lift, including persons with spasticity of the soft palate, hypersensitivity to touch, and hyperactive gag reflexes. For those individuals, Daniel suggested a palatal desensitization program before palatal lift fitting. In the program, someone other than the speaker applies pressure in a rubbing motion on the alveolar ridge with cotton placed on the index finger. Gradually, the hard palate is stimulated at the midline further and further posteriorly. When the speaker feels the urge to gag, he or she is instructed to utter a sound and the posterior progression of the stimulating finger is stopped and lateral movements begun. After 30 seconds of lateral massage, a 15-second rest period is provided. The stimulation pattern then begins again. Daniel suggested that exercises should be completed for 5 minutes, four times per day, 7 days per week, and that desensitization, if it is going to occur, usually takes 2 or 3 weeks.

Grand and colleagues (1988) attempted to fit a palatal lift for a person with TBI. This individual experienced lift retention problems as he continuously dislodged the device from attachments to the teeth. Traditional desensitization treatment was unsuccessful. In an effort to reduce sensory feedback, topical anesthetic lidocaine gel was applied to the upper surface of the prosthesis. The authors report dramatic results in that the lift was retained for up to 3 or 4 hours per application.

Decisions regarding the *timing* of palatal lift fitting are often difficult in the TBI population because of the potential for improvement in neurologic status that may be accompanied by return of velopharyngeal function. During the past 10 years the authors have fitted approximately 40 TBI individuals with palatal lifts. The general guidelines for timing of lift fitting have developed as a result of that experience. Various centers through the country have different guidelines for the timing of intervention.

At the authors' center, we do not require good oral articulation or respiratory function before proceeding with a palatal lift fitting for stable or gradually recovering speakers. A number of TBI individuals were initially evaluated years after onset. The velopharyngeal dysfunction of these individuals was not managed early in the course of recovery, and, unfortunately, velopharyngeal function did not return to normal spontaneously. Failure to manage these individuals early may have contributed to a number of "preventable" problems. First, these individuals often appear to "give up" the use of natural speech and depend exclusively on augmentative communication systems. This is quite predictable because their attempts to speak were usually effortful and unsuccessful. Indeed, they may often fail to use their residual speech capability to their maximum potential. For example, individuals may fail to produce oral articulatory gestures when speaking despite relatively preserved lip and tongue movement. It is as if the velopharyngeal incompetency so distorts whatever signal is produced that the speaker begins to ignore the oral articulatory movement capability. Finally, unmanaged velopharyngeal incompetency may also encourage the development of other bad habits. Perhaps the most common of these is respiratory overdrive. Thus, when considering the timing of palatal lift fitting, the authors do not require good oral articulation. However, they do not typically recommend palatal lifts for individuals who are unable to achieve consistent, voluntary phonation because of a severely compromised phonatory-respiratory system. Other contraindications for palatal lift fitting are agitation and severe swallowing disorders.

One of the questions most frequently asked at the time of palatal lift fitting is "Will I need to wear this lift permanently?" Answering this legitimate question with any degree of certainty is very difficult. No one has followed enough young, severely dysarthric, TBI individuals to understand the usual pattern, timing, and extent of recovery. Until research provides clinicians with more information regarding the natural course of recovery from TBI, limited experience must provide the answers. The authors have had the opportunity to follow a small number of cases over a number of years. Three cases in which TBI individuals were fitted with palatal lifts and followed for an extended period are reported elsewhere (Yorkston and colleagues, 1989). A typical pattern seen in their clinical experience is one in which the lift is worn for an extended time. Although some recovery occurs during that period, the speaker continues to benefit from the palatal lift. Figure 9-4 illustrates the results of a phoneme identification task recorded with and without the palatal lift at the time of initial lift fitting (23 months after onset), after 2 months of speech intervention (25 months after onset), and after long-term followup (85 months after onset). Note that gains in pressure consonant production were achieved at the initial lift fitting. After a period of treatment and accommodation, improvement was also noted in the patient's ability to produce nasals and glides with the lift in place. Five years later results of measures obtained during a followup visit indicated that although some overall improvement had occurred, the pattern of articulatory error was similar to the one seen at 25 months after onset. The pattern just described is perhaps the most typical one. However, the authors have also seen cases in which palatal lifts, fitted when severe velopharyngeal incompetence had

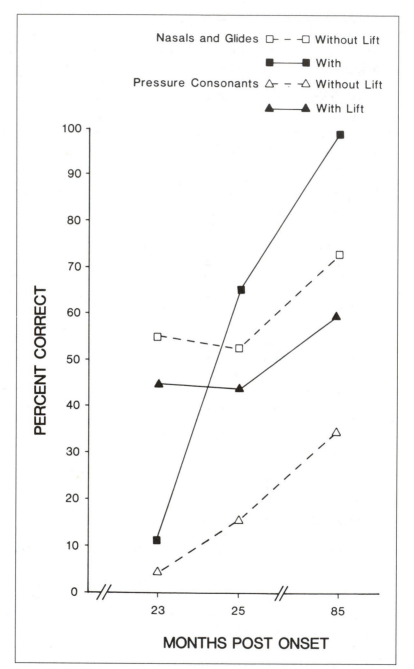

Figure 9-4. Measures of perceived articulatory adequacy (with and without the palatal lift) for a TBI speaker. Measures were obtained at the initial lift fitting (23 months postonset [MPO]), after 2 months of

stabilized, proved to be of temporary benefit and could be eliminated after adequate velopharyngeal function returned. Better understanding of the natural course of recovery from severe dysarthria is a pressing need. Until that research is available, patients and families should realize that many recovery courses are possible.

Surgical Treatment of Velopharyngeal Dysfunction. Surgical procedures are rarely reported with persons who exhibit velopharyngeal dysfunction after TBI. Surgical procedures tend to be permanent, and the potential of recovery in TBI individuals makes such intervention unattractive. Two surgical procedures have been used in the past to alter velopharyngeal dysfunction. Teflon injections have been reported by Lewy and colleagues (1965), who injected a Teflon and glycerine mixture into the area of Passavant's line in patients with neurologically based dysfunction. The pharyngeal flap has also been used to manage velopharyngeal incompetence in persons with dysarthria. This procedure is reviewed by Johns (1985). There are no reports in the literature of pharyngeal flaps being used with persons who have velopharyngeal dysfunction as a result of TBI.

ORAL ARTICULATION

Articulation can be defined as the movement of speech structures employed in producing the sounds of speech. The oral articulatory components of speech provide an excellent illustration of the interdependencies among various speech components. For example, Hardy (1967) described a 24-year-old man who was evaluated 2 years after TBI. His unintelligible speech was characterized by extremely rapid rate with an initial "explosive" burst followed by rapidly decreasing loudness. Cinefluorographic films revealed "gross immobility of the tongue" at habitual speaking rates. However, an increase in the extent of lingual and palatal movement was noted at reduced speaking rates. This case illustrates an incidence where severely restricted movement of the oral articulators may not have been the direct result of damage to the neuromotor control of these structures. Rather, these severely restricted movements may have been the consequence of a poorly controlled respiratory system in an attempt to compensate for that impairment.

Figure 9-4 (continued). speech treatment (25 MPO), and after long-term followup (85 MPO). From Yorkston, K.M., Honsinger, M.J., Beukelman, D.R., and Taylor, T.D. (1989). The effects of palatal lift fitting on the perceived articulatory adequacy of dysarthric speakers. In K.M. Yorkston and D.R. Beukelman (Eds.) *Recent advances in dysarthria.* Boston: College-Hill Press.

An understanding of the nature and variety of articulatory disorders seen in dysarthria following TBI is essential for planning appropriate treatment, since impairment in oral articulator function is almost a universal characteristic of dysarthria. The articulatory patterns associated with the dysarthria associated following TBI have received minimal research attention. This probably occurred because of the mixed nature of the neurologic impairment resulting from TBI. In most cases, the research has tended to focus on those etiology groups in which the neurologic deficit is more clearly defined (Parkinson's disease and cerebellar lesions).

Assessment

The assessment approach that speech-language pathologists use when attempting to understand the oral articulatory aspects of dysarthria following TBI is similar in process to that used with the other speech components. First, they perceptually rate oral articulatory performance. At this point, general questions are asked by the clinician. They include:

Is there an oral articulatory impairment?
If so, how severe is it?
How does the severity of the articulatory impairment compare with the
    respiratory, phonatory or velopharyngeal impairment?

The administration of traditional articulatory inventories or less formal word lists that sample all speech sounds appear not to have been accepted as a routine part of the clinical assessment of the dysarthric speakers. It is not clear why clinicians have not chosen to use these procedures. It is possible that the pattern of articulatory errors in dysarthria has contributed to this decision. The most prevalent articulatory error in dysarthria is the distortion, with many fewer substitutions and omissions. Because most traditional articulation tests measure the presence but not the severity of distortion, it is possible that a TBI individual with a high proportion of distortions can improve oral articulation considerably by diminishing the distortions. However, these changes will not be reflected during traditional articulation testing. It will be necessary to attempt to develop a system for more reliably scoring the severity of distortions for perceptual measures of articulatory performance to be useful in this population (Yorkston and colleagues, 1986).

Treatment

The treatment of articulatory disorders in dysarthria may take many forms. Generally, these approaches and techniques can be divided into those that attempt to normalize function by reducing the impairment, such as medical management, biofeedback training, or strengthening exercises, and those which are compensatory. Compensatory techniques use behavioral training or prosthetic management to assist the individual to compensate for motor impairment.

Normalizing Function. An attempt can be made to normalize function or reduce overall impairment in a number of ways. In the presence of abnormal muscle tone, Netsell and Cleeland (1973) reported the use of a biofeedback procedure to reduce the extent of bilateral lip retraction in a woman with a 15-year history of Parkinson's disease. Attempts have also been made to reduce tone through medication. No detailed research has been reported about the efficacy of this approach in TBI. Results are mixed. Commonly the levels of medication required to reduce the tone in the oral musculature has tended to be so excessive that it interfered with the swallowing performance of patients or diminished their overall alertness.

For persons with muscle weakness, function can be normalized with attempts to strengthen the oral musculature. Weakness is by no means universally present in dysarthria. One should be careful to demonstrate the presence of weakness before the articulatory impairment is approached with strengthening procedures. A fundamental question is "Does the weakness interfere with speech function?" The presence of weakness in the oral structures does not necessarily imply a speech disability. Speech is a skilled motor task that is much more demanding in terms of movement and precision than in terms of strength. In fact, Barlow and Abbs (1983) report that speech requires only 10 to 20 percent of the maximal force of lip movement. Thus, if a person demonstrates limitations in maximal lip strength, these limitations probably will not interfere with speech. However, if weakness is present and appears to interfere with speech production in a dysarthric individual with TBI, attempts to improve the strength of lips and tongue are appropriate. Rosenbek and LaPointe (1985) caution against other abuses of strengthening exercises, including delaying of other intervention approaches until strengthening is "finished" and increasing strength of certain muscles so that they overwhelm the efforts of others.

Compensation for the Impairment. Because dysarthria is often associated with chronic neuromotor impairment, a common goal to improve articulatory performance is to teach the dysarthric speaker to compensate for motor limitations. The authors have used contrastive productions and intelligibility drills to assist the speaker to modify production depending on the adequacy of the final speech end product. These approaches do not attempt to train the speaker to change specific movement patterns. Rather, general information about the adequacy of speech is provided. Thus it is assumed that the speaker will make the necessary changes to change the final outcome. DeFeo and Shaefer (1983) have provided an excellent example of compensatory adjustments made by an individual with neurologic impairment specific to certain speech components. Although this child had Moebius syndrome rather than TBI, their report illustrates the approach very nicely.

The authors will often use intelligibility drills, in which the individual is asked to produce a variety of sounds or words depending on the severity of dysarthria. The listeners then are asked to report their perceptions of the sound or word that has been spoken. Examples of word lists for intelligibility drills are presented in Table 9-6. If the listener is unable to identify correctly the sound or word produced, the dysarthric speaker is asked to attempt to modify the production approach in an effort to compensate for motor impairment and make the utterance more understandable.

Intelligibility drills provide a useful framework for treatment of articulatory disorders for a number of reasons. First, they do not require specific instruction about how to produce a sound. Rather, they depend on the speaker's ability to compensate for motor impairment and to find ways to produce perceptually acceptable sounds. In the clinical setting, the clinician rarely has detailed information about movement control and movement patterns of various articulators. If such information were available, it might not make a difference in clinical practice. For example, a speaker simply may not be able to modify a severely impaired lip movement and instead may need to compensate for such movements by making a complex series of adjustments in the movements of other structures. Tasks such as the intelligibility drills allow the speaker to attempt compensation in the presence of perhaps the most important

Table 9-6. Examples of word lists for intelligibility drills

Vowels			Initial consonants			Final consonants		
mail	hole	feel	ban	Paul	beer	lab	map	rub
Mell	heal	file	pan	ball	tear	lack	mat	rut
mall	hail	foil	tan	tall	dear	lag	mad	Russ
mule	hall	fowl	Dan	call	gear	lap	Mack	rust
mole	hill	fuel	can	stall	fear	lad	mass	rough
mile	Hal	fill	ran	fall	mere	lass	mash	run
mill	who'll	fall	Stan	mall	near	last	match	rum
meal	hell	fail	span	shall	we're	lash	mast	rush
mull	howl	fool	man	small	cheer	latch	Madge	rug
			fan	hall	shear	laugh	ma'am	runs

Source: Yorkston, K.M., Beukelman, D.R., and Bell, K.R. (1988). *Clinical management of dysarthric speakers.* Boston: College-Hill Press.

kind of feedback—knowledge of whether the listener has understood his or her attempt.

The second aspect of intelligibility drills that makes them practical and useful in the clinical setting is that the difficulty of the task can be easily adjusted to meet the needs of the individual dysarthric speaker. If a target accuracy of 80 to 90 percent is the goal, then the clinician can select phonemes and a list length to achieve target accuracy. Intelligibility drills may be used with the most severely involved dysarthric speaker as the first practice in speaking by having the speaker attempt to produce vowel sounds so that they can be differentiated by the listener. The third clinical advantage of intelligibility drills is that they allow early training in communication breakdown resolution strategies. The dysarthric speaker first learns to signal to the listener whether the listener's perception was correct. If it was not correct, then the speaker must resolve the communication breakdown, either by producing the word more precisely or by using an alternative communication strategy such as spelling. Thus, intervention activities are placed within a communication context.

RATE CONTROL

Rate control is an important strategy in treatment of dysarthric individuals with TBI. Ataxia is a frequent component of the motor dysfunction seen following TBI. This, coupled with the sudden onset of the disorder and poor monitoring associated with reduced cognitive functioning, make rate control an important aspect of early efforts to establish intelligible speech in TBI patients. Reducing an individual's speaking rate may improve intelligibility for a number of reasons. First, the overall slowing of movement rates may allow individuals to achieve articulatory targets more accurately. Second, a slow speaking rate may reduce the number of irregular articulatory breakdowns that are typical in ataxic dysarthria. Finally, rate control may be of benefit to the listener, giving him or her slightly more processing time and thus increasing speech intelligibility.

Assessment

Assessment in the area of rate control has a number of purposes. The obvious first question is, "Would slowing this speaker's rate improve speech intelligibility?" If the speaker's habitual rate is not the optimal one, then the speech-language pathologist also must ask, "What speaking rate is optimal, and how should that optimal rate be achieved?" The most straightforward way to answer these and related questions is to try various speaking rates and measure the impact of rate modification on speech intelligibility and judgments of naturalness. Clinically one does this by measuring the rate of habitual speech (Yorkston and colleagues,

1984), then slowing the speaker's rate using software (Beukelman and colleagues, 1988) that presents standard sentence material at any rate the speech-language pathologists selects. Comparing the intelligibility of habitual and slowed speech gives a clear indication of whether rate control is a fruitful avenue for exploration.

As in so many aspects of clinical management, finding the optimal speaking rate for a dysarthric individual is often a compromise. Typically, clinicians select rates that are slow enough to improve intelligibility yet not slow enough to markedly reduce speech naturalness. In the case of TBI, where rate control techniques are frequently used early in recovery, the optimal rate may change over time. Figure 9-5 contains data

Figure 9-5. Sentence intelligibility and speaking rates obtained over a period of recovery from TBI. From Yorkston, K., and Beukelman, D., (1981b). Ataxic dysarthria: Treatment sequences based on intelligibility and prosodic considerations. *Journal of Speech and Hearing Disorders, 46,* 398–404.

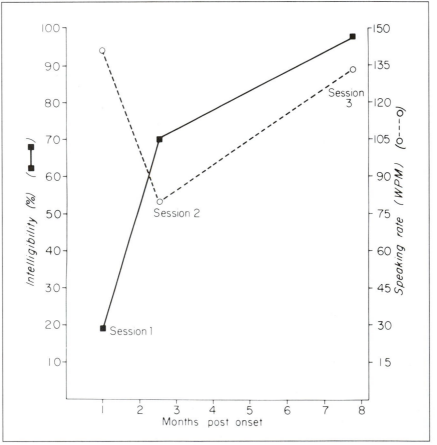

illustrating the recovery pattern of an ataxic dysarthric speaker with TBI (Yorkston and Beukelman, 1981b). At 1 month after onset, when the patient was speaking at 137 wpm, intelligibility was low, approximately 20 percent. At that point, a rate control training program was initiated. By the second recording session, this patient had reduced his rate to 80 wpm with an accompanying increase in speech intelligibility to approximately 70 percent. As the speaker continued to improve, this target speaking rate was systematically increased. By 8 months after onset, he was nearly completely intelligible at a speaking rate of over 130 wpm. Thus, the target speaking rate must continue to change as long as the speaker is able to maintain an acceptable level of intelligibility. Once intelligibility has been achieved at a particular rate, treatment can appropriately focus on increasing the rate and naturalness of speech.

Treatment

In attempting to select the most appropriate rate control technique, a number of issues must be considered. These are reviewed in more detail elsewhere (Yorkston and colleagues, 1988a). First, of course, is the effectiveness of the rate control strategy. Does the technique consistently and effectively allow the speaker to achieve the target rate? The second important question in selecting a particular rate control technique is, "Are the training requirements reasonable considering the speaker's level of cognitive function, communication needs, and availability of training time?" Some of the rate control techniques that will be described below require little training, while others require extensive practice. Another consideration is, "What are the potential negative consequences of using the technique?" For example, some techniques encourage a one-word-at-a-time speaking style. This style may not only reduce speech naturalness but also enhance the development of abnormal respiratory habits.

The following section reviews some of the rate-control techniques that have been reported in the clinical and research literature as being effective in the management of TBI. They will be presented in sequence roughly based on the amount of control needed to achieve the desired speaking rate. Generally, the more rigid the control technique, the more unnatural the resulting speech. However, the rigid rate-control techniques serve the important function of slowing rate when other techniques are ineffective.

Alphabet Supplementation. The alphabet supplementation approach described earlier in this chapter not only provides the listeners with extra information in the form of the first letter of each word, but also forces speakers into a slowed rate as they locate and point to the letters of the alphabet. Advantages of this technique include minimal training time and marked reductions in speaking rate. Disadvantages include a reduction in speech naturalness and the potential for development of poor respiratory habits that may persist even after the technique is no longer being used.

Computer Pacing. Frequently the goal of intervention is to train the individual to speak at the desired rate without the aid of a prosthesis such as an alphabet board. Learning to consistently use a speaking rate that is different from habitual usually requires extensive practice. Computerization of the practice process appears to be beneficial in allowing the TBI patient sufficient practice to reestablish a speaking rate that is appropriate for the level of motor control. A software program PACER (Beukelman and colleagues, 1988) presents text stimuli on the monitor of any Apple II series computer at a rate and in a format specified by the clinician. The dysarthric speaker then practices reading that passage at a controlled rate.

Speaking Rate Feedback. Once a dysarthric speaker with TBI has established and practiced reading passages using the computer pacing program described above, generalization of the new speaking rate is accomplished in two phases. First, the patient is asked to maintain the target speaking rate while reading without pacing. This is accomplished by asking the speaker to read a printed copy of the same passages that had been practiced using the PACER software. The speaking rate can be confirmed using TALLY (Beukelman and colleagues, 1988), a counting and calculation software program that allows the clinician to tally speaking rate online and provide specific feedback regarding speaking rate to the dysarthric individual. Once the speaker is able to maintain an appropriate target rate on written passages without cueing, then the final phase of training can be initiated. During the second phase of treatment, the new speaking rate is generalized to spontaneous speech. The dysarthric individual is asked to prepare and present short monologues. Using the TALLY software, the clinician can produce feedback regarding actual speaking achieved during this monologue. The ability to provide such immediate feedback on speaking rate is valuable in generalizing appropriate speaking rates to natural communication situations.

MAXIMIZING SPEECH NATURALNESS

For individuals with mild motor speech disorders, speech naturalness often remains a concern even after problems with speech intelligibility have been resolved. Intervention to improve the speech naturalness of mildly dysarthric individuals is an important but poorly understood area. To achieve natural-sounding speech, attention must be paid to the prosodic aspects of speech production. These aspects induce stress patterning, intonation, and rate-rhythm. Although prosody can be viewed as the melodic component of motor speech, the prosodic code carries its own meaning. Prosodic features indicate to the listener whether an utterance is a statement or a question, which words in the utterance are the most important, and what the mood of the speaker may be. Because prosodic features break the utterance into small units of meaningful information, they are also important in the overall organization of discourse. Clinicians who seek to improve the naturalness of their clients find themselves working both within the motor and cognitive domains. Speech naturalness can be viewed from a motor production viewpoint. That is, what is the speaker doing in terms of breath grouping, adjusting fundamental frequency intensity and pausal aspect of speech production? However, speech naturalness can also be viewed from a cognitive perspective. What nuances of meaning is the speaker wishing to convey? Intervention in the realm of speech naturalness for the mildly dysarthric TBI speaker is particularly challenging because deficit may be apparent in both the motor production and cognitive-organization aspects of speech production.

Prosodic Abnormalities in Dysarthria

Prosodic abnormalities are a frequent characteristic of dysarthric speech. Dysarthric speech can be unnatural or bizarre for a number of reasons that usually involve complex and incompletely understood interaction between prosodic features. The contributors to bizarreness generally fall into three categories (Yorkston and colleagues, 1988a). The first is monotony. Monotony may be the result of an excessively even rhythmic patterning of syllables, an evenness of stress patterning, a minimizing of intonation contours, or a combination of all these features. The second important contributors to bizarreness are syntactic mismatches. This occurs when the prosodic features do not coincide with the syntactic structure of the utterance. Normal speakers have sufficient respiratory support to breath only at syntactically appropriate boundaries so that prosodic features reinforce syntactic structures. When, for physiologic or cognitive reasons, prosodic and syntactic features no longer overlap, speech is perceived as unnatural. The final contributor to bizarreness is inconsistency across features. This occurs when various prosodic features conflict with one another. Although normal speakers send consistent prosodic signals, dysarthric speakers may produce utterances with peak fundamental frequency on one syllable, peak intensity on another, and maximum duration on still another.

Intervention Planning

Clinical treatment planning for the prosodic aspects of dysarthric speech is accomplished to a large extent by making perceptual judgments of speech adequacy. A detailed model of this assessment process can be found elsewhere (Yorkston, 1988). Although no standard assessment protocol exists on which to base decisions, assessment usually involves a series of questions. By answering these questions in a sequential fashion, the clinician describes the disability and identifies an appropriate starting place for intervention.

The following sequence may serve as a guide for management of prosodic aspects of dysarthria.

1. *Cognitive appreciation of utterance meaning.* The first phase in assessment of prosodic aspects of dysarthric speech is to confirm the speaker's understanding of the task. This is particularly important when attempting to understand the prosodic features of the TBI speaker. Because prosodic patterns are used to signal meaning, clinicians should verify the speaker's cognitive appreciation of the message.

2. *Identification of habitual and modified breath group units.* The second phase of assessment is to evaluate the breath group lengths produced by the speaker. Clinically, it is useful to consider the breath group as the unit of prosody. Thus, features such as intonation and stress patterning are first examined within the breath group unit. Recall from the discussion of respiratory support for speech that the poor respiratory support may make it physiologically impossible for some severely dysarthric individuals to produce long breath group units. However, other dysarthric speakers appear to have developed maladaptive breath patterning habits, such as taking breaths at syntactically "illegal" locations. Thus, when assessing the group unit, the clinician should assess what the speaker is doing habitually, then what the speaker can do when asked to modify habitual production. Typically one can conduct this part of the assessment by video-recording speakers reading a written passage. In reviewing the tape, locations of pauses and breaths can be identified and compared with the breath grouping characteristic of normal production of the passage. Figure 9-6 contains the text of the Mt. Rainier passage. Included in the text are slashes to indicate locations at which breaths were taken by at least some of the normal speakers who read the passage. Also indicated in the figure are the locations at which one of our mildly dysarthric speakers took breaths. This TBI speaker appears to have the respiratory support to produce normal breath group length in that she was able to

Believe me, // my goal is not to perfect [B] your knowledge of nature // or any of its [B] attributes, // [B] but let's// record the story // of Sam's first day on the mountain.//[B] Unbelievably// [B], this was the first time [B] that he had seen Mount [B] Rainier.// [B] It was a perfect day.// [B] I didn't know what to [B] show [B] him first//, "Show Sam some [B] snow,"// someone said// I pointed to the mountain [B] covered with snow// but someone said// [B], don't try to show him [B] all that snow // [B], "Show Sam some snow.// [B]" I picked a handful of snow [B] and began to show everyone//, but they [B] interrupted [B] again and said//, "Show Sam some snow.// [B]" Pretending to be angry// [B] I questioned//, "Show [B] Sam some snow?//" What a ridiculous idea.//

Figure 9-6. Mt. Rainier Passage with indications of locations at which normal speakers took breaths "//" and where a mildly dysarthric individual took breaths, "[B]."

sustain phonation for 20 seconds and could produce long utterances when requested to do so. Note that she took a breath 24 times as she read this passage. Eleven of the 24 breaths (46 percent) were at locations that normal speakers never took breaths, for example, between the words "its" and "attributes" in the phrase "any of its attributes." This mismatch between the syntax and meaning of the passage and breath patterning was an important contributor to this speaker's reduced naturalness. This speaker is typical of other TBI individuals we have treated in that once she grouped words more appropriately, naturalness improved. Thus it was not the intonation patterns or the ability to signal stress that was abnormal but abnormal phrase or poor selection of breath group units.

3. *Intonation and stress patterning within breath groups.* After the breath group units have been identified, then the assessment questions can turn to such issues as the accuracy and naturalness of stress patterning within a breath group. Typically habitual performance and modified performance are compared. The features associated with the most natural productions are identified and the speaker is trained to consistently use those features. In training for naturalness, a "normal" model is rarely used because suprasegmental fea-

tures used by normal speakers are so complex, and subtle and require such a high level of motor control that it may not be reasonable to expect such performances in dysarthric speakers. Rather than normalcy, the goal should be "the best possible speech."

4. *Generalization to spontaneous speech*. The final phase of intervention for individuals with prosodic disruption involves generalization of the strategies learned during highly structured tasks to more natural communication situations. Video-taped monologues are helpful during this generalization phase. Figure 9-7 contains a portion of the transcript from a mildly dysarthric TBI speaker. Before injury this individual had been a loan officer in a bank. Although his fund of information related to financial matters was excellent and his discourse organization adequate, his presentation style distracted from the overall quality. Terms such as *cluttered* and *too rapid* were used to describe his presentation. In the 32 samples contained in the figure, there were no occurrences of pauses without breaths. The speaker often took a breath at syntactically impermissible locations. He had the tendency to use fillers such as "uh" when he appeared to be formulating messages. Although his overall rate was 170 words per minute, his lack of appropriate pausing contributed to the perception of the unnaturalness of his speech. A careful review of the transcript also reveals that he made grammatical and word selection errors. Treatment focused on slowing his overall rate to 130 words per minute by encouraging him to use appropriate

Figure 9-7. A portion of the monologue produced by a mildly dysarthric traumatically brain injured speaker. [B] indicates that the speaker took a breath at this location.

Uh another term that you might find associated with a uh

[B] uh mortgage lending are C CD's or certificates of

deposit I'm sure you're all familiar with their uh them   [B]

it's you can buy them from any investment institution uh

you go down and give a [B] lump sum of money for a

stipulated period of time and you earn a uh [B] a yield on

that money it's fairly straight forward your investment up

to one hundred thousand is protected by the government

through the FDIC [B] uh so its a relatively again uh safe

instrument [B] uh along the line of money market funds

although a little differ in nature [B].. .

---

pauses to formulate his message. Slowing his rate not only reduced the perceptual of "clutteredness" but also appeared to reduce other grammatic and word selection error, presumably by giving him slightly more processing time. This case illustrates a situation in which clinical goals and practice behaviors were based on principle of motor speech production, but in effect the clinical process was directed as both cognitive-organizational and motor production aspects of speech.

Acknowledgment. This chapter was supported in part by Grant #133B80081 from the National Institute of Disability and Rehabilitation Research, Department of Education, Washington, DC.

REFERENCES

Aronson, A. (1980). *Clinical voice disorders: An interdisciplinary approach.* New York: Thieme-Stratton, Inc.

Barlow, S. M., and Abbs, J. H. (1983). Force transducers for the valuation of labial, lingual, and mandibular function in dysarthria. *Journal of Speech and Hearing Research, 26,* 616–621.

Bauer, B., Gerstenbrand, R., and Rump, E. (1979). Varieties of locked-in syndrome. *Journal of Neurology, 221,* 77–91.

Bellaire, K., Yorkston, K. M., and Beukelman, D. R. (1986). Modification of breath patterning to increase naturalness of a mildly dysarthric speaker. *Journal of Communication Disorders, 19,* 271–280.

Bettinghaus, M. C. (1980). International standards for a system of disability classification. Paper presented at the Annual Meeting of the American Psychological association, Montreal.

Beukelman, D.R., and Yorkston, K.M. (1977). A communication system for the severely dysarthric speaker with an intact language system. *Journal of Speech and Hearing Disorders, 42,* 265–270.

Beukelman, D., Yorkston, K., and Tice, R. (1988). *PACER/TALLY.* Tucson: Communication Skill Builders.

Bray, L., Carlson, F., Humphrey, R., Mastrilli, J., and Valko, A. (1987). Physical Rehabilitation. In M. Ylvisaker & E. Gobble (Eds.), *Community re-entry for head injured adults.* Boston: College-Hill Publication.

Collins, M., Rosenbek, J., and Donahue, E. (1982). The effects of posture on speech in ataxic dysarthria. *ASHA, 24,* 767.

Crow, E., and Enderby, P. (1989). The effects of an alphabet chart on the speaking rate and intelligibility of speakers with dysarthria. In K.M. Yorkston and D.R. Beukelman (Eds.), *Recent advances in dysarthria.* (pp. 99–108) Boston: College-Hill Press.

Daniel, B. (1982). A soft palate desensitization procedure for patients requiring palatal lift prostheses. *Journal of Prosthetic Dentistry, 48,* 565–566.

Darley, F.L. (1969). Aphasia: Input and output disturbances in speech and language processing. Paper presented in dual session on aphasia to the American Speech and Hearing Association, Chicago.

Darley, F., Aronson, A., and Brown, J. (1969). Differential diagnosis patterns of dysarthria. *Journal of Speech and Hearing Research, 12,* 246–269.

DeFeo, A., and Shaefer, C. (1983). Bilateral facial paralysis in a preschool child: Oral-facial and articulatory characteristics (a case study). In W. R. Berry (Ed.), *Clinical dysarthria.* Boston: College-Hill Press.

Dresser, A.C., Meirowsky, A.M., Weiss, G.H., McNeel, M.L., Simon, G.A., and Caveness, W.F. (1973). Gainful employment following head injury: Prognostic factors. *Archives of Neurology, 29*(2), 111–116.

Dworkin, J. P., and Johns, D. F. (1980). Management of velopharyngeal incompetence in dysarthria: A historical review. *Clinical Otolaryngology, 5,* 61–74.

Ewing-Cobbs, L., Fletcher, J.M., and Levin, H.S. (1986). Neurobehavorial sequelae following head injury in children: Educational implications. *Journal of Head Trauma Rehabilitation, 1* 57–65.

Folkins, J. W., and Kuehn, D. P. (1982). Speech production. In N. J. Lass, L. V. McReynolds, J. Northern, and D. Yoder (Eds.), *Speech, language and hearing* (Vol. 1). *Normal Processes.* Philadelphia: Saunders.

Froeschels, E. (1943). A contribution to pathology and therapy of dysarthria due to certain cerebral lesions. *Journal of Speech Disorders, 8,* 301–321.

Froeschels, E., Kastein, S., and Weiss, D. A. (1955). A method of therapy for paralytic conditions of the mechanisms of phonation, respiration, and glutination. *Journal of Speech and Hearing Disorders, 20,* 365–370.

Gonzales, J., and Aronson, A. (1970). Palatal lift prosthesis for treatment of anatomic and neurologic palatopharyngeal insufficiency. *Cleft Palate Journal, 7,* 91–104.

Grand H., Matsko, T., and Avart, H. (1988). Speech prosthesis retention problems in dysarthria: Case report. *Archives of Physical Medicine and Rehabilitation. 69,* 213–214.

Groher, M. (1977). Language and memory disorders following closed head trauma. *Journal of Speech and Hearing Research, 20,* 212.

Groher, M. (1983). Communication disorders. In M. Rosenthal, E. Griffith, M. Bond, & J.D. Miller (Eds.), *Rehabilitation of the head injured adult.* Philadelphia: Davis.

Hagen, C., Malkmus, D., and Durham, P. (1979). Levels of cognitive functioning. In *Rehabilitation of the Head Injured Adult: Comprehensive Physical Management.* Downey, CA: Professional Staff Association of Rancho Los Amigos Hospital, Inc.

Hardy, J. (1967). Suggestions for physiological research in dysarthria. *Cortex, 3,* 128–156.

Hardy, J. (1983). *Cerebral palsy.* Englewood Cliffs, NJ: Prentice-Hall.

Hirano, M., Koike, Y., and von Leden, H. (1968). Maximum phonation time and air usage during phonation. *Folia Phoniatrica, 20,* 185.

Hixon, T. (1973). Respiratory function in speech. In F. Minifie, T. Hixon, and F. Williams (Eds.), *Normal aspects of speech, hearing, and language* (pp. 73–126). Englewood Cliffs, NJ: Prentice-Hall.

Hixon, T. J. (1987). *Respiratory function in speech and song.* Boston: College-Hill Press.

Hixon, T. J., Mead, J., and Goldman, M. (1976). Dynamics of the chest wall during speech production: Function of the thorax, rib cage, diaphragm, and abdomen. *Journal of Speech and Hearing Disorders, 48,* 315–327.

Hixon, T., Hawley, J., and Wilson J. (1982). An around-the-house device for the clinical determination of respiratory driving pressure: A note on making simple even simpler. *Journal of Speech and Hearing Disorders, 47,* 413.

Hunker, C., Bless, D., and Weismer, G. (1981). Respiratory inductive plethysmography: A clinical technique for assessing respiratory function for speech. Paper presented at the Annual Convention of the American Speech-Language-Hearing Association, Los Angeles.

Jennet, W. B., and Plum, F. (1972). The persistent vegetative state: A syndrome in search of a name. *Lancet, 1,* 734.

Johns, D. (Ed.). (1985). *Clinical management of neurogenic communication disorders.* Boston: Little, Brown.

Kennedy, J.G., and Kent, R.D. (1985). Anatomy and physiology of deglutition and related functions. In J. Logemann (Ed.), *Seminars in speech and language.* (pp. 257–274). New York: Thieme-Stratton.

Kuehn, D. P. (1982). Assessment of resonance disorders. In N. Lass, L. McReynolds, J. Northern, and D. Yoder (Eds.), *Speech, language and hearing* (Vol. III). *Pathologies of speech and language.* Philadelphia: Saunders.

Larson, C. (1985). Neuro-physiology of speech and swallowing. In J. Logemann (Ed.), *Seminars in speech and language.* (pp. 275–290). New York: Thieme-Stratton.

Levin, H., Madison, C., Bailey, C., Meyer, C., Eisenberg, H., and Gunito, F. (1983). Mutism after closed head injury. *Archives of Neurology, 40,* 601–606.

Lewy, R., Cole, R., and Wepman, J. (1965). Teflon injection in the correction of velopharyngeal insufficiency. *Annuals of Otology, Rhinology, and Laryngology, 78,* 874.

Light, J., Beesley, M., and Collier, B. (1988). Transition through multiple augmentative communication systems: A three-year case study of a head injured adolescent. *Augmentative and Alternative Communication, 4,* 2–14.

McClean, M.D. (1988). Neuromotorspects of speech production and dysarthria. In K.M. Yorkston, D.R. Beukelman, & K.R. Bell (Eds.), *Clinical management of dysarthric speakers.* Boston: College-Hill Press.

Nagi, S. (1965). Some conceptual issues in disability and rehabilitation. In M. D. Sussman (Ed.), *Sociology and rehabilitation.* American Sociological Association in cooperation with the Vocational Rehabilitation Administration. Washington, DC: U.S. Department of Health, Education, and Welfare.

Nagi, S. (1969). *Disability and rehabilitation: Legal, clinical and self concepts and measurements.* Columbus: Ohio State University Press.

Nagi, S (1976). An epidemiology of disability among adults in the United States. In Health and Society. *Milback Memorial Fund Quarterly, 54,* 439–467.

Nagi S. (1977). The disabled and rehabilitation services: A national overview. *American Rehabilitation, 2,* 26–33.

Netsell, R. (1969). Subglottal and intraoral air pressures during the intervocalic contrast of /t/ and /d/. *Phonetica, 20,* 68–73.

Netsell, R., and Cleeland, C. (1973). Modification of lip hypotonia in dysarthria using EMG feedback. *Journal of Speech and Hearing Disorders, 40,* 170–178.

Netsell, R. and Daniel, B. (1979). Dysarthria in adults: Physiologic approach to rehabilitation. *Archives of Physical Medicine and Rehabilitation, 60,* 502–508.

Netsell, R. and Hixon, T., (1978). A noninvasive method for clinically estimating subglottal air pressure. *Journal of Speech and Hearing Disorders, 43,* 326–330.

Netsell, R., and Rosenbek, J. C. (1985). Treating the dysarthrias. In *Speech and language evaluation in neurology: Adult disorders.* New York: Grune & Stratton.

Netsell, R., Lotz, W., and Shaughnessy, A. L. (1984). Laryngeal aerodynamics associated with selected voice disorders. *American Journal of Otolaryngology, 5,* 397–403.

Netsell, R., Lotz, W., and Barlow, S. (1989). A speech physiology examination for individuals with dysarthria. In K.M. Yorkston & D.R. Beukelman (Eds.), *Recent advances in dysarthria*. Boston: College-Hill Press.

Plum, F., and Poser, J. (1980). *Diagnosis of stupor and coma* (ed. 3). Philadelphia: Davis.

Prator, R. J., and Swift, R. W. (1984). *Manual of voice therapy*. Boston: Little, Brown.

Putnam, A., and Hixon, T. J. (1984). Respiratory kinematics in speakers with motor neuron disease. In M. McNeil, J. Rosenbek, and A. Aronson (Eds.), *The dysarthrias*. Boston: College-Hill Press.

Rosenbek, J. (1985). Treating apraxia of speech. In D. Johns (Ed.), *Clinical management of neurogenic communicative disorders* (pp. 267–312). Boston: Little, Brown.

Rosenbek, J., Kent, R., and LaPointe, L. (1984). Apraxia of speech: An overview and some perspectives. In J. Rosenbek, M. McNeil, and A. Aronson (Eds.), *Apraxia of Speech: Physiology, Acoustics, Linquistics, Management.* (pp. 1–72). Boston: College Hill Press.

Rosenbek, J. C., and LaPointe, L. L. (1985). The dysarthrias: Description, diagnosis, and treatment. In D. F. Johns (Ed.), *Clinical management of neurogenic communication disorders*. Boston: Little, Brown.

Rusk, H., Block, J., and Lowman, E. (1969). Rehabilitation of the brain injured patient: A report of 157 cases with long term follow-up of 118. In E. Walker, W. Caveness, and M. Critchley (Eds.), *The late effects of head injury*. Springfield, IL: Charles C. Thomas.

Sapir, S., and Aronson, A. (1985). Aphonica after closed head injury: Aetiologic considerations. *British Journal of Disorders of Communication, 20,* 289–296.

Sarno, M., Buanaguro, A., and Levita, E. (1986). Characteristics of verbal impairment in closed head injured patients. *Archives of Physical Medicine and Rehabilitation, 67,* 400–405.

Simmons, N. (1983). Acoustic analysis of ataxic dysarthria: An approach to monitoring treatment. In W. Berry (Ed.), *Clinical dysarthria*. Boston: College-Hill Press.

Smitheran, J., and Hixon, T. (1981). A clinical method for estimating laryngeal airway resistance during vowel production. *Journal of Speech and Hearing Research, 46,* 138–146.

Thompsen, V. (1983). Standardized methods of assessing and predicting outcome. In M. Rosenthal, E. Griffith, M. Bond, and J. Mill (Eds.), *Rehabilitation of the head injured adult*. Philadelphia: Davis.

Von Cramon, D. (1981). Traumatic mutism and the subsequent reorganization of speech functions. *Neuropsychologia, 19,* 801–805.

Warren, D. W. (1975). The determination of velopharyngeal competence by aerodynamic and acoustic techniques. *Clinical Plastic Surgery, 2,* 299–304.

Weismer, G. (1985). Speech breathing: Contemporary views and findings. In R. Daniloff (Ed.), *Speech science: Recent advances*. San Diego: College-Hill Press.

Wertz, T. (1985). Neuropathologies of speech and language: An introduction to patient management. In D. Johns (Ed)., *Clinical management of neurogenic communicative disorders.* (pp. 1–96). Boston: Little Brown.

Wertz, R., LaPointe, L., and Rosenbek, J. (1984). *Apraxia of speech in adults: The disorder and its management*. New York: Grune & Stratton.

Wood, P. (1980). Appreciating the consequences of disease—the classification of impairments, disability, and handicaps. *The WHO Chronicle, 43,* 376–380.

Workinger, M., and Netsell, R. (1988). Restoration of intelligible speech 13 years post-head injury (in preparation).

Yanagihara, N., Koike, Y., and von Leden, H. (1966). Phonation and respiration: Function study in normal subjects. *Folia Phoniatrica, 18,* 323.

Yorkston, K.M. (1988). Prosody in the adult. In D. Yoder, and R. Kent (Eds.), *Decision making in speech-language pathology.* Toronto: Decker.

Yorkston, K., and Beukelman, D. (1981a). *Assessment of intelligibility of dysarthric speech.* Austin, TX: Pro-Ed.

Yorkston, K., and Beukelman, D. (1981b). Ataxic dysarthria: Treatment sequences based on intelligibility and prosodic considerations. *Journal of Speech and Hearing Disorders, 46,* 398–404.

Yorkston, K.M., Beukelman, D.R., and Bell, K.R. (1988a). *Clinical management of dysarthric speakers.* Boston: College-Hill Press.

Yorkston, K.M., Beukelman, D.R., Honsinger, M.J., and Mitsuda, P.M. (1989a). Perceived articulatory adequacy and velopharyngeal function in dysarthric speakers. *Archives of Physical Medicine and Rehabilitation 70,* 313–317.

Yorkston, K.M., Beukelman D.R., and Traynor, C.D. (1984). *Computerized assessment of intelligibility of dysarthric speech.* Austin TX: Pro-Ed.

Yorkston, K., Beukelman, D., Minifie, F., and Sapir, S. (1984). Assessment of stress patterning in dysarthric speakers. In M. McNeil, A. Aronson, and J. Rosenbek, (Eds.). *The dysarthrias: Physiology, acoustics, perception, management.* Boston: College-Hill Press.

Yorkston, K.M., Beukelman, D.R., and Traynor, C.D. (1988b). Articulatory adequacy in dysarthric speakers: A comparison of judging formats. *Journal of Communication Disorders, 21,* 351–361.

Yorkston, K. M., Dowden, P. A., Beukelman, D. R., and Traynor, C. D. (1986). *A phoneme identification task as a measure of perceived articulatory adequacy.* Paper presented at the third biennial Clinical Dysarthria Conference, Tucson, AZ.

Yorkston, K.M., Honsinger, M.J., Beukelman, D.R., and Taylor, T.D. (1989b). The effects of palatal lift fitting on the perceived articulatory adequacy of dysarthric speakers. In K.M. Yorkston and D.R. Beukelman (Eds.), *Recent advances in dysarthria* (pp. 85–98). Boston: College-Hill Press.

Yorkston, K.M., Honsinger, M.J., Mitsuda, P.M., and Hammen, V. (1989c). The relationship between speech and swallowing disorders in head injured patients. J. Logemann (Ed.), *Journal of Head Trauma Rehabilitation* 4(4), 1–16.

CHAPTER 10

*Augmentative Communication
Following Traumatic Brain Injury*

FRANK DERUYTER
MARY R. T. KENNEDY

Because the patient can only answer simple questions and respond to simple commands, I do not feel that he has the ability to communicate effectively and subsequently cannot do testing or recommend treatment.

Nonspeaking TBI Patient
Medical Record (1987)

Over the past few years, many clinicians have become skilled in the areas of brain injury and augmentative communication. However, working with the individual who is both nonspeaking and brain injured creates havoc for many. Statements like the one above are repeatedly entered into the medical records and reports of nonspeaking traumatic brain–injured (TBI) individuals by clinicians who are to serve them. The difficulty in working with this particular population is not unique to speech-language pathologists but encompasses numerous other professionals, including neuropsychologists, occupational therapists, ophthalmologists, physiatrists, physical therapists, and psychologists. As a result, the assessment and management of nonspeaking TBI individuals is frequently compromised due to the limited knowledge base on the part of clinicians.

This chapter will assist the clinician in becoming proficient at decision making and management of nonspeaking TBI individuals. Specifically, this chapter will focus on three specific issues: (1) identifying TBI nonspeaking individuals and their communication needs and capabilities at various cognitive levels, (2) assessing what can be done for these nonspeaking TBI individuals, and (3) providing the necessary services to these individuals.

IDENTIFICATION OF THE NONSPEAKING POPULATION WITH TRAUMATIC BRAIN INJURY

NONSPEAKING POPULATION AT LARGE

Until recently, the demographic information on the nonspeaking population reflected data about the school-aged individual (Bureau of Education for the Handicapped, 1976; Aiello, 1980; Matas and colleagues, 1985). These reports, although useful, provided only limited information about the nonspeaking population at large. In 1985, in an attempt to describe further the demographic and clinical characteristics of the nonspeaking population, a database study presented information on 200 successive nonspeaking individuals with various etiologies (DeRuyter and Lafontaine, 1985). This report was based on nonspeaking individuals seen in the Augmentative Communication Center at Rancho Los Amigos Medical Center between September 1983 and June 1985. A team approach (speech-

Table 10-1. Categorization of nonspeaking
individuals by primary medical diagnosis

Primary medical diagnosis	N = 200	
	Number	Percent
Brain injury	63	31.5
Cerebral palsy	66	33.0
Cerebral vascular accident	33	16.5
Progressive neuromuscular disease	27	13.5
Other	11	5.5
Total	200	100.0

Source: DeRuyter, F., and Lafontaine, L.M. (1985). *Relational data-base report of the nonspeaking population.* Paper presented to the American Speech-Language-Hearing Association, Washington, DC.

language pathologist, occupational and physical therapists, and rehabilitation engineer) was used. All 200 nonspeaking individuals participated in a five-phase assessment and management program that consisted of (1) referral and screening, (2) communication and functional assessment, (3) system selection, (4) system management and training, and, (5) followup. These nonspeaking individuals were then classified into one of five primary medical diagnostic categories: brain injury, cerebral palsy, progressive neuromuscular disease, stroke, or other. The percentage of nonspeaking individuals in each category is displayed in Table 10-1. Of particular interest to this chapter will be the findings related to the 31.5 percent (n=63) of the population sample that included the nonspeaking brain injured.

NONSPEAKING BRAIN INJURED

Immediately following TBI, the severely injured individual's need to communicate is usually minimal or nonexistent. As vital functions stabilize, communication assumes greater importance. However, because of the nature of TBI, the resultant communication disorder greatly compromises the individual's expressive communicative ability. It is generally accepted that following TBI the communicative disorder as well as the amount and rate of communicative recovery may assume a variety of types and combinations (Hagen, 1984). These depend predominantly on the nature of the lesion and any associated premorbid factors. The types of injury vary greatly and range from generalized to focal, temporary to permanent, shearing of neuronal axons, to swelling of brain tissue. Premorbid factors, on the other hand, may include aspects such as psychological status, presence of learning disabilities, and cultural differences.

It is because of the nature of the lesion and the associated premorbid factors that the resultant communicative disorders can include general cognitive-language disorganization, specific language disorders, motor speech disorders, and hearing impairment. Specific reference to the types and combinations of injury as well as to associated premorbid factors are well documented throughout the literature and elsewhere in this text (see Chapt. 2). There are instances, however, when the severity of the communicative disorder is great enough that communication recovery is not possible without some method of either temporary or permanent communication augmentation. Fortunately, the increased awareness and knowledge base within the area of brain injury as well as the explosion of technologic advances in augmentative communication have dramatically expanded the options available to augment expressive communication for nonspeaking TBI individuals.

Demographic Characteristics

Just as there have been no demographic studies that have identified the incidence, prevalence, or recovery patterns of severe speaking and writing impairments following TBI, the percentage or estimates of the TBI individuals who are nonspeaking is not known. The information available about the TBI nonspeaking individual is based on the larger database report mentioned earlier (DeRuyter and LaFontaine, 1985). Of 200 nonspeaking individuals included in that report, persons with brain injury made up 31.4 percent (n=63) of the database sample population. Categorizing these 63 nonspeaking brain-injured individuals according to their type of injury, it was noted that 68.3 percent (n=43) of the injuries were the result of traumatic closed head injuries, 22.2 percent (n=14) were due to global brain injuries such as anoxia and infections, and 9.5 percent (n=6) resulted from traumatic open head injuries that penetrated the dura (DeRuyter and Lafontaine, 1987).

An important observation in the database report was the remarkable similarity of the demographic characteristics of the nonspeaking TBI individuals to those noted with the TBI population at large (Anderson and McLaurin, 1980; Annegers and colleagues, 1980; Jennett and Mac-Millan, 1981; Levin and colleagues, 1982). As illustrated in Table 10-2, males accounted for almost 70 percent of the nonspeaking brain-injured population sample, which is consistent with the male to female ratio in TBI demographic investigations at large. Their age ranged from 6 years to 61 years, with the mean age noted at 24.8 years. Males exhibited a slightly lower mean age than females, which, along with the reported age range distribution for the population sample, is very similar to that reported in the literature for the TBI population at large. Further information from the database report will be presented throughout this chapter as it applies to the relevant sections.

**Table 10-2. Sex distribution and age characteristics
of nonspeaking individuals with traumatic brain injury**

Sex	Number	Percentage	Age range	Mean age
Males	44	69.8	6–47	23.7
Females	19	30.2	7–61	27.3
Total	63	100.0	6–61	24.8

Source: DeRuyter, F., and Lafontaine, L.M. (1987). The nonspeaking brain-injured: A clinical and demographic database report. *Augmentative and Alternative Communication, 3,* 18–25.

Communicative Needs

Identifying communication needs in the nonspeaking population has recently been reviewed (Light, 1988); however the communicative needs of the nonspeaking TBI individual have been largely ignored. To date, assessments of nonspeaking individuals' communication needs, irrespective of etiology, have only emphasized the surface structure of the interactions and the nature of the messages required. The nonspeaking are typically provided with augmentative systems that allow them to communicate needs and wants for items that they are often already able to indicate through some other means or by limited interaction. Augmentative systems usually include vocabulary that encourages some form of socialization, although observation of functional usage is rare because the individuals using the system primarily occupy a respondent role in their interactions.

It has been suggested that interaction for communicative needs might be better considered by examining the broader agendas or social purposes for an individual's interactions (Light, 1988). The expression of needs and wants, information transfer, social closeness, and social etiquette are all purposes or agenda that are fulfilled within any communicative interaction. The nature and importance of these characteristics of communicative interaction also appear to vary across an individual's life span (Beukelman, 1987). By the same token, it would be reasonable to assume that the importance of these characteristics also varies among the etiologies of various nonspeaking individuals, including the nonspeaking TBI.

The authors recently began to address the issues of the nonspeaking TBI individual's communication interaction needs by comparing adult interactive needs with those of the nonspeaking TBI client functioning at various stages on the Rancho Los Amigos Medical Center Levels of Cognitive Functioning Scale (LOCF) (Hagen and colleagues, 1979). As illustrated in Table 10-3, one notes specific differences when comparing

Table 10-3. Anticipated interactive needs: The normal adult compared with each cognitive level in nonspeaking individuals with traumatic brain injury

Interaction purposes	Cognitive level						
	Adult	*III*	*IV*	*V*	*VI*	*VII*	*VIII*
Wants and needs	−	−/+	−/+	−/+	+	+/−	−
Sharing information	+	−	−	−/+	−/+	+	+
Social closeness	+	−	−	−	−/+	+	+
Social etiquette	+	−	−	−	−/+	−/+	+

− = low need; + = high need; −/+ = emerging need; +/− = decreasing need

Source: DeRuyter, F., Becker, M.R., and Doyle, M. (1987). *Assessment and intervention strategies for the nonspeaking brain injured.* Short courses presented to the American Speech-Language-Hearing Association, New Orleans.

the anticipated interactive needs for a normal adult with those that would be expected of the TBI individual at each LOCF. By acknowledging the different interactive needs for the nonspeaking TBI individual at each cognitive level, clinicians are provided with a guideline in the various selection dilemmas they are faced with when choosing such things as an appropriate augmentative system, vocabulary, and intervention strategies. This enhances goal setting and treatment interventions as they relate to the specific rehabilitation program and beyond. The interactive needs focus also allows clinicians to expand on the traditional methods from which they have operated in the past.

To discuss the nonspeaking TBI population adequately, clinicians must understand that most communication deficits that exist in the speaking TBI population are also noted in the nonspeaking TBI individual. As such, the assessment and management of these individuals is similar to that of the speaking TBI population. However, with the nonspeaking TBI population, the assessment and recovery processes are typically slower because the injury is usually more severe. Before addressing how to evaluate and manage, it is worthy to indicate the ways that the nonspeaking TBI individual can benefit from services.

WHAT CAN BE DONE FOR THE NONSPEAKING POPULATION WITH TRAUMATIC BRAIN INJURY

SYSTEMS ACCORDING TO COGNITIVE LEVEL

In a recent retrospective study of nonspeaking TBI individuals, the authors demonstrated that there is a direct relationship between the LOCF and the primary type of augmentative system selected and used. Records were examined on nonspeaking TBI individuals functioning from LOCF II through LOCF VIII. The findings revealed that augmentative systems were provided in a hierarchy in which the lower the LOCF, the more basic the system selected. Specifically, yes or no as a primary system may be used as early as LOCF III; however its use as a primary system decreases as cognitive level increases. Communication boards can be introduced as early as LOCF V but do not become primary systems until LOCF VI. Dedicated devices (such as the Canon, Casio, or SpeechPac), that are used to perform a predesignated function and serve a specific purpose such as communication, may be introduced at LOCF VI but do not become primary systems until LOCF VII. Finally, multipurpose systems (such as the LightTalker, Equalizer II, or Scanwriter), which are designed to change functions easily and serve a variety of purposes such as communicative, educational, vocational, and recreational, are usually not introduced until LOCF VII. How these systems are best introduced, used, and modified in the treatment regimen is a question that can be addressed by examining the nonspeakers' interactive needs.

SYSTEMS ACCORDING TO INTERACTIVE NEEDS

As mentioned earlier, it has been suggested that interaction for communicative needs appears to vary across an individual's life span and can be examined through the expression of needs and wants, information transfer, social closeness, and social etiquette (Beukelman, 1987; Light, 1988). These are all purposes or agendas that are fulfilled within any communicative interaction.

The importance of these characteristics appears to vary among the various nonspeaking etiologies. This has been illustrated by the authors in Table 10-3, which compares the adults' interactive needs to those of the nonspeaking TBI at each LOCF. It is important for clinicians to examine the communicative interaction categories in this manner to expand on the traditional methods of system selection and usage in addition to determining whether the system will be used for assessment, communication, rehabilitation, integration into the outside environment, or a combination of these. As a result, nonspeaking TBI individuals are less likely to be set up for failure because the selection and intervention process takes into account their unique interactive needs according to their cognitive status. This has implications for professionals when they are faced with clinical dilemmas such as choosing an appropriate augmentative system, vocabulary, or intervention strategies. To demonstrate this concept further, one can examine its applicability to two different nonspeaking TBI individuals.

In examining a LOCF V to VI TBI individual (see Table 10-3), one notes emerging but inconsistent communicative interaction needs in all four categories. Typically, due to their cognitive impairments, these TBI individuals are more concerned about self-comfort and self-needs rather than including others into the communication process through social closeness or etiquette. When asked to assist in vocabulary selection, these individuals have difficulty indicating what they need, and clinicians often end up eliminating many choices because they are inappropriate. On the other hand, examining a LOCF VII to VIII TBI individual, one observes communicative interaction needs that begin to exhibit similarities to those of the normal speaking adult. These individuals are beginning to exhibit less egocentricity and typically request specific vocabulary for their systems. They are also beginning to realize the need and potential of their augmentative system through the sharing of information and obtaining social closeness. As such, the focus of system use is very different than that for the lower LOCF individual.

A note of caution for the clinician when using Table 10-3. Cognitively, the table reflects those behaviors that individuals can do. Because of the type of injury, the individual's impaired flexibility of thought, or changing cognitive status, some individuals may still have difficulty with specific behaviors (tasks) in various communicative settings or situations. In addition, the severe physical involvement in some individuals may require additional communicative need categories not included in Table 10-3. The table therefore demonstrates a "trend" in recovery of interaction abilities rather than distinctive behaviors at each cognitive level. Nevertheless, it is important for clinicians to consider the nonspeaking TBI individuals' communicative needs during the assessment, selection, establishment, and training of augmentative systems.

INFLUENCE OF COGNITION ON SYSTEMS

The authors have observed that frequently nonspeaking TBI individuals who are referred for reassessment appear with multiple primary systems rather than a primary and a backup system, as would typically be provided to other types of nonspeakers. Individuals at the higher LOCF, who are more than 1 year after injury, are often observed with three and four different systems that they are trying to use simultaneously for communicative purposes. These systems are usually less than optimal and typically do not meet the individuals' communicative needs. On occasion this has occurred because the nonspeaking individual was unwilling to incorporate an existing system into a new system when modifications were made. More often than not, however, clinicians appeared unable to provide for an optimal system. This was supported by a recent survey that asked speech-language pathologists, who had provided augmentative services to the nonspeaking TBI for at least 2 years, what they perceived as the primary followup problem in the provision of their services (DeRuyter and colleagues, 1989). It was reported by 82 percent (n=23) of the respondents that the lack of available qualified personnel to upgrade systems and to provide the necessary followup services was the primary and most frequent problem encountered. A total of 64 percent (n=18) specifically indicated that clinicians appear to lack an understanding of the influence of cognition on system selection and training.

The authors have long hypothesized that performance on various cognitive-language processes influences system selection in the nonspeaking TBI population. However, it is only recently that the relationship between cognitive-language and behavioral deficits, and how they relate to system selection and usage, has been documented (DeRuyter and Becker, 1988). For that reason, the processes and behaviors manifested by the nonspeaker should be understood as completely as possible before the system is selected.

INVOLVING NONSPEAKING INDIVIDUALS WITH TRAUMATIC BRAIN INJURY IN DECISIONS

Traditionally, nonspeakers have been included in the system selection decision-making process. However, with nonspeaking TBI individuals, it is recommended that the system selection decision be made without the individuals' input, except in those instances where the nonspeaker is functioning at the higher LOCF (VII or VIII). This is primarily due to the lack of insight on the TBI individual's part until this cognitive level is reached. The severely cognitively impaired nonspeaking TBI individual often is not capable of making an appropriate system selection because the future implications of system usage cannot be fully understood. It has been our clinical experience that when TBI individuals, at the lower cognitive levels, are included in the selection process, they usually opt for inappropriate systems that are too basic and serve no real purpose in the communication and cognitive-language recovery process.

Excluding the low LOCF nonspeaking individual from the system selection process may be a difficult concept for some clinicians to accept. However, it is important to remember that TBI individuals do not view themselves as being any different from their premorbid status despite their communication problem. As one nonspeaking TBI individual indicated: "with an alphabet board I never have to change or program anything and I don't have 'another thing' to carry around or worry about." This is quite contrary to many cognitively intact nonspeaking cerebral palsied individuals, who often prefer high-technology, multipurpose augmentative systems.

It should become obvious that nonspeaking TBI individuals can benefit from the delivery of augmentative services. The issues confronting the clinician at this stage are how to go about the assessment, system selection, and management of these individuals.

HOW TO PROVIDE THE NECESSARY SERVICES

Before discussing specific assessment, system selection, and intervention strategies, it is important to discuss the service delivery philosophy that the author's work follows, important factors in TBI, and some special issues that are considered unique to this specific nonspeaking population.

SERVICE DELIVERY PHILOSOPHY

Assessment of and intervention with the TBI individual may be based on "behavioral" and "process" models. Strategies for the assessment of cognitive-language functions are traditionally based on the premise that language is a behavioral product subserved by cognitive functioning (Hagen, 1984; Adamovich and colleagues, 1985). However, a process approach through the use of task analysis allows the examiner to define accurately the underlying cause for the communicative breakdown. This is described in significantly greater detail in Chapter 7 as well as documented throughout the speech-language pathology and psychology-neuropsychology literature.

Specific to the augmentative field are three primary intervention models. These have been referred to as the communication processes model, the communication participation model, and the communication needs model. The reader is referred to the following reference for further discussion of these models (Beukelman and Garrett, 1988). The communication needs model has undergone numerous additions over the past few years, but it continues to remain the most appropriate for adults with acquired severe communication disorders, including the nonspeaking TBI population. Components of this model are used by the authors.

In recent years, application of the process assessment model within the rehabilitation setting has been supplemented with a "functional" or needs component. This allows the assessment process, within this functional component, to examine performance by an individual on various activities within the environment (Beukelman and colleagues, 1984). The functional component to the assessment process may be viewed in two ways. The first is the "capability-need evaluation," which analyzes an individual's cognitive-language, physical, and visuoperceptual needs in a variety of settings and environments. The other aspect is the "performance evaluation," which measures and analyzes the performance of an individual in a variety of settings and environments that may be either natural or simulated (Beukelman and Yorkston, 1980). Recently it was suggested that these two components allow clinicians to assess along three parallel lines: communication needs, residual capabilities, and external constraints. (Beukelman and Garrett, 1988). These three areas have particular importance in assessment of an intervention with the nonspeaking TBI individual.

Clinicians must give serious consideration to the type of service delivery model used with the nonspeaking TBI population. Of importance is how the delivery of augmentative services to the TBI population differs from the provision of services to nonspeaking individuals with other disorders. Clearly, the needs of the nonspeaking TBI individual differ from the needs of an individual who is nonspeaking because of a congenital condition or progressive neurologic disease. As such, the service delivery models used for each etiology differ. However, the services to the TBI population are provided in a wide variety of settings that can include acute care medical centers, rehabilitation hospitals, transitional living centers, outpatient clinics, home health agencies, and skilled nursing facilities. In each of these settings, the nonspeaking TBI individual will be at varying stages of recovery and have different augmentative communication needs. Consequently, one must consider whether services to these individuals should be delivered from a center-based or a community-based program. Unfortunately, it still must be determined which type of program is more effective for the various types of settings in which nonspeaking TBI individuals may be encountered

IMPORTANT FACTORS IN TRAUMATIC BRAIN INJURY

It has been well documented and agreed on that cognitive, memory, and linguistic deficits result from TBI. Specific cognitive deficits identified as being present in diffuse TBI have included (1) impaired arousal and attention (vigilance, selective attention, and attention span); (2) delayed and disordered information processing; (3) thought disorganization; (4) disorders of sequential analysis and problem solving; (5) disorders of memory (particularly storage and retrieval of new information); (6) impaired mental shifting; (7) slowing of motor responses; and (8) impaired reasoning and integration (Ben-Yishay and colleagues, 1979; Levin and colleagues, 1982; Hagen, 1984; Meyer, 1984; Prigatano and colleagues, 1984). As a result of these cognitive deficits, behaviors such as (1) disorientation and confusion, (2) confabulation, (3) poor concentration, (4) disorganized verbal and nonverbal behavior, (5) reduced learning potential, (6) reduced initiation or inhibition, (7) poor mental shifting, (8) incompleteness of thought and activity, and (9) poor reasoning and problem solving have all become associated with TBI (Luria, 1973; Malkmus, 1980; Cummings, 1985). Which behaviors remain impaired, which behaviors resolve, and the rate at which they resolve depends largely on the individual's premorbid personality, the extent of injury, and the type of injury. This is true irrespective of speaking status.

Language disorders commonly associated with TBI (with or without cognitive disruption) include impaired word fluency and retrieval, delayed auditory processing and comprehension (associated with temporal lobe contusions), dysnomia, and mild aphasia (including reading and writing impairments) (Heilman and colleagues, 1971; Thomsen, 1975; Groher, 1977; Levin and colleagues, 1979). In addition to these disorders, pragmatic disturbances have been identified as a long-term behavioral residual following TBI. These disturbances often contribute and lead to social isolation that can include the loss of friends and family as well as difficulties in returning to school or work (Kodimer and Styzens, 1980; Jacobs, 1984). All these disorders compound the problem of nonspeaking for the TBI individual.

Motor speech impairments associated with TBI can be correlated with the locus of injury. However, because of the sensory deficits and cognitive disruption in the individual with TBI, it is often difficult to assess the motor speech processes (Becker and Malkmus, 1982). Although verbal apraxias are infrequent, it has been reported that all closed-head-injured individuals continue to demonstrate some type of verbal impairment 1 year after injury and that one third of the individuals who were in a coma lasting anywhere from 15 minutes to 6 months exhibited dysarthric speech (Sarno, 1980, 1984). The types of dysarthria have not been reported. Other observed "speech" disorders, such as echolalia, pallalia, whispered speech, and dysprosody, appear to be associated with reductions in self-monitoring and delayed auditory processing rather than with disorders of the motor speech system (Hagen and colleages, 1979; Ross, 1981; Adamovich and colleagues, 1985). Given the lack of data identifying the types of dysarthrias or the rate of pattern of recovery following TBI, assessment and management of the nonspeaking TBI individual becomes even more complicated.

In recent years, research efforts in TBI have focused on identifying cognitive and linguistic predictors for long-term recovery (Levin and colleagues, 1979; Roberts, 1980; Levin and colleagues, 1982; Brooks and colleagues, 1986). Various behavioral measures have been suggested for use during the acute medical and rehabilitation recovery phases as predictors of overall recovery outcome. Neuropsychological and linguistic assessment batteries have been administered at various intervals of recovery, resulting in a wealth of "possible" outcome predictors. Rating scales have been included in the assessment process because they provide a common referent vocabulary, view behavior in an organized manner, and provide baseline behavioral information to evaluate progress. In addition to serving as outcome predictors, many of these behavioral measures have become useful for treatment planning and behavioral research on therapy effectiveness. Even though predictors of recovery have proved helpful, caution must be taken in generalizing the conclusions. This is especially so when the complication of a motor speech impairment or nonspeakingness is present, for which very little long-term information is currently available.

SPECIAL ISSUES RELATED TO THE NONSPEAKING POPULATION WITH TRAUMATIC BRAIN INJURY

Several issues unique to the nonspeaking TBI individual must be understood by clinicians before they address assessment, system selection, and intervention issues. These issues include professional involvement, reimbursement for services, funding for augmentative systems, and long-term outcomes and ethics.

Professional Involvement

There should be no doubt that providing services to the TBI and nonspeaking populations necessitates some degree of specialization on the part of clinicians. Traditionally, services provided to these populations have consisted of multidisciplinary or, in some instances, interdisciplinary team approaches. However, given the uniqueness of nonspeaking TBI individuals and the various needs these individuals have within the different types of clinical settings, the level and type of professional involvement in the assessment and intervention process must be considered. It has been suggested that professional involvement be considered at one of three levels (Yorkston and Karlan, 1986). First is the primary level, where the professional serves as a generalist who provides basic brain injury and augmentative services. A secondary level exists, whereby the professional serves as a specialist working specifically with the nonspeaking TBI population. The third level is a tertiary level, whereby services are provided by a highly specialized team serving in a resource capacity at a major augmentative center. In each instance, the service delivery model and the patient setting will dictate the level of professional involvement required.

Reimbursement for Services

A major concern must be the allocation of resources for reimbursement of services. As health care funding continues to shrink and reimbursement for rehabilitation appears to be changing to a prospective payment or managed care system, one must be concerned about how the delivery of services to the nonspeaking TBI population will be affected. Clinicians must begin concerning themselves with how and whether they are going to be reimbursed for providing augmentative services in the future. With so much of the assessment and management of the TBI population being done at an interdisciplinary level, agencies are likely to begin questioning multiple-discipline reimbursement for cognitive-language services. One must only ask under which heading is nonspeaking reimbursement going to be considered, especially in light of present health care reimbursement issues. Clinicians must remain proactive in the reimbursement process and educate third-party intermediaries about the importance of the services.

Funding for Augmentative Systems

In addition to concern about reimbursement for services provided, it is equally important for clinicians to be concerned about how the actual augmentative systems for these individuals are going to be funded. Despite the improvements in system selection criteria, clinicians continue to experience tremendous difficulty in the funding of systems. It has been documented that approximately 75 percent of the devices and systems recommended for TBI individuals are funded (Beukelman and colleagues, 1985; DeRuyter and Lafontaine, 1987). Closer examination of these data, however, indicate that in many instances funding came from sources other than third-party payers. In one report, only 25 percent of the systems were actually funded by these sources, with the majority purchased by families (DeRuyter and Lafontaine, 1987). This should alarm clinicians, since the value of the services provided to the nonspeaker has increased; however, the funding for systems has decreased. Consequently, there exists a gap between what clinicians are able to do and who will be funded.

Long-Term Outcomes and Ethics

The final consideration revolves around the issues of outcome and ethics. Although it has been demonstrated that the provision of augmentative services appears to enhance the nonspeaking TBI individual's abilities, little data to support this contention exists. Clinical observation can demonstrate that augmentative systems are beneficial and assist individuals in the treatment process; however, long-term outcomes and the benefits of systems have not been documented. Initial data from a preliminary followup study that the authors have completed on 25 nonspeaking TBI individuals who received their systems between 1983 and 1985 reveals that only 56 percent of the nonspeakers were actually using their systems in the manner for which they were designed 1 year after discharge from the augmentative program. Of those not using their systems, 24 percent had totally discarded their systems and the remaining 20 percent were only using their systems in certain environments (e.g., outpatient therapy).

Although many advances in assessment and management have occurred over the past 5 years, clinicians must remember that there are members of the TBI population who may never return to society as functional members. With the changes in health care reimbursement, clinicians must be prepared to answer whether the expenses associated with the nonspeaker justify the benefits. This will require accurate documentation regarding the assessment and provision of augmentative services as well as the outcomes.

Assessment

The primary objective of the assessment process is to gather as much information as possible on which to base system selection and intervention decisions. For the TBI individual, this includes determining the individual's overall communicative and physical needs. Because technology has allowed for the compensation of many severe physical problems, it is the cognitive-language problems that interfere the most when the clinician attempts to evaluate and determine a nonspeaking TBI individual's success with an augmentative system. Therefore, assessment should be viewed as an ongoing process, in which "assessment triggers or critical decision-making points" occur as the individual's communicative and physical needs change (Yorkston and Karlan, 1986). This is particularly true for nonspeaking TBI individuals because their recovery process varies so greatly.

To ensure that the most appropriate augmentative system is selected and modified as recovery occurs, ongoing evaluation of cognition, language structures and use, behavior, positioning, motor access site, and visual abilities is necessary. As such, assessment can be divided into communication and physical evaluation areas.

Communication Evaluation

Strategies to assess communicative function in the TBI population have been well documented (Hagen, 1984; Adamovich and colleagues, 1985). However, the assessment procedures for the nonspeaking TBI population are not clearly delineated in the literature and are at times seemingly random (DeRuyter and colleagues, 1988). Assessment of cognitive-language functioning within the TBI population can be problematic for clinicians and is compounded by a number of factors. First, the clinician must identify the cognitive-language deficits and their underlying causes. Second, he or she must determine how the deficits will influence the selection and use of an augmentative system. Finally, the individual's cognitive-language status must be reevaluated during system use in an effort to obtain more detailed information about the deficits.

Assessment of the communication processes in the nonspeaking TBI individual should include four specific areas: cognition, language, motor speech, and symbol system. The difficulty that clinicians experience in assessing nonspeaking TBI individuals was illustrated in the previously mentioned database study, which revealed that over 90 percent of the nonspeaking population with brain injury, who had received thorough communicative assessments and were referred to our center for further assessment, required further evaluation in at least three of the four areas mentioned above (DeRuyter and Lafontaine, 1987). The specific processes most frequently requiring additional assessment included memory, sequencing, reading, writing, and symbol system selection. This finding is further supported by a recent study that indicated that 64 percent (n=18) of the clinicians surveyed consider cognitive-language functioning the most difficult area to evaluate (DeRuyter and colleagues, 1989).

Basic Considerations and Underlying Issues

With the nonspeaking TBI population, several issues directly affect the information obtained in the assessment process. These issues will have an impact on system selection and management of the nonspeaking individual. They include population factors, interdisciplinary roles, test instrumentation, nonspeaking status and system, and the potential for speech. On careful consideration of these basic underlying issues, the clinician should be able to address communicative function within the nonspeaking TBI individual.

Population Factors. It has been well documented that various types of brain injury result in a great variety of specific impairments. When the variable of speaking status is added, a number of factors will influence the assessment process. The primary factor is the recovery pattern. The nonspeaking TBI individual usually represents the more severely injured population and is often included in the slow-to-recover category. As such, tremendous variability in recovery is observed within the nonspeaking TBI population. These variations are noted in terms of the performance and recovery of cognitive-language functioning. Because it is not always possible to depend on the TBI individual's cooperation during the recovery process, clinicians experience even greater fluctuations in performance when working with the nonspeaking TBI individual. In addition to the varied types of injury and recovery patterns, other issues are unique to the TBI population. These include premorbid factors such as behavioral problems, learning disabilities, and cultural differences. All can have a significant impact on the assessment process and the results obtained.

Interdisciplinary Roles. A second underlying issue is the specific role of the speech-language pathologist in providing services to the TBI population. In the past, the speech-language pathologist's role in the delivery of services to the neurogenically disordered population was well accepted. However, as the delivery of services has expanded, it has required other professionals once again to expand their view of the speech-language pathologist's professional role. This has been especially noticeable in the areas of augmentation, cognition, and pragmatics. Sensitivity to professional roles must obviously be demonstrated, but not at the expense of high-quality service delivery. A variety of service delivery models exist in which the roles of interdisciplinary team members vary greatly. It is important when interdisciplinary service delivery models are used that professional roles are clearly delineated so that team building, communication, and good working relationships can be established and maintained.

Test Instrumentation. In many instances, the assessment tools that have been used with the TBI population are traditional instruments. Many of these tools were standardized on patient populations other than TBI individuals and are based on categorical disturbances that tend to isolate communication, especially language, into component parts. As a result, this has led to inaccurate as well as inappropriate assessments of the TBI population, since some individuals perform normally on tests even though they have difficulty organizing and using language concepts (Becker and Malkmus, 1982). This assessment problem is compounded when the TBI individual is nonspeaking and the completeness of test responses may be severely abbreviated.

As with other types of nonspeaking individuals, an assortment of assessment tools is often used when clinicians evaluate the nonspeaking TBI individual. These tools consist of rating scales, standardized tests, nonstandardized procedures, and observational information, all of which will be discussed in more detail later in this chapter. However, an important consideration with the nonspeaking TBI individual, compared with other nonspeaking individuals, is that the specific tools used will vary according to factors unique to the TBI population. These include the individual's stability with respect to cognitive recovery, ability to cooperate, and communicative needs. As a result, the clinician must be sensitive to these factors, since they do influence the assessment variables that ultimately assist in the system selection process.

Nonspeaking Status and System. The nonspeaking TBI individual can be categorized as either a temporary or permanent augmentative communication system user, depending on the individual's communicative needs at any given time (DeRuyter and Lafontaine, 1987). Temporary users are those who require systems for short periods during the initial recovery and rehabilitation phase. Individuals who require systems beyond the initial assessment or treatment regimen, including those who appear to require a system for the rest of their lives, are usually categorized as permanent system users. Although early determination of nonspeaking status would greatly assist in the system selection process and any subsequent management, caution must be used in labeling the status of the nonspeaking TBI individual. This is due to the variety of settings in which nonspeaking TBI individuals are found, the general lack of knowledge on how many brain-injured persons are nonspeaking, and the lack of information regarding recovery patterns following brain injury. Clinicians should be encouraged to focus on areas other than nonspeaking status or type of system with the nonspeaking TBI population. As a general rule, all individuals should be considered temporarily nonspeaking and simply in need of temporary systems.

The importance of the above statement is realized as one follows the sequence of events of the nonspeaking TBI individual. Immediately following TBI, medical care is focused on obtaining and maintaining vital cardiopulmonary and neurologic functions. During this time, a severely injured individual's need to communicate is minimal or even nonexistent. As cardiopulmonary and neurologic functions stabilize, the need to communicate begins to assume a greater importance. This, of course, depends somewhat on the individual's cognitive status. At this early stage, temporary augmentative systems can be explored and provided when they are appropriate. Depending on the individual's cognitive status, these temporary systems can in some instances be used to communicate basic needs, wants, and desires that are essential for appropriate care (Beukelman and Yorkston, 1982). More important, these temporary systems can be developed to assist in assessing cognitive-language status (DeRuyter and Becker, 1988). Following the cognitive-language assessment process, the temporary systems can assist the individual in becoming an active participant in the rehabilitation program.

Frequently, the nature of the recovery pattern is such that one can capitalize on the individual's verbal output abilities and phase out a temporary system at about the time the individual shifts from the acute medical to the rehabilitation phase of the program (DeRuyter and Becker, 1988). That is not to say, however, that there are not instances where spasticity and speech motor control problems are so severe that they require a more long-term or permanent system. In these instances, the augmentative systems must not only be integrated into the rehabilitation regimen of communication, reassessment, and treatment, but they must also be evaluated in light of future educational, vocational, recreational, and environmental aspects of that individual's life (DeRuyter and Becker, 1988).

Potential for Speech. Primary to the potential success of any augmentative system with the nonspeaking TBI population is an assessment of the individual's cognitive-language status. (DeRuyter and David, 1982). The strategies for assessing communicative function in the speaking brain-injured population has been well documented. However, the assessment procedures for the nonspeaking TBI population have not been clearly delineated in the literature and are at times seemingly random (DeRuyter and colleagues, 1988). For the nonspeaking TBI population, the cognitive-language deficits must be first identified to determine how they will influence augmentative system selection and usage. As the temporary system becomes functional, its use becomes vital in re-evaluating cognitive-language processes for more detailed information. It is at this stage that one must begin to examine the nonspeaking individual's potential for speech. The authors have followed TBI individuals who have remained nonspeaking for up to 7 years only to become oral communicators. Although these individuals' speech is slow, imprecise, and deliberate, it is often intelligible enough to communicate with strangers who have a general idea of the topic. Often at this stage nonspeakers will consider themselves an oral communicator despite the inefficiency of their communicative abilities (DeRuyter and colleagues, 1987).

Assessment and prognosis of the potential for speech in the nonspeaking TBI individual is frequently ignored. This appears to be due to the difficulty in addressing three specific questions:

1. What is the individual's speech production status at present?
2. Does the speech impairment reflect other physical impairments, or does it reflect the individual's overall cognitive status?
3. Based on the speed of recovery and other prognostic indicators, does it appear that speech will emerge?

Clinicians can address each of these questions in the following manner. When determining the nonspeaking individual's current speech production status, they should describe the functionality of the speech with respect to its presence, efficiency, and intelligibility in various environments and with various listeners. If the individual is able to participate, formal assessment using standardized measures may be administered. More often than not, however, the clinician must rely on clinical observation and other team members (e.g., physical therapist adjusting body position) to examine speech production and intelligibility. The second question requires determination of whether the non-speakingness reflects other physical deficits or overall cognitive status (e.g., the inability to monitor speech output). Although the literature has identified some speech impairments in association with cognitive deficits, the types and severity of dysarthrias associated with TBI have not been described. However, the fact that the observed dysarthrias do not appear in isolation reflects the diffuse nature of the injury and implies that cognitive-language deficits interfere with usage of the oral-motor musculature.

The degree to which this occurs is not clearly understood and, as such, often makes it difficult to address the third quetion, which is whether speech will emerge based on the speed of recovery and other prognostic indicators. Addressing this question requires close monitoring of the individual's cognitive status to note any improvement in the presence of persistent oral reflexes as well as any changes in tone or posture or the selective control of other muscle groups. In addition, prognostic factors such as the type and site of injury, severity of injury, the individual's age, and speed of recovery should all be considered when the clinician addresses the question of whether speech will emerge.

Communication Evaluation for LOCF II and III (Generalized and Localized Levels of Response)

All TBI individuals functioning at LOCF II and III (generalized and localized levels of response) should have a comprehensive communication evaluation irrespective of whether they are speaking or nonspeaking. Unfortunately, because of their severe cognitive involvement in the areas of alertness and attention, these individuals are unable to initiate communication. Nevertheless, assessment is possible and should be completed.

Paramount to the assessment of the individual at this level is a reliable response mode by which responses to assessment tasks can be communicated. The nature of the cognitive-language, physical, and visual involvement following TBI almost indicates that a response mode be considered. In some instances, individuals at LOCF III will vocalize, but usually only in response to pain. Although individuals at this level do not initiate communication, they will frequently respond to communication by indicating through some type of yes and no system. For the nonspeaking individual, an appropriate nonverbal mode must be established as a response mode.

Yes-No Response Mode. The initial consideration of clinicians should be whether the nonspeaking individual can use an alternative yes and no system. The authors have noted repeatedly that individuals at LOCF III can learn alternative yes and no systems. The training, however, does require frequent repetition, redirection, and structuring of the environment to limit any external distractions.

The greatest consideration must be given to the type of yes and no system that is to be used. This requires two basic skills on the part of nonspeaking TBI individuals. First, they must be able to localize to people or objects; second, there must be an identifiable mode by which to indicate a response. Once established, the yes and no system can be very functional for the very low cognitive level patient. Our clinical experience indicates that there is a hierarchy of yes and no response modes applicable to the nonspeaking TBI population that differs from those used with other nonspeaking populations. The hierarchy is illustrated in Table 10-4. Specifically, the more natural the movement (e.g., head nods, gestures) or the more visible the system (e.g., color-coded cards), the more successful the system will be. It is important to note that because of the cognitive impairment, the TBI individual frequently requires some form of external feedback cue within the visual field when responding in a manner that is unnatural and other than speech. As a result, eye blinks and gaze and buzzer systems are the least successful types of yes and no response modes for TBI individuals in contrast to their success with individuals with other etiologies such as cerebral palsy, progressive neurologic disease, or spinal injury.

Communication Evaluation. TBI individuals at LOCF II and III typically require maximum assistance for activities of daily living, position-

Table 10-4. Hierarchy of yes-no response modes for nonspeaking individuals with traumatic brain injury

Functionality	Response mode
Most	Head nods
	Gestures
	Colored cards
	Eye blinks
Least	Buzzer

Source: DeRuyter, F., Becker, M.R., and Doyle, M. (1987). *Assessment and intervention strategies for the nonspeaking brain injured.* Short course presented to the American Speech-Language-Hearing Association, New Orleans.

ing, and ranging. As a result, an interdisciplinary team approach should be used to obtain information specific to cognitive status as it relates to the various disciplines. Nonstandardized procedures and clinical observation are typically used in the assessment process.

With respect to cognitive-language function, nonstandardized stimuli should be organized, used, and presented in a systematic manner. The specific processes to examine include (1) alertness, (2) arousability, (3) modality responses (auditory, gustatory, kinesthetic, olfactory, tactile, visual), (4) communication (expressive and receptive), (5) reflexes (oral, body), (6) balance (head control, limb alignment, posture, sitting, standing), (7) arm-hand function (gestures, grasping, pointing, reaching), and (8) tone (at rest, in motion, positional) (Donoghue and Reimer, 1987). The amount, complexity, duration, rate, and repetition of stimuli should be altered during presentation so that performance variables such as delay, endurance, recovery time, and type of response may be observed (Malkmus and colleagues, 1980). From these observations one can begin systematically to compare information obtained by other team members on other tasks so that the evaluation allows patterns of behavior to emerge. This allows one to begin answering the three questions raised earlier regarding prognosis for speech. As a general rule, if the nonspeaking status is a function of the individual's cognitive status, then speech will emerge as alertness and activity increase, which would occur as the individual progresses to LOCF IV and V.

It is also possible, at LOCF III, to begin addressing the individual's potential use of an augmentative system. As mentioned earlier, it is possible to establish use of a system through repetition and structure and by frequently redirecting the individual to the task. Carryover, however, should not be expected.

Communication Evaluation For LOCF V through VIII (Confused-Inappropriate to Purposeful-Appropriate)

The components used in the communication evaluation for nonspeaking TBI individuals functioning from LOCF V (confused-inappropriate) to LOCF VIII (purposeful-appropriate) are similar to those used for assessing speaking TBI individuals. The assessment process is best accomplished through the combined use of rating scales, standardized tests, nonstandardized procedures, and clinical observations (Malkmus, 1980; Hagen, 1984; DeRuyter and Becker, 1988). An understanding of the nonspeaking individual's cognitive-language status is primary to the potential success of any augmentative system.

Rating Scales With the Nonspeaking TBI. The use of rating scales for the scaling of responses has been demonstrated to be very useful in the systematic identification of behaviors and treatment planning without requiring the TBI individual's participation. Two rating scales widely used with the brain injured are the Rancho Levels of Cognitive Functioning (LOCF) (Hagen and colleagues, 1979), which may be used for tracking behavior or program planning, and the Disability Rating Scale (Rappaport and colleagues, 1982; Gouvier and colleagues, 1987), which may be used for monitoring physical and motor recovery.

With the nonspeaking TBI individual who exhibits severe physical impairment, either of these rating scales can be extremely helpful; however, there are two reasons why they should be used cautiously. First, rating scales can categorize an individual with severe physical limitations inappropriately because of that individual's inability to "act out" the specific behavior. Second, when measured on a broad scale, recovery by a severely physically involved nonspeaking TBI individual may be poorly reflected. Although for treatment planning purposes it is important to acknowledge cognitive level, it is of greater importance to identify accurately specific deficits in conjunction with the scaling of responses. This allows the small increments of improvement to be noted and described. It is this information that assists in determining the amount and complexity of stimulus material to be used with the augmentative system.

Standardized Tests. The use of standardized assessment batteries to evaluate communicative processes following TBI has been well described in the literature (Hagen, 1984; Adamovich and colleagues, 1985). By using a task analysis and process approach, various subtests from standardized batteries can yield vital information on various cognitive deficiencies ranging from attention to organization to problem solving. With the nonspeaking population, it is not uncommon to adapt subtests from standardized assessment batteries to the nonspeaking individuals' mode of expression (Yorkston and Karlan, 1986).

Adaptation of standardized batteries may be done in a number of ways. Open-ended tasks can be changed to a question format through the use of multiple choice or yes and no questions. However, by doing this, one builds cues into the tasks, thereby providing more structure and predictability to the question. This, in turn, decreases the individual's chance for error. As a result, it is important to be mindful that when standardized batteries are adapted, the rules of standardized assessment are violated, and therefore caution must be used in interpreting the results. Despite the ability to use existing standardized batteries, the need exists for the development of a formal assessment protocol that is useful specifically for the severely disabled nonspeaking TBI individual (DeRuyter and Becker, 1988).

Nonstandardized Procedures. Nonstandardized tasks have been adopted as an acceptable part of the assessment process in both the brain-injured and nonspeaking populations at large (Vanderheiden and Grilley, 1976; Malkmus, 1980; Hagen, 1984; Adamovich and colleagues, 1985). The use of these procedures allows the clinician to manipulate the amount, complexity, modality (input and output), rate, and duration of stimuli presented. Frequently, nonstandardized tasks provide information that standardized tests are not sensitive enough to measure.

The use of nonstandardized procedures is most helpful when assessing either the low or high LOCF nonspeaking TBI individual. It has been noted that a number of cognitive processes can influence system selection, modification, and usage (DeRuyter and colleagues, 1988). Therefore, the process of sequencing, organization, reasoning, memory, problem solving, abstraction, and integration must be carefully examined. Failure to do so may result in inaccurate assessment, as was demonstrated by a nonspeaking TBI individual who had a significant prospective memory loss but had the procedural memory capability to operate a system that had a memory component for message storage. Had the memory deficits not been carefully examined, one would have assumed that this patient was "confused" and incapable of operating such a system.

Clinical Observation. In the nonspeaking TBI individual, clinical observation of behaviors identifies performance in various environments and situations much the same way as it does for speaking brain-injured individuals. The frequent observation of altered organization and use of language in context is the result of a lack of integration of cognitive-language, emotional, and social components. It has been well documented that poor social communication skills in the brain-injured population contribute to social isolation and stress in the family of the individual (Katz and Lyerly, 1963; Brooks, 1984). These rules of conversation, commonly referred to as pragmatics, are usually retained by nonspeaking adults with etiologies other than brain injury. However, the nonspeaking TBI individual must relearn these rules of interaction (Beukelman and Yorkston, 1982).

The authors use two organized approaches to collecting observational data on interaction behaviors. They are the *Interaction Checklist for Augmentative Communication* (INCH) (Bolton and Dashiell, 1984) and the *Pragmatic Inventory for Brain Injury* (PIBI) (Kennedy and colleagues, 1989). Selection of the instrument depends on the desired information to be obtained. The INCH, which was specifically designed for the overall nonspeaking population, examines behaviors in the categories of initiation, facilitation, regulation, and termination. The PIBI, which was designed for the TBI population, examines pragmatic behaviors grouped into categories of content and interaction, cohesion, fluency, and nonverbal aspects. In each approach, the systematic observation and collection of data allows the clinician to identify patterns of behavior in the respective areas.

Although pragmatic behaviors have been documented in the brain-injured population, few data have been collected on pragmatic behavior and its recovery in the nonspeaking TBI population. In a preliminary study, the authors have observed that nonspeaking TBI individuals who demonstrate behavioral initiation deficits have difficulty providing feedback to their listeners when communication breakdowns occur. These same individuals are the ones who will inconsistently respond to social greetings without any prompting. Furthermore, the nonspeaking disinhibited TBI individual using an alphabet-word board will not terminate message transmission even after the listener has determined the message. In many instances, these nonspeakers insist on the methodical elaboration of messages, which reflects mental flexibility. These findings are consistent across individuals, irrespective of their LOCF. The use of advanced pragmatic skills is only demonstrated by those nonspeakers functioning at LOCF VIII or those who have used their augmentative system for a number of years after injury.

Clinicians must keep in mind that there is no one overall strategy or cookbook approach to assess the nonspeaking TBI individual. This is what makes the evaluation appear so difficult for clinicians. Instead, clinicians should capitalize on all available resources to assess these individuals accurately.

Physical Evaluation

Physical deficits following brain injury can range from very mild to extremely severe and include any number of neuromuscular disorders. Involvement can be unilateral or bilateral and may be compounded by sensory impairments such as visual and auditory deficits. Functional physical changes can occur long after injury and rehabilitation even though the underlying neuromotor functioning appears unchanged (Garland, 1982; Botte and Moore, 1987). Such involvement impairs independent function, which obviously can greatly affect augmentative system selection and usage.

The importance of using an interdisciplinary approach to physical evaluation cannot be overemphasized. It has been reported that a team evaluation was required to assess physical status in over 65 percent of the nonspeaking brain-injured population (DeRuyter and Lafontaine, 1987). When asked to indicate the most difficult area to evaluate within the nonspeaking TBI population, 36 percent (n=10) of the speech-language pathologists surveyed identified physical status as being the most difficult area (DeRuyter and colleagues, 1989). Consequently, a team evaluation by the speech-language pathologist, occupational therapist, physical therapist, and rehabilitation engineer should be performed whenever a physically involved nonspeaking TBI individual is encountered. The evaluation should focus on three specfic areas: (1) seating and positioning, (2) motor access site, and (3) visuoperceptual and acuity skills.

Seating and Positioning. Proper seating and positioning assists in minimizing reflex activity, excessive tone, and other body movements that may interfere with verbal communication or augmentative system usage. Traditional evaluation methods and attempts to provide a stable base of support for the body are usually not possible or of a high priority with nonambulatory TBI individuals during early recovery. This is primarily due to the acute medical and physical problems associated with the injury. However, during the rehabilitation phase, seating and positioning must be addressed to ensure effective use and control of the motor access site during augmentative communication system usage (DeRuyter and David, 1982). Because it is not uncommon to observe changes in an individual's physical abilities years after injury, positioning should be continuously reevaluated during all followup visits (Bray and colleagues, 1987).

Frequently, clinicians will only examine the nonspeaking TBI individual's positioning as it relates to postural seating systems. It is important, however, to examine other potential positioning environments. Positioning, as it relates to static postural seating systems, is typically examined by the physical therapist in the following areas: proximal joint position and stability, alignment of head on body, orientation and position of head in space, distal joint position, alignment of the body, and interaction of the individual with the environment and equipment such as a lapboard or wheelchair control (Norgard, 1986).

With the nonspeaking TBI individual, it is equally important to examine other potential positioning environments as they relate to augmentative system usage. These environments may include various positions (supine, elevated), positioning in various bed styles, positioning in arm restraints if the patient is at LOCF III or IV, positioning within the confines of medical equipment, and positioning as it relates to other forms of mobility. One method of examining positioning environments in this area is through a needs assessment, which is typically conducted on all nonspeaking individuals. Many such needs assessment protocols are available throughout the literature, and the reader is referred to the following references for more specific information (Beukelman and colleagues, 1985; Munson and colleagues; 1987; Porter and colleagues, 1988).

The overall seating and positioning goal during the early rehabilitation phase should be to provide for a structurally appropriate and functional position in which minimal or no pain is encountered. This enables the team to then examine the effective use and control of possible motor access sites to access potential augmentative communication systems. At the later stages of recovery, the goal becomes one of reevaluation to note any changes in physical abilities that may have occurred and that could affect system usage.

Motor Access Site. In conjunction with seating and positioning, potential motor access sites should be examined to identify the source that will allow the individual to interface with an augmentative system. Typically this evaluation is completed in conjunction with or immediately after optimal positioning has been obtained. Access sites should be examined with respect to accuracy and reliability of movement, range of control, speed of movement, and endurance (Lehman, 1986). This examination is often done in conjunction with an occupational therapist. Evaluation of the motor access site will assist the clinician in identifying the method of indication, the specific motor movement as well as body part to be used in accessing the augmentative system, and whether adaptation will be required to access an existing system. The reader is directed to the following references for more specific information related to motor assessment of the upper extremities for augmentative communication (Yorkston and Karlan, 1986; Stowers and colleagues, 1988).

Through the motor access site evaluation, the technique by which message elements are selected and transmitted by the nonspeaker can be determined. Two primary methods of indication—direct selection and scanning—can be identified. Direct selection requires the nonspeaker to indicate directly all the desired choices from the selection display. This may be done through pointing with a body part (finger, hand, foot, eyes, etc.) or with some specific interface (headpointer, mouthstick, lightpointer). Scanning, on the other hand, requires the nonspeaker to select the desired choice from a selection display in which items are typically presented one at a time. There are a variety of modes by which message elements are offered through the scanning method of indication: row-column–multidimensional scanning, linear-circular scanning, and directed scanning. In some instances, a commercially available switch may serve as an interface between the nonspeaker and a scanning augmentative system. Often reference is made to a third method of indication called encoding. This method of selecting message elements was designed to increase the speed and the number of choices available for communication by the nonspeaker. However, in actuality, encoding techniques are used in conjunction with direct selection and scanning and should not be considered a separate technique. The reader is directed to the following references for more specific information related to method of indication (Beukelman and colleagues, 1985; Vanderheiden and Lloyd, 1986).

Despite the high incidence of physical problems in the brain-injured population at large, it has been reported that over 77 percent (n=49) of the nonspeaking brain injured are able to select message elements directly. The remainder of the population sample used scanning or directed scanning methods to select message elements. It was further reported that almost 75 percent (n=47) of the nonspeaking brain injured used either their finger or hand as the motor site to access their augmentative system. The remainder of the individuals used either head or eye movements. Only 6 percent (n=3) of the brain-injured population sample required some type of switch to interface with their system (DeRuyter and Lafontaine, 1987).

Despite the importance of the motor access site assessment, it is unclear whether there is a progression of motor access response modes that the nonspeaking TBI individual goes through during physical recovery. The authors have noted, however, that severely physically involved nonspeaking TBI individuals, functioning at the lower cognitive levels and unaware of their sensory deficits, usually require extensive training and redirection to reestablish motor movements. On the other hand, severely physically involved nonspeaking TBI individuals, functioning at the higher cognitive levels, must have the cognitive capability to understand that to communicate, they must learn to compensate for their motor and sensory deficits as well as learn to express themselves through their motor access site. It should be evident that the identification and training of the motor access site requires use of an interdisciplinary approach.

Another important facet related to the motor access site during recovery and rehabilitation is to ensure that the nonspeaking individual's response mode is not unnecessarily compromised at the expense of orthopedic management (DeRuyter and colleagues, 1987). An active role should be taken in providing input when any orthopedic management is being considered for the nonspeaking TBI individual (Donoghue, 1988). In instances where the response modality will be affected by orthopedic management, a secondary or backup modality should be established before any surgical involvement. The importance of having a backup system is illustrated by a nonspeaking TBI individual at LOCF V who undergoes an active nerve block and serial casting program. For this particular individual, before orthopedic management, an established gesture system (thumbs up or down) for yes and no responses existed, and the nonspeaker was actively involved in a comprehensive rehabilitation program. A secondary head nod system was established before surgery as a backup response mode. As a result of postsurgical pain, the individual was unable to participate in any treatment program or bedside activities and was having difficulty concentrating on previously learned tasks. Team members, however, were able to interact with the individual through the backup yes and no system (head nods) so that appropriate pain management could be carried out (DeRuyter and Donoghue, 1989). This nonspeaker would have suffered unnecessarily if there had been no backup modality. Unfortunately, the provision of a backup system to persons with TBI is not as routine as it should be.

Visuoperceptual and Acuity Skills. Visual disturbances are also common in brain injury. As a result, visual perception and acuity should be accurately assessed in the nonspeaking TBI individual because of the importance that these skills play in augmentative system usage.

These skills are typically difficult to evaluate and should also be assessed using an interdisciplinary team approach. During the early recovery phase, assessment is typically a clinical judgment. It is based on any apparent degree of observed impairment, such as figure-ground and spatial relations problems, noted during the individual's responses to various stimuli within the environment. As recovery continues, visuoperceptual skills can be examined more formally. This is done in a hierarchy that ranges from easy gross table activities (e.g., puzzles, objects) to more difficult traditional paper and pencil assessment batteries.

Although the assessment emphasizes the individual's visuoperceptual skills, any visual acuity difficulties (e.g., field cuts, double and blurred vision) should be noted as early as possible. With the nonspeaking TBI individual functioning at the lower LOCF, this can be done by observing the individual's responses to threat, gross focus, and tracking when using a bright object or familiar face. Clinicians should always observe for any possible visual field cut with individuals at the lower cognitive levels. At the higher LOCF, the presence of visual field cut or blurred or double vision can all be detected through traditional assessments performed by an ophthalmologist.

Since it is unclear whether there is a progression to the recovery pattern of visual disturbances, the clinician should accompany the nonspeaker when a formal visuoperceptual or acuity assessment is being conducted. This provides the nonspeaker with an advocate in case any communication breakdowns should occur and allows any emerging difficulties to be pointed out to the ophthalmologist or occupational therapist. Furthermore, it ensures that the assessment examines those areas important for communication and augmentative system usage. For further information on the vision assessment of persons with TBI, the reader is referred to Chapter 8.

Interrelationship Among Assessment Components

The interrelationship and clinical implications among the assessment components discussed should be readily apparent. With the TBI individual a comprehensive and integrated rehabilitative approach is used because of the problems interrelated among the communicative, cognitive, and physical deficits (Bray and colleagues, 1987). Unfortunately, these problems are compounded when that TBI individual is also nonspeaking.

In the nonspeaking TBI individual, functional limitations due to physical impairments can be exaggerated by any number of cognitive deficits. These interfere with physical assessment in activities such as positioning and the selection of motor access sites. The nonspeaking individual's inability to monitor behaviors can result in the inability to habituate appropriate motor patterns that influence the selection and usage of an augmentative system. Conversely, cognitive impairments can be exaggerated by the physical impairments. A nonspeaking TBI individual with limited attentional abilities would appear to have significant difficulty if required to minimize an upper extremity tremor before accessing an augmentative system through the use of some fine motor movement. This type of impairment would appear to limit the types of communicative options available. The ability to access an augmentative system would be of no benefit to the nonspeaker if that individual did not have the perceptual or learning skills required to use the system or did not recognize the need to communicate effectively because of impaired awareness and monitoring skills. Finally, communicative deficits can exaggerate the effects of cognitive and physical impairments. The compensatory strategies that a speaking TBI individual might use to overcome cognitive and physical deficits would be ineffective if they could not be communicated effectively, as is the case with the nonspeaking TBI individual.

The major point for clinicians to always remember is that problems do not exist in isolation in the nonspeaking TBI individual. The interrelationship among physical, cognitive, and communicative deficits as well as the subsequent clinical implications are apparent. However, it is still not clearly understood how the cognitive deficits affect an individual's ability to use an augmentative system. To determine the interrelationships, followup conducted over a number of years is required. When working with the nonspeaking TBI individual, the clinician must include all aspects of the assessment process. It is from the assessment results that clinicians can begin considering what type of augmentative system to use.

SYSTEM SELECTION

The process involved in selecting augmentative communication systems for nonspeaking individuals have been thoroughly described in the literature (Vanderheiden and Grilley, 1976; Silverman, 1979; Harris and Vanderheiden, 1980; Shane and Bashir, 1980; Beukelman and colleagues,

1985). Although the procedures outlined in the literature vary slightly from one another, they all have the common goal of selecting systems that augment, enhance, and support communication for the nonspeaking individual.

Cognitive Factors Influencing System Selection

The principles applied in selecting a system for the nonspeaking TBI individual are very similar to those used for nonspeaking individuals with other etiologies. However, one factor must always be considered when selecting systems for the nonspeaking TBI individual: The augmentative systems selected must be flexible enough to undergo frequent modifications to keep up with the cognitive-language and physical changes that occur as these individuals continue to recover. The system selection process must therefore always be considered an ongoing and dynamic process rather than a static or one-time event.

The type of system selected depends largely on the rate of recovery of the individual's cognitive and physical deficits. Typically, the initial consideration is positioning and motor access site. As soon as these issues have been adequately addressed, the individual's cognitive-language status becomes and remains the primary consideration in the system selection process. In a recent survey, 68 percent (n=19) of speech-language pathologists providing services to the nonspeaking TBI population indicated that cognitive functioning was the primary critical indicator used to determine augmentative system candidacy. Therefore, the selection process will obviously be greatly influenced by nonspeakers' impairments on various cognitive-language processes (DeRuyter and colleagues, 1988; DeRuyter and Becker, 1988).

Cognitive deficits can influence the selection process in the following manner. An individual's selective attention and visuoperceptual impairments make focusing on the relevant and necessary stimuli difficult. This necessitates that stimuli on communication boards be limited in amount, type, and complexity and placed in highly visible locations to promote self-cuing. The use of certain types of systems is precluded by categorization deficits that influence the nonspeaker's memory processes. Sequencing impairments can interfere with the organization, structuring, and order of stimuli presentation to the degree that only simple communication systems can be used. Depending on the type and degree of impairment, memory deficits can also interfere with the nonspeaker's ability to complete multistage steps, which are often required to use the more sophisticated type of systems. Retrieval deficits, on the other hand, typically do not have a major effect on the system selection process, since cuing devices and strategies can be designed and incorporated into system usage. The nonspeaker with integration deficits in all likelihood will experience difficulty using a system in unfamiliar and unstructured environments. This would preclude the use of certain systems and require that role playing be incorporated into any system training process.

Linguistic deficits also influence the system selection process. The nonspeaker's reading and writing abilities must be appropriate for the system selected. It has been demonstrated that the nonspeaking TBI population used more alphabet and word based systems than other neurologically involved nonspeaking individuals (DeRuyter and colleagues, 1988). Impairments in auditory comprehension or processing would necessitate use of systems with very simple language structures to minimize confusion for the nonspeaker. When disorganized language is present, systems must be designed to provide the nonspeaker with adequate structure. This would necessitate the use of strategies such as color coding, limited choices, careful placement of stimuli, and preprogrammed messages.

Behavioral impairments manifested in the nonspeaking TBI individual can also influence the system selection and usage process. Initiation deficits typically result in the inability to begin conversations and places the communication interaction responsibility completely on the listener. Excessive impulsiveness and expansiveness in the communicative act by the nonspeaker are usually the result of disinhibition and impulsiveness. Perseveration of thought by the nonspeaker would be exhibited on an ideational level through the tendency to repeat messages and the inability to shift topics. Severe confusion and confabulation would require that the nonspeaker use simple communication systems that rely on remote memory or old learning (DeRuyter and Becker, 1988).

The influence of the nonspeaker's performance on each of the various cognitive, language, and behavioral processes must obviously be considered in the system selection process. Many other factors can influence the system selection process and require the clinician to be flexible and innovative. These include factors such as severe physical impairments that require extensive orthopedic management, agitation and uncooperative behaviors (LOCF IV) during cognitive recovery, and uncertainty of the potential for speech. These factors should be considered, but they should not preclude initiation of the system selection process.

Approaches to Communication Augmentation

The approaches to communication augmentation are varied and have been classified in a variety of ways. The various types of systems (e.g., unaided and aided, temporary and permanent) may be classified into one of three categories (Cohen and DeRuyter, 1982). This categorization has been helpful in the system selection process for nonspeaking TBI individuals (DeRuyter and colleagues, 1988). The three categories are (1) simple systems (including communication boards [picture, symbol, alphabet, word], gestures, yes-no [20 questions], and writing), (2) dedicated devices (such as the Canon, Casio, or SpeechPac, which are used to perform a predesignated function and serve a specific purpose such as communication), and (3) multipurpose systems (such as the Light Talker, Equalizer II, or Scanwriter, which are designed to change functions easily and serve a variety of purposes such as communicative, educational, vocational, and recreational activities). Generally, temporary systems include the simple systems and dedicated devices. Permanent systems can constitute any one or combination of simple, dedicated, or multipurpose devices.

It has been reported that the majority of nonspeaking brain-injured individuals can be classified as simple system users (DeRuyter and Lafontaine, 1987). Over 76 percent of the nonspeaking TBI population used simple augmentative communication systems rather than dedicated or multipurpose systems. Of all the different types of simple systems used, 77 percent were communication boards, with 65 percent being alphabet or word boards.

Purpose of the System

When clinicians begin working with nonspeaking TBI individuals, they often feel compelled to determine whether a temporary or permanent system will be required for the nonspeaker. Although determining this issue is often appropriate for individuals with other etiologies, all systems for the nonspeaking TBI individual should be temporary at least throughout the early recovery and rehabilitation phases. This allows for greater modification to the system as cognitive-language and physical changes occur. It is also the authors' experience that the TBI nonspeakers and their families often initially reject systems; however, they can be persuaded to accept a system that is considered temporary. Certain specific issues are related to the system selection process that clinicians should consider.

As opposed to other etiologies, establishing the purpose of the system is important early in the selection process. Determining whether the system is to be used for assessment, reassessment, communication, rehabilitation, integration into the outside environment, or a combination of these factors greatly influences the design of the system to be selected. This includes not only the organization and selection of vocabulary but also the physical setup and placement of the system. Findings obtained in the communicative and physical assessment should provide the necessary information regarding the selection, amount, and complexity of vocabulary. This information, along with the vocabulary requested by the family and team members, must be considered. In a recent survey, it was revealed that 93 percent (n=26) of speech-language pathologists used either environmental surveys or patient-family-therapist lists as the primary vocabulary selection techniques (DeRuyter and colleagues, 1989). For the higher LOCF nonspeaker, the completion of a needs inventory can assist in further determination of the specific system and communicative needs within various environments. There are numerous examples of these inventories cited in the literature (Beukelman and Yorkston, 1982; Bray and colleagues, 1987; Gobble and colleagues, 1987). As previously mentioned, the emphasis on temporary systems allows the greatest flexibility in addressing communicative needs and modifying systems as cognitive levels change during recovery.

INTEGRATION OF THE SYSTEM INTO THE INTERVENTION PROCESS

Integrating the nonspeaking TBI individual with an augmentative system into the overall intervention process poses one of the greatest challenges for the clinician. System usage strategies must be designed so that they promote, facilitate, and improve communication as well as impaired cognitive-language processes. When they were asked the most difficult area to treat in the nonspeaking TBI population, 64 percent (n=18) of the speech-language pathologists surveyed indicated that cognitive-language deficits were the most difficult, and 18 percent (n=5) indicated communication.

It is important to view integration as an ongoing process in which reevaluation and system modification are the norm rather than the exception. Integrating the augmentative system into the intervention process is a three-stage process that includes (1) training in proper system usage, (2) incorporating the system into all aspects of the recovery and rehabilitation program, and (3) using the system beyond the treatment environment (DeRuyter and colleagues, 1987; DeRuyter and Becker, 1988).

Training Proper System Usage

Training the nonspeaker how to use an augmentative system is a difficult task. This difficulty is further compounded by any cognitive-language deficits. Two erroneous assumptions are sometimes made, which add to the difficulty in the training of system usage (DeRuyter and Becker, 1988). The first assumption is that nonspeaking TBI individuals will not learn to generalize usage of the system within various contexts because of the deficits in basic cognitive processes (i.e., decreased learning and confusion due to memory loss). The other assumption is just the opposite. If the nonspeaking TBI individual presents with the basic cognitive processes, then that individual will be able to use a dedicated device or multipurpose system in a variety of settings. Neither can be assumed, and both require systematic training.

An augmentative system should be introduced as early as possible in the recovery or rehabilitation process. Systems can be provided in any number of settings, including intensive care units, rehabilitation centers, outpatient settings, skilled nursing facilities, and home. Irrespective of the setting, the ultimate goal is to have the nonspeaking TBI individual use the system independently. Systems should be introduced in highly structured environments, although the nonspeaker's cognitive status and communicative needs will ultimately determine the dependence on structure. In instances where a system is provided at bedside, all family and staff directly associated with the individual should be trained in use of the system. This training facilitates repetition, consistency, and carry-over of system usage. When systems are provided to nonspeakers capable of participating in different activities throughout the day, the systems should be introduced in a situational hierarchy reflecting the individual's cognitive abilities.

Other issues to consider include system training in multiple settings, provision of vocabulary relevant to various situations, reducing reliance on structure, modifying systems to meet specific needs and capabilities, mounting systems so they are always available, encouraging multimodality communication, and providing backup systems. The first task at hand, however, is acceptance of the augmentative system.

Acceptance of the Augmentative System

It is often difficult for the nonspeaker and family to realize the benefits of an augmentative system. Clinicians should address this issue early in the training process to facilitate acceptance and alleviate concerns that the system will interfere with the recovery of natural speech. In a recent survey, 54 percent (n=15) of speech-language pathologists reported that patient-family acceptance was the primary prognostic indicator for successful system usage (DeRuyter and colleagues, 1989).

The nonspeaking TBI individual's difficulty accepting a system is the result of that individual's self-concept, which is based on premorbid abilities and attitudes. With the resultant impaired insight following an injury, the nonspeaker has difficulty acknowledging the deficits, let alone realizing the benefits associated with facilitatory and compensatory techniques. However, acceptance of the augmentative system can be facilitated through counseling, establishing goals, and providing support systems for the individual. Specifically, it should be emphasized to the individual that the system is temporary and that it will increase communication, facilitate speech, and increase independence through the environment. Goals that are concrete and attainable are identified for the individual and reviewed daily. Interaction and treatment with the system should be structured so that the individual experiences success to realize the benefits of the system. Immediate reinforcement should be provided. In group treatment sessions, composed of both speaking and nonspeaking individuals, the purpose of the system and how it is used can be openly discussed. In addition, nonspeaking TBI individuals who are using systems should at times be grouped together for treatment sessions, social and recreational activities, and housing to facilitate support systems. Although grouping provides tremendous benefits for system acceptance, the clinician can encounter decreased system usage when a nonspeaking individual advances to a different treatment group or is discharged.

Family or caregiver acceptance of the system largely depends on the TBI individual's LOCF and the type of system provided. With an individual functioning at LOCF III and utilizing a yes-no system, acceptance is less of a problem because the family can readily observe the benefits of the system. However, with individuals at the higher LOCF (V through VIII), the family will often view the system as interfering with the recovery of speech. Consequently, the family or caregiver must be counseled on the same issues that were addressed with the nonspeaker to gain acceptance. Included are that the system is temporary at this stage and will increase communication, facilitate speech, and increase independence throughout the environment. In addition, these counseling sessions can serve as excellent training sessions for the family to become incorporated into the system usage regimen. Issues such as the types of questions to ask and the type and amount of cueing to provide should all be discussed with the family. The importance of practice and repetition should also be discussed to facilitate generalization of system usage. By having the nonspeaking TBI individual demonstrate the system in the presence of the family, it is possible to discuss the components of the system as well as mention potential modifications as recovery occurs. Finally, by observing how performance deteriorates as the complexity of the task increases, the family observes the impact of the cognitive deficits. This usually causes the family to become an active participant in the system usage process.

It is imperative that the nonspeaker experience a degree of success with the system during the introduction phase to facilitate integration into the intervention process. It is after the introduction phase that actual training is initiated. By using a treatment hierarchy that includes situations, tasks and cuing-prompting, the process begins.

Situational Components. The situational components include those related to the setting and environment as well as the receiver. Because

TBI individuals frequently have difficulty retaining and generalizing new information, it is very important that clinicians use a situational hierarchy when training the nonspeaking TBI individual in proper system usage. This is contrary to what is often done with nonspeaking individuals with disorders other than TBI.

System training should be initiated in a structured, quiet treatment room or environment. The minimal distractions within the environment assist in compensating for the individual's impaired selective attention abilities as well as for the difficulty in learning and retaining new information. As performance in system usage improves, structure is gradually decreased and distractions are gradually increased. This requires the clinician to begin introducing the system in other familiar environments, such as in a group therapy situation, which has potential distractions with other patients and a different clinician. Throughout this process the family should be encouraged to participate actively in the training and use of the system. This assists in the facilitation of repetition, consistency, and carryover of system usage.

As the nonspeaking TBI individual begins to demonstrate success in usage, the system can be used in different and multiple environments throughout the day. Once again, the system should be introduced in each setting in a situational hierarchy, progressing from the most to the least structure. At this level of intervention, cotreatment and team interaction are critical during the training phase to facilitate acceptance and generalization. For example, the initiation of communication might be facilitated if the occupational therapist and speech-language pathologist perform the nonspeaker's morning care routine together while using the augmentative system.

As the individual becomes reliable in system usage in different but familiar environments, training should be transferred to less familiar settings. For the nonspeaker in a medical center, this may include the cafeteria, gift shop, or snack bar. If the individual is living at home, less familiar settings can include a restaurant, market, or other environment outside the living setting. Frequently, nonspeaking TBI individuals reaching LOCF VII exhibit difficulty initiating communication in the less familiar setting and consequently require extensive repetition. These individuals also have difficulty preventing and repairing communicative breakdowns, especially with less familiar listeners such as store clerks. As a result of the residual deficits, many nonspeaking TBI individuals are unable to proceed independently in system usage beyond this stage.

Task Components. Like situational components, treatment tasks should be presented in a hierarchy. The initial task in the treatment hierarchy of initiating a reliable system response should be automatic and natural. Typically this is done through a gross body movement such as indicating yes or no or pointing to a specific picture. As soon as the response is consistent, one can proceed to posing simple questions for response. These initial tasks should use automatic and overlearned information that relies on the nonspeaker's remote memory and does not interfere with learning the actual response. The use of automatic and overlearned information also allows further familiarization and success of system usage. This is important for ensuring acceptance and usage of the system.

As the nonspeaker begins to demonstrate reliable responses for overlearned information, simple but concrete questions related to daily activities (e.g., shaving and dressing routines) should be introduced. After that, hypothetical and open-ended communication situation tasks should be presented. The initial questions should be automatic (e.g., What did you eat this morning?) but become more functional as responses become more reliable (e.g., How would you tell your doctor that your cast hurts?). Because open-ended questions require retrieval, organization, and formulation skills, it is important to begin at the automatic level to ensure success in system usage. The hierarchy progression then leads to role playing and communicative situations in familiar settings.

As the treatment task moves into familiar settings and role playing, the communicative task required of the nonspeaking TBI individual also changes. Specifically, the demands placed on the nonspeaker change from simply responding to questions to initiating and responding to communication. As such, the tasks required are those of providing messages and initiating communication to other staff, family, and peers.

Although the initiation of effective communication in all situations and environments is the desired result, it is typically at the initiation stage that many nonspeaking TBI individuals experience difficulty and breakdown. This greatly limits effective use of their system. Although the task of initiating communication is difficult for many nonspeakers, it is a skill that can be learned. However, as with any task for the TBI individual, it requires presentation in a hierarchy to be learned effectively.

At the most basic level, nonspeakers should be expected to use their systems to greet all staff and peers whom they come into contact with during all therapies. Often it is beneficial to put social phrases (e.g., Hi! How are you? What's new? Let's talk.) on communication boards or have them preprogrammed into a dedicated device. This increases the speed of communication while reducing perseverative interactions that can occur with the TBI individual. Next, treatment sessions should be structured so that the nonspeaker initiates topics for discussion or selects activities at the beginning of each session. The final level is role playing various communicative interactions in an unfamiliar setting before going on outings to the actual settings.

Although the emphasis is on effective use of the augmentative system, the nonspeaking individual should be encouraged and reinforced for using any modality that will effectively communicate the message. This can include pointing, gestures, facial expressions, and speech. The length of time spent on each task will vary according to many factors. These can include the individual's accuracy of response, length of time required to prepare and deliver messages, and the time required to respond to messages. As a result, variables such as the amount and complexity of information and stimulus rate and its duration may all require modification to increase the difficulty of task presentation for effective system usage.

Cuing Components. Typically, the cognitive deficits of TBI individuals are severe enough that to achieve functional usage with the augmentative system, various levels of cuing are required. The nonspeaking TBI individual's cognitive and physical abilities as well as the type of system provided determine the type and extent of cuing required. As a general rule, the more severe the cognitive manifestations, the greater the reliance the nonspeaker places on the listener to direct the communicative act. Consequently, the goal should be the gradual reduction of the individual's reliance on prompts to achieve independence in communication. This is done through the teaching of self-cuing strategies or by altering the system to compensate for the cognitive deficits.

For the nonspeaking TBI individual, it is more appropriate to simplify the task so that it only requires minimal cuing for an accurate response than to provide a difficult task that requires extensive cuing. In the same manner that the situational and task components were addressed, cuing should also be facilitated using a hierarchy.

The hierarchy begins with the physical cue, which is the most basic form of cuing. This requires the clinician to guide the individual through the motor response. This is followed by gestural cuing, which relies on the individual's visual attention abilities. Typically, the physical and gestural cues are coupled with verbal cuing, which can vary from descriptions to simple questions for clarification (e.g., Are you sure you want to give me that finger?). Next in the hierarchy is nonverbal cuing (paralinguistic, proxemic, and kinesic). Use of nonverbal cues requires the individual to have more finely tuned attention and interpretation skills. With the nonspeaking TBI individual, impairment of these skills can influence independence of communication. The highest level of cuing is self-cuing, which requires the individual to have initiation skills. This is typically observed in those individuals functioning at the higher LOCF (VII or VIII).

The authors have noted that nonspeaking TBI individuals rely heavily on cues throughout the intervention training process. As a result, it is important to maintain accurate frequency counts during training to facilitate decreasing the number of cues while moving through the hierarchy. It is also helpful to mount the system on a lap tray, arm rest, or bedrail so that it is always available within the individual's visual field irrespective of the individual's cognitive level. Finally, for the higher LOCF (VI through VIII) individual's written cue cards for self-cuing have proved helpful.

Controlling Interactions and Repairing Breakdowns

The communicative process involves answering questions, requesting information, controlling interactions, and resolving communication breakdowns. The reduced rate of communication, common to all nonspeakers, affects many aspects of the communicative events. Included are missed or restricted communicative opportunities, misunderstood messages, and difficulty introducing new topics (Beukelman and colleagues, 1985; Kraat, 1986). In addition, the nonspeaker is interrupted by listeners who are attempting to predict the message. For the nonspeaking TBI individual, these interruptions can be quite distracting and at times disastrous to the communicative event. The interruptions require the nonspeaker to shift from a mode of formulating responses to a mode of answering questions, usually a series of yes or no questions. The nonspeaker's reduced flexibility of thought and difficulty adapting to new situations and reduced flexibility virtually eliminate any possibility for regaining control of the conversation. This results in a communication breakdown. The clinician must therefore provide the nonspeaker with strategies to control interactions and repair breakdowns.

Communication breakdowns in the nonspeaking TBI population can be prevented (DeRuyter and colleagues, 1987). Specific strategies can be listed in a hierarchy, as illustrated in Table 10-5. As the table reflects, the nonspeaking TBI augmentative communication user has access to a greater number of strategies to prevent communication breakdowns as the system becomes more sophisticated. Specifically, the simplest manner is through educating staff, family, and peers on how to interact with a particular nonspeaker. The education must be based on the nonspeaker's interactive style. Unfortunately, the training is of little assistance when new listeners are brought into the communicative process. The education process also does not resolve breakdowns that are caused by system limitations (e.g., inadequate vocabulary).

Another strategy to prevent breakdowns is to provide the listener with a set of rules on how to interact with the nonspeaker and the system. Messages written on cue cards handed to listeners or mounted on lap trays, wheelchair arm rests, and bedrails have been used to forewarn listeners about the nonspeaker's particular communicative needs and

Table 10-5. Prevention and repair strategies for the nonspeaking individual with traumatic brain injury according to type of augmentative system

	Augmentative system		
Strategy	Boards	Dedicated	Multipurpose
Listener training	X	X	X
Nonverbal behaviors	X	X	X
Written cue cards	X	X	X
Conversational control phrases	X	X	X
Continuous feedback		X	X
Preprogrammed messages		X	X
Encoding		X	X
Abbreviation expansion		X	X
Word prediction			X

Source: Doyle, M., and DeRuyter, F. (1989). *Vocabulary selection and expansion in the nonspeaking traumatic brain injured.* Paper submitted to RESNA, New Orleans.

strategies. With some systems, messages can be incorporated into the system. These usually request that the listener be patient and wait until the nonspeaker's message is completed before interrupting. Additional techniques to prevent communication breakdowns include creating systems that enable faster communication. This has included encoding techniques, preprogramming of frequently used messages, and preparing standard responses that provide the listener with more rapid and continuous feedback. The acceleration features of newer dedicated and multipurpose systems have been helpful for TBI individuals at the higher cognitive levels.

To repair breakdowns and take control of the interaction process, conversational control phrases (e.g., please wait, you misunderstood, shut up) can be made part of the system's vocabulary. Probably the most effective method, with the nonspeaking TBI population, is to reduce the effect that the individual's behavioral problems has on system usage.

Behavioral problems such as confabulation, disinhibition, egocentricity, and perseveration during system usage are treated in the same manner that they are with the speaking TBI individual. The clinician or listener can structure the interaction by pausing between tasks, monitoring the complexity of the input, and redirecting the nonspeaker. Frequently the nonspeaker will perseverate on certain topics or vocabulary items. If association, recent memory, and learning skills are adequate, the clinician can circle those topics or vocabulary items on which the individual perseverates. The circles serve as a self-cuing strategy for the nonspeaker to pick another topic or word.

Inflexibility on the nonspeaker's part is often manifested by reliance on only one mode of communication and by not using the most appropriate system or acceleration techniques. This is most commonly demonstrated by the nonspeaking TBI individual who chooses to spell everything, even though many of the words or phrases are already listed on the communication board or programmed in the dedicated or multipurpose system. This behavioral problem compromises the rate of communication by failing to use the system's built-in acceleration features. In instances where a word or phrase board is being used, it is necessary to remove the alphabet from the board to overcome this problem. This requires the nonspeaker to scan the board for the appropriate word before the alphabet board can be requested. Then, by selecting an appropriate phrase (e.g., It's not on my board; I need to spell), an alphabet board can be provided. Although this strategy requires a greater dependency on the listener, it is usually only temporary. In extreme cases of inflexibility, the authors have observed individuals who spell messages by using the letters of the words and phrases on the communication board. In these instances, the above-mentioned strategy is obviously ineffective. At that point, it is recommended that the nonspeaking individual be provided with only an alphabet board since words on the system will only create confusion for the listener.

Another common behavioral problem that frequently influences augmentative system usage is initiation. This problem is not unique to the nonspeaking TBI individual, but, given the cognitive component, it does require some alternative strategies. Specific techniques to manage this were discussed earlier. As proper system usage begins to emerge, the augmentative system can begin to be used to integrate the nonspeaker into an appropriate treatment program.

Incorporating the System Into the Treatment Program

The nonspeaker should be integrated into the appropriate treatment program as soon as possible. This requires incorporating the augmentative system into the program, which often involves adapting and modifying the system so that the nonspeaker can respond appropriately. Integrating into the treatment program allows for the blending of cognitive rehabilitation, system training, and communication. As a result, interaction becomes the expected behavior during individual and group treatment sessions as well as during such activities as transportation between therapies, meals, and any social activities. The integration process further assists in acceptance and generalization of system usage.

The type of intervention depends on the type and severity of the individual's cognitive deficit. Typically, the principles of cognitive rehabilitation and behavioral management used in the treatment of TBI are incorporated but modified for the nonspeaking TBI individual. For convenience, incorporation of the system into the intervention process can be divided into three stages based on the individual's cognitive level: stimulation (LOCF II and III), structured (LOCF IV to VI), community (LOCF VII to VIII).

Stimulation Stage (LOCF II and III). At the lower LOCF, the treatment strategies used for the nonspeaking TBI individual are similar to those used with the speaking individual. Isolated stimuli are selectively presented in an effort to establish the yes-no response. For the nonspeaking individual, the tasks must be modified to elicit and establish the nonverbal yes-no response.

Structured Stage (LOCF IV to VI). At the structured stage, the clinician can begin to use the system to improve the nonspeaking individual's specific cognitive-language deficits. It is at this stage that the augmentative system begins to be integrated into the intervention process.

At LOCF IV, where the nonspeaking individual is in transition through the agitation stage, it is important for clinicians and family to be sensitive to the individual's inability to express confusion. This confusion may present itself in various forms, including nonpurposeful behavior. Attempts should be made to use the established nonverbal yes-no response mode to attend selectively to the nonspeaking individual's confusion.

At LOCF V, the augmentative system begins to serve a major role in the treatment program. At this stage, a simple system is introduced to facilitate recovery of the cognitive-language deficits as well as to serve communication purposes. Specific cognitive skills that may be worked on using the augmentative system include categorization, discrimination, immediate memory, orientation, selective attention, and sequencing. With communication boards, vocabulary can be categorized and sequenced according to color to improve discrimination. Training system usage assists in increasing selective attention abilities. Daily schedules can be incorporated into the system to aid in orientation skills. The system should also be used to facilitate motor speech output by encouraging the nonspeaker to attempt to vocalize or verbalize each message selection. Language impairments, including auditory comprehension, sentence formulation, and word retrieval, are treated as they would be with the speaking TBI individual, except that the tasks are modified to allow the nonspeaking individual to respond using the augmentative system.

At LOCF VI, most nonspeaking TBI individuals are using simple systems in the treatment program. In some instances, a dedicated device is being considered or has been introduced. Just as in the previous stage, the system is used to facilitate cognitive-language functions as well as communicative purposes. Specific cognitive goals at this level include categorization, discrimination, orientation, recent memory, selective attention, and sequencing. In addition to the strategies used in the previous stage, the system should be made more complex with increased vocabulary, further categorization of stimuli, and other system enhancements. In many instances, specific visuoperceptual and acuity deficits become more prominent, requiring marginal color or tactile cues to assist discrimination. Increasing the complexity of the system with new vocabulary or the development of miniboards for specific topics, therapies, or projects assists in improving recent memory abilities. This also assists in orientation, interaction, and integration of the system into other settings. Whenever possible at this level, the nonspeaking individual should assist in modifying the system. By having the individual select new vocabulary and decide on placement, it is possible to facilitate specific categorization and sequencing deficits.

In addition to using the system to improve cognitive functioning, nonspeakers at LOCF VI should continue to use their systems to improve language and motor speech impairments. Treatment strategies for language activities are the same as those used with the speaking TBI individual, except that tasks should be modified to allow responses with the augmentative system. Speech output is strongly encouraged in conjunction with the selection of message elements. This is designed to facilitate the motor speech mechanism as well as promote self-monitoring skills. The observation of poor self-monitoring skills in the TBI individual has often been contributed to decreased intellect. Consequently, at this level it is imperative that listeners be instructed to repeat verbally the elements selected to provide the nonspeaker with feedback. This effort often enhances the nonspeaker's self-monitoring skills.

Community Stage (LOCF VII and VIII). By the time the nonspeaking TBI individual has reached the community stage, other issues related to augmentative communication begin to emerge. Individuals at this level can use simple, dedicated, or multipurpose systems and, in some instances, multiple systems. In most cases, the system has taken on a sense of permanence for the family and nonspeaker. There is often acknowledgement that the system will be required in the home and community. Although the system continues to be used for communication as well as to improve cognitive-language abilities, other issues that will require the individual to adapt to the outside environment become the major focus. These issues include compensatory strategies for the residual deficits, long-term educational or vocational goals, and discharge planning. Consequently, use of the system to address these issues becomes a major component of the intervention process. Typically, use of the augmentative system to address these issues can be accomplished during the cognitive-language and communicative intervention process.

SUMMARY

The provision of services to the nonspeaking TBI individual poses many challenges for the clinician. This chapter has identified the population, indicated what can be done for these individuals, and provided direction on how to provide the necessary services to nonspeaking TBI individuals. The clinician should remember that there is no one way to provide services to this unique population. Rather, the assessment, system selection, and intervention processes pose many challenges for the clinician. Although at times monumental, these challenges are by no means insurmountable. As clinicians continue to enhance their skills and expertise with this unique population and the augmentative communication field, the nonspeaking TBI individual will be afforded with access to quality services, a means to communicate, and, one hopes, the ability to become a functional member of society once again.

Acknowledgements. The authors wish to thank Debbie David, Molly Doyle, and Linda Lafontaine for their program development and work with the nonspeaking population that led to this manuscript. They would also like to acknowledge Ann, Paul, Ron, P.J., and Rhonda for their assistance. Finally, they wish to thank David and Kathy for their encouragement, advice, and support and for making them understand that "the weakest ink is better than the strongest memory."

REFERENCES

Adamovich, B.B., Henderson, J.A., and Auerbach, S. (1985). *Cognitive rehabilitation of closed head injured patients: A dynamic approach.* Boston: College-Hill Press.

Aiello, S.C. (1980).*Non-oral communication survey: A one-county needs assessment and demographic study.* Unpublished educational study, Plavan School, Fountain Valley, CA.

Anderson, D.W., and McLaurin, R.L. (1980). The national head and spinal cord injury survey. *Journal of Neurosurgery, 53,* s1–s43.

Annegers, J.F., Grabow, J.D., Kurland, L.T., and Laws, E.R. (1980). The incidence, causes, and secular trends of head trauma in Olmsted County, Minnesota, 1935–1974. *Neurology, 30,* 912–919.

Becker, M., and DeRuyter, F. (1989). AAC systems for the nonspeaking traumatic brain injured according to cognitive level. Unpublished paper.

Becker, M., and Malkmus, D. (1982). Nonstandardized cognitive-linguistic assessment of the adult. In *Rehabilitation of the head injured child and adult: Selected problems.* Downey, CA: Professional Staff Association of Rancho Los Amigos Hospital, Inc.

Ben-Yishay, Y., Rattok, J., and Diller, L. (1979). A clinical strategy for the systematic amelioration of attentional disturbances in severe head trauma patients. *Institute of Rehabilitation Monograph,* New York: New York Medical Center.

Beukelman, D.R. (1987). *Augmentative communication. . . . Working together.* Paper presented to the American Speech-Language-Hearing Foundation Conference, Denver, CO.

Beukelman, D.R., and Garrett, K.L. (1988). Augmentative and alternative communication for adults with acquired severe communication disorders. *Augmentative and Alternative Communication, 4,* 104–121.

Beukelman, D.R., and Yorkston, K.M. (1980). Nonvocal communication: Performance evaluation. *Archives of Physical and Medical Rehabilitation, 61,* 272–275.

Beukelman, D.R., and Yorkston, K.M. (1982). Communication interaction of adult communication augmentation system use. *Topics in Language Disorders, 2,* 39–53.

Beukelman, D.R., Yorkston, K.M., and Dowden, P.A. (1985). *Communication augmentation: A casebook of clinical management.* Boston: College-Hill Press.

Beukelman, D.R., Yorkston, K.M., and Lossing, C.A. (1984). Functional communication assessment of adults with neurogenic disorders. In A.S. Halper and M.J. Fuhrer (Eds.), *Functional assessment in rehabilitation.* Baltimore: Paul H. Brookes Publishing.

Beukelman, D.R., Yorkston, K.M., and Smith, K. (1985). Third-party payer response to requests for purchase of communication augmentation systems: A study of Washington state. *Augmentative and Alternative Communication, 1,* 5–9.

Bolton, S.O., and Dashiell, S.E. (1984). *Interaction checklist for augmentative communication.* Huntington Beach, CA: INCH Associates.

Botte, M., and Moore, T. (1987). The orthopedic management of extremity injuries in head trauma. *Journal of Head Trauma Rehabilitation, 2,* 13–27.

Bray, L.J., Carlson, F., Humphrey, R., Mastrilli, J.P., and Valko, A.S. (1987). Physical rehabilitation. In M. Ylvisaker and E.M.R. Gobble (Eds.), *Community re-entry for head injured adults.* Boston: College-Hill Press.

Brooks, N. (1984). *Closed head injury: Psychological, social, and family consequences.* New York: Oxford University Press.

Brooks, N., Hosie, J., Bond, M.R., Jennett, B., and Aughton, M. (1986). Cognitive sequelae of severe head injury in relation to the Glasgow Outcome Scale. *Journal of Neurology, Neurosurgery, and Psychiatry, 49,* 549–553.

Bureau of Education for the Handicapped. (1976). *Conference on communication aids for non-vocal severely physically handicapped persons,* December 7–8. Alexandria, VA: Bureau of Education for the Handicapped.

Cohen, C.G., and DeRuyter, F. (1982). Technology for the communicatively impaired: A perspective for future clinicians. *Journal of the National Student Speech-Language-Hearing Association, 10,* 67–76.

Cummings, J. (1985). Behavioral disorders associated with frontal lobe injury. *Clinical Neuropsychiatry,* 57–67.

DeRuyter, F., and Becker, M.R. (1988). Augmentative communication: Assessment, system selection, and usage. *The Journal of Head Trauma Rehabilitation, 3,* 35–44,

DeRuyter, F., and David, D.S. (1982). *Transitional and permanent usage of augmentative communication with the head injured.* Short course presented to the American Speech-Language-Hearing Association, Toronto.

DeRuyter, F., and Donoghue, K.A. (1989). Communication and traumatic brain injury: A case study. *Augmentative and Alternative Communication, 4,* 49–54.

DeRuyter, F., and Lafontaine, L.M. (1985). *Relational data-base report of the nonspeaking population.* Paper presented to the American Speech-Language-Hearing Association, Washington, DC.

DeRuyter, F., and Lafontaine, L.M. (1987). The nonspeaking brain-injured: A clinical and demographic database report. *Augmentative and Alternative Communication, 3,* 18–25.

DeRuyter, F, Becker, M.R., and Doyle, M. (1987). *Assessment and intervention strategies for the nonspeaking brain injured.* Short course presented to the American Speech-Language-Hearing Association, New Orleans.

DeRuyter, F., Doyle, M., and Becker, M.R. (1989). *Provision of services to the nonspeaking TBI: A survey.* Unpublished paper.

DeRuyter, F., Lafontaine, L.M., and Becker, M.R. (1988). The patient with traumatic brain injury versus stroke. In D.E. Yoder and R.D. Kent (Eds.), *Decision making in speech-language pathology.* Ontario, Decker.

Donoghue, K. (1988). *Speech-language pathology's role in the orthopedic management of nonspeaking brain injured individuals.* Paper presented to the International Society for Alternative and Augmentative Communication, Anaheim, CA.

Donoghue, K., and Reimer, T.J. (1987). *The speech pathologist's role in the stimulation of the low level brain injured patient.* Paper presented to the California Speech-Language-Hearing Association, San Diego, CA.

Doyle, M., and DeRuyter, R. (1989). *Vocabulary selection and expansion in the nonspeaking traumatic brain injured.* Paper submitted to Rehabilitation Engineering Society of North America, New Orleans.

Garland, D.E. (1982). Head injuries in adults. In Nickel, V. (Ed.), *Orthopedic rehabilitation.* New York: Churchill Livingstone.

Gobble, E.M.R., Dunson, L., Szekeres, S.F., and Cornwall, J. (1987). Avocational programming for the severely impaired head injured individual. In M. Ylvisaker and E.M.R. Gobble (Eds.), *Community re-entry for head injured adults.* Boston: College-Hill Press.

Gouvier, W.D., Blanton, P.N., LaPorte, K.K., and Nepomuceno, C. (1987). Reliability and validity of the Disability Rating Scale and the levels of cognitive functioning scale in monitoring recovery from severe head injury. *Archives of Physical and Medical Rehabilitation, 68,* 94–97.

Groher, M. (1977). Language and memory disorders following closed head trauma. *Journal of Speech and Hearing Research, 20,* 212–223.

Hagen, C. (1984). Language disorders in head trauma. In E. Holland (Ed.), *Language disorders in adults: Recent advances.* Boston: College-Hill Press.

Hagen, C., Malkmus, D., and Durham, P. (1979). Levels of cognitive functions. In *Rehabilitation of the head injured adult: Comprehensive physical management.* Downey, CA: Professional Staff Association of Rancho Los Amigos Hospital, Inc.

Heilman, K.M., Safran, A., and Geschwin, N. (1971). Closed head trauma and aphasia. *Journal of Neurology, Neurosurgery, and Psychiatry, 34,* 265–269.

Harris, D., and Vanderheiden, G.C. (1980). Augmentative communication techniques. In R.L. Schiefelbusch (Ed.), *Nonspeech language and communication: Analysis and intervention.* Baltimore: University Park Press.

Jacobs, H. (1984). The family as a therapeutic agent: Long term rehabilitation for traumatic head injury patients, final report. Washington, D.C. *National Institute of Handicapped Research.*

Jennett, B., and MacMillan, R. (1981). Epidemiology of head injury. *British Medical Journal, 282,* 101–104.

Katz, M.M., and Lyerly, S.B. (1963). Methods for measuring adjustment and social behavior in the community. *Psychology Reports, 13,* 503–535.

Kennedy, M.R., Reimer, T.J., Burton, W., Lawson, A., Crabtree, R., Doyle, M., and Dobeck, C. (1989). *Pragmatic inventory for brain injury (PIBI).* Unpublished assessment battery.

Kodimer, C., and Styzens, S. (1980). The psychology of the head injured adult. In *Rehabilitation of the head injured adult: Comprehensive management.* Downey, CA: Professional Staff Association of Rancho Los Amigos Hospital, Inc.

Kraat, A. (1986). Develop intervention goals. In S.W. Blackstone (Ed.), Augmentative communication: An introduction. Rockville, MD: American Speech-Language-Hearing Association.

Lehman, M. (1986). *Nonspeaking communication boards.* Workshop presented at Rancho Los Amigos Medical Center, Inc., Downey, CA.

Levin, H.S., Benton, A.L., and Grossman, R.G. (1982). *Neurobehavioral consequences of closed head injury.* New York: Oxford University Press.

Levin, H.S., Grossman, R.G., Rose, J.E., and Teasdale, G. (1979). Long-term neuropsychological outcome of closed head injury. *Journal of Neurosurgery, 50,* 412–422.

Light, J. (1988). Interaction involving individuals using augmentative communication systems: State of the art and future directions. *Augmentative and Alternative Communication, 4,* 66–82.

Luria, A.R. (1973). *The working brain.* New York: Basic Books.

Malkmus, D. (1980). Cognitive assessment and goal setting. In *Rehabilitation of the head injured adult: Comprehensive management.* Downey, CA: Professional Staff Association of Rancho Los Amigos Hospital, Inc.

Malkmus, D., Booth, B.J., and Kodimer, C. (1980). *Rehabilitation of the head injured adult: Comprehensive management.* Downey, CA: Professional Staff Association of Rancho Los Amigos Hospital, Inc.

Matas, J.A., Mathy-Laikko, P., Beukelman, D.R., and Legresley, K. (1985). Identifying the nonspeaking population: A demographic study. *Augmentative and Alternative Communication, 1,* 17–31.

Meyer, A. (1984). The anatomical facts and clinical varieties of traumatic insanity. *American Journal of Insanity, 660,* 373–441. See also Wilson and Moffatt (Eds.), *Clinical management of memory problems.* Rockville: Aspen Systems Corp.

Munson, J.H., Nordquist, C.L., and Thuma-Rew, S.L. (1987). *Communication systems for persons with severe neuromotor impairment.* Iowa City: The University of Iowa.

Norgard, M. (1986). Seating and positioning. *Pegasus 1,* 1–4.

Porter, P.B., Wurth, B., and Stowers, S. (1988). Seating and positioning for communication. In D.E. Yoder and R.D. Kent (Eds.), *Decision making in speech-language pathology.* Ontario: Decker.

Prigatano, G.P., Fordyce, D.J., Zeiner, H.K., Roueche, J.R., Pepping, M., and Wood, B.C. (1984). Neuropsychological rehabilitation after closed head injury in young adults. *Journal of Neurology, Neurosurgery, and Psychiatry, 47,* 505–513.

Rappaport, M., Hall, K.M., Hopkins, K., Belleza, T., and Cope, D.N. (1982). Disability Rating Scale for severe head trauma: Coma to community. *Archives of Physical and Medical Rehabilitation, 63,* 118–123.

Roberts, A.H. (1980). *Severe Accidental Head Injuries: An Assessment of Long-term Prognosis.* Baltimore: University Park Press.

Ross, E.D. (1981). The aprosodias. *Archives of Neurology, 38,* 561–569.

Sarno, M.T. (1980). The nature of verbal impairment after closed head injury. *Journal of Nervous and Mental Disease, 168,* 685–692.

Sarno, M.T. (1984). Verbal impairment after closed head injury. *Journal of Nervous and Mental Disease, 172,* 475–479.

Shane, H.C., and Bashir, A.S. (1980). Election criteria for the adoption of an augmentative communication system: Preliminary considerations. *Journal of Speech and Hearing Disorders, 45,* 408–414.

Silverman, F.H. (1979). *Communication for the speechless.* Englewood Cliffs, NJ: Prentice-Hall.

Stowers, S., Altheide, M.R., and Porter, P.B. (1988). Motor assessment of the upper extremities for augmentative communication. In D.E. Yoder and R.D. Kent (Eds.), *Decision making in speech-language pathology.* Ontario: Decker.

Thomsen, I.V. (1975). Evaluation and outcome of aphasia in patients with severe closed head trauma. *Journal of Neurology, Neurosurgery, and Psychiatry, 38,* 713–718.

Vanderheiden, G.C., and Grilley, K. (1976). *Non-vocal communication techniques and aids for the severely physically handicapped.* Baltimore: University Park Press.

Vanderheiden, G.C., and Lloyd, L.L. (1986). Communication systems and their components. In S.W. Blackstone (Ed.), *Augmentative communication: An introduction.* Rockville, MD: American Speech-Language-Hearing Association.

Vanderheiden, G.C., and Yoder, D.E. (1986). Overview. In S.W. Blackstone, (Ed.), *Augmentative communication: An introduction.* Rockville, MD: American Speech-Language-Hearing Association.

Yorkston, K.M., and Karlan, G. (1986). Assessment procedures. In S.W. Blackstone (Ed.), *Augmentative communication: An introduction.* Rockville, MD: American Speech-Language-Hearing Association.

CHAPTER 11

Diagnosis and Management of Swallowing Disorders in Traumatic Brain Injury

CATHY L. LAZARUS

Professionals have become increasingly aware of the high incidence of dysphagia and the need for swallowing programs within hospital and rehabilitation settings (Groher, 1986). Winstein (1983) found that
approximately 27 percent of the traumatically brain-injured (TBI) individuals admitted to a rehabilitation facility over a 1-year period demonstrated swallowing problems on admission. Although dysphagia is a
known sequela in the TBI population, it is only recently that clinicians
have begun to incorporate dysphagia programs into the overall management of these individuals. Early identification of dysphagia and appropriate intervention are important in safe oral feeding and improved quality
of life for the TBI individual.

SWALLOWING DISORDERS

ORAL PREPARATORY AND ORAL PHASE

Lips

Dysfunction of swallowing during the oral preparatory phase of the
swallow can occur when lip, tongue, and jaw functioning are impaired.
Reduced lip closure can cause leakage of secretions or food and liquids
out of the mouth. Drooling of saliva is a common problem, particularly if
the head is positioned in a downward and forward posture, since gravity will cause secretions to accumulate in the anterior oral cavity. Drooling has also been shown to be correlated with reduced or discoordinated
voluntary swallowing frequency, as observed in the pediatric cerebral
palsy population. Discoordination between swallowing and respiration
was also found in children who drooled (Sochaniwskyj and colleagues,
1986). Inadequate lip tone can cause material to slip within the lower
anterior alveolar sulcus during oral preparation, chewing, or during
bolus formation for preparation to swallow. Reduced buccal tension can
cause stasis of food or liquid within the lower lateral sulci (Kilman and
Goyal, 1976; Logemann, 1983). In addition, reduced buccal tension can
interfere with the flow of food posteriorly through the oral cavity during
oral transit.

Tongue

Lingual dysfunction, particularly reduced range of motion, can affect
various aspects of the oral preparatory and oral phases of the swallow
(Kilman and Goyal, 1976; Logemann, 1983). Reduced lingual lateralization will create difficulties in trafficking the food over the teeth for

chewing and reduced ability to retrieve the food back onto the mid-dorsum of the tongue. Reduced tongue lateralization also interferes with retrieval of food that has lodged within the lower lateral sulcus, the space between the buccal mucosa and the lateral teeth. Reduced tongue tip and mid-tongue elevation impair ability to seal a bolus against the hard palate in preparation for the swallow. Often, when tongue functioning is reduced, the bolus is held anteriorly against the central incisors during chewing and during holding of the bolus before initiation of the swallow. This is frequently seen in individuals with Parkinson's disease or amyotrophic lateral sclerosis, whom often demonstrate lingual dysfunction (Blonsky and colleagues, 1975; Robbins and colleagues, 1986). Reduced vertical range of the posterior tongue can lead to spillage of material over the tongue base into the pharynx before initiation of the pharyngeal swallow.

Overall reduction in fine tongue control also contributes to loss of the bolus over the tongue base into the pharynx. Reduced fine tongue shaping or cupping leads to reduced ability to seal the bolus against the palate, since the lateral margins of the tongue normally contact the upper lateral alveolar ridges, while the mid-portion of the tongue is grooved to hold the bolus. Reduced vertical tongue range will interfere with propulsion of the bolus into the pharynx, since tongue propulsion requires a peristaltic squeezing of the bolus against the hard and soft palate. Reduced vertical range, particularly of the back of the tongue, will also interfere with triggering of the pharyngeal swallow, since sensory and proprioceptive input to the faucial arches is reduced. Reduced anterior-posterior tongue range will impair ability both to propel the bolus and to initiate the pharyngeal swallow. A generalized reduction in tongue control can create poor manipulation of the bolus.

Jaw

Reduced vertical, lateral, and rotary range of jaw motion can interfere with chewing. A munching of the bolus is often seen, with small, repeated up-and-down movements of the jaw during chewing attempts.

PHARYNGEAL STAGE

Pharyngeal Swallow Delay

A delay in the triggering of the pharyngeal swallow occurs when all the neuromuscular components of the pharyngeal swallow do not occur in a smooth and timely fashion. The tongue propels the bolus into the pharynx; however, there is a hesitation of the bolus within the pharynx.

Thus, the bolus may fall into the velleculae, the space formed by the tongue base and epiglottis, or the bolus may continue the descent through the pharynx into the pyriform sinuses, the cavities formed between the inferior constrictor musculature and the larynx. A pharyngeal delay is often accompanied by reduced tongue functioning to initiate the swallow. The delay may be seen as only a slight hesitation of the bolus within the pharynx before trigger of the pharyngeal swallow, the bolus may sit within the pharynx for several seconds before the pharyngeal swallow occurs. A pharyngeal swallow is defined as absent if no pharyngeal response occurs or if a pharyngeal response occurs after 30 seconds (Logemann, 1983).

Reduced Pharyngeal Peristalsis

Reduced pharyngeal peristalsis occurs when the pharyngeal constrictor musculature functioning is reduced. Material does not clear the pharynx but remains within the pharynx after the swallow. Material can remain within the velleculae, along the aryepiglottic folds, within the pyriform sinuses, or along the posterior pharyngeal wall, or it can be situated within the entire pharynx. Some of this material may slip down into the laryngeal vestibule or may continue down through the larynx and be aspirated into the trachea. Generalized residue within the pharynx usually indicates a bilateral pharyngeal disorder. Material that tends to be located along one side of the pharynx indicates a unilateral pharyngeal paresis or paralysis. Material is often situated within one pyriform sinus. Sensation can often be reduced, such that the dysphagic individual does not spontaneously attempt to reswallow to clear this residue from the pharynx.

Reduced Laryngeal Elevation

Reduced laryngeal elevation can contribute to reduced ability to clear material from the pharynx, causing residue within the pharynx after the swallow. Reduced laryngeal elevation can also contribute to reduced opening of the cricopharyngeus during the swallow, since the upward and forward pull of the larynx creates anterior stretch on the cricopharyngeus muscle (Dodds and colleagues, 1988; Curtis and colleagues, 1985).

Reduced Laryngeal Closure

Reduced laryngeal closure occurs when there is incomplete adduction of the true vocal cords during the swallow. This can be due to a unilateral or bilateral vocal cord paralysis or paresis. Reduced laryngeal closure can be seen as penetration of material through the larynx below the level of the true vocal cords during the swallow.

Cricopharyngeal Dysfunction

Cricopharyngeal dysfunction occurs when the cricopharyngeus muscle does not relax and open sufficiently to allow the bolus to pass through into the esophagus during the swallow. Very small amounts of the bolus may pass through the segment during swallow attempts. If the cricopharyngeal dysfunction is severe, none of the bolus will enter the esophagus and will remain in the pyriform sinuses after the swallow. Cricopharyngeal dysfunction is related to several variables. The segment may be relaxing but not opening, since relaxation and opening are two distinct components (Kahrilas and colleagues, 1988). Cricopharyngeal opening can be impaired due to reduced laryngeal elevation or reduced pressures from above to propel the bolus through the segment. In the latter case, reduced pressures within the pharynx may be caused by reduced tongue functioning to exert posterior and downward thrust onto the bolus (McConnel, 1988). Reduced cricopharyngeal relaxation can be caused by reduced innervation to the cricopharyngeus muscle (Kirchner, 1986).

ESOPHAGEAL STAGE

The presence of a tracheo-esophageal (t-e) fistula should be considered as a possible cause of dysphagia when the oropharyngeal swallow appears to be otherwise normal. T-e fistulae can occur when chest and laryngeal trauma are present. The fistula is often identified on videofluorographic examination (VFG) when material is coughed out of the airway without prior aspiration of material into the trachea from above. The fluoroscopic tube should then be focused lower, within the lower cervical and upper thoracic esophagus to identify the fistula. Esophageal reflux can cause dysphagia when cricopharyngeal functioning is reduced and material refluxes out of the esophagus and into the pharynx. Similarly, the presence of a diverticulum, or outpouching within the cervical esophagus, can lead to aspiration if cricopharyngeal functioning is reduced. Material that has spilled out of the diverticulum upward and out into the pharynx can be aspirated.

SWALLOWING DISORDERS IN THE TRAUMATICALLY BRAIN INJURED POPULATION

PATTERNS OF SWALLOWING DISORDERS

Although dysphagic individuals with TBI demonstrate many of the previously mentioned types of swallowing disorders, few studies have examined the nature of swallowing disorders in the TBI population. Ekedahl (1974) found a high incidence of drooling within the TBI population. Lazarus and Logemann (1987b) examined the frequency and co-occurrence of swallowing motility disorders and found nine distinct swallowing motility disorders in a group of 53 TBI individuals (38 men and 15 women) ranging in age from 4 to 69 years (mean age of 29). These individuals sustained a head injury within an average of 16 months of the VFG examination. Forty-one individuals had computed tomographic (CT) scans. In this study, no attempt was made to correlate lesion site to the nature of the swallowing disorder because many subjects only exhibited diffuse cortical atrophy. All subjects were undergoing some type of swallow therapy prior to their VFG study.

Twenty-four subjects (45%) were seen for the videographic study before receiving oral feeding or were seen within 2 months following commencement of oral intake. At the time of their radiographic study, six subjects ate by mouth while 11 subjects were fed through nasogastric tubes. Eighteen underwent gastrostomy or jejeunostomy for primary or supplemental nutrition. Only one subject with a nasogastric tube and two subjects who had gastrostomies were ingesting oral diets and were receiving supplemental nutrition through their tubes. None of the fourteen subjects with tracheostomy tubes at the time of their swallow evaluations demonstrated swallowing problems directly related to the tracheostomy tube placement. Only one individual exhibited a laryngeal elevation disorder, and that person had sustained laryngeal trauma at the time of his head injury.

The severity of each subject's swallowing problem was evaluated against three parameters: (1) increase in oral transit times, indicating reduction in tongue functioning during the oral stage of swallowing (*mild* being a 1- to 5-second increase in oral transit, *moderate* being a 5- to 10-second increase, and *severe* being over 10 seconds to complete oral transit); (2) length of delay in triggering of the swallow reflex (*mild* being 0 to 5 seconds delayed, *moderate* being 5 to 10 seconds delayed, and *severe* being over 10 seconds delayed); and (3) severity of aspiration (*mild* being trace to less than 20% of the bolus aspirated, *moderate* being 20% to 30% aspirated, and *severe* being greater than 30% of the bolus aspirated).

If any subject demonstrated at least one rating of severe in any of the three categories, the swallowing problem was labeled severe. If two of the three ratings were moderate, the patient's swallowing problem was labeled moderate. If two or all three ratings were mild, the patient was labeled as having a mild swallowing problem.

Results of this study revealed that severity of swallowing problem increased for subjects who had been comatose. In addition, greater severity of swallowing problems was observed as the duration of coma increased. However, some subjects with severe swallowing problems had not been comatose or had been comatose for only short periods. In addition, there were subjects who had not been comatose or had been comatose for extended periods who demonstrated only mild swallowing difficulties.

Duration of nonoral feeding, whether gastrostomy or nasogastric tube, did not correspond with swallowing problem severity. No observed swallowing problems were related to the presence of the nasogastric tube. Eight subjects who took nutrition orally at the time of their VFG study demonstrated moderate to severe swallowing problems or were aspirating. Four of these subjects subsequently underwent gastrostomy of nasogastric tube placement for primary nutrition while they received swallowing therapy.

Within each lesion type, severity of swallowing problems was examined in relation to coma duration. There was a tendency for subjects in coma for longer than 24 hours to exhibit more severe swallowing problems than patients whose coma lasted less than 24 hours.

There were nine swallowing motility problems exhibited by these 53 head trauma subjects. As can be seen on Table 11-1, the most frequently occurring motility disorders were a delayed triggering of the pharyngeal swallow (seen in 81%) and reduced tongue control (seen in 53%). Thirty-two percent exhibited reduced pharyngeal peristalsis. Only a few individuals (14%) showed disorders involving the larynx, including reduced closure, elevation, or spasm. One of the individuals with reduced laryngeal closure had sustained laryngeal trauma concurrent with his injury. Few persons demonstrated cricopharyngeal disorders (6%).

Table 11-1. Frequency of swallowing motility disorders in 53 subjects who sustained closed head trauma

Swallowing motility	Subjects	
	Number	Percentage (%) of total
Swallowing reflex problem	43	81
Delayed reflex	(37)	(70)
Absent reflex	(6)	(11)
Reduced lingual control	28	53
Reduced peristalsis	17	32
Reduced laryngeal closure	3	6
Reduced laryngeal elevation	2	4
Spasm in larynx	2	4
Cricopharyngeal dysfunction	3	6
Could not test	1	2
Normal swallow	1	2
Esophageal stricture	1	2

When examining co-occurrence of swallowing motility disorders, Lazarus and Logemann (1987b) reported that the majority of these 53 individuals demonstrated two-component swallowing disorders. The two most frequently occurring combinations of two-component problems were reduced tongue control with delayed or absent swallow (22%) and delayed pharyngeal swallow with reduced pharyngeal peristalsis (17%). Twenty-one percent of the individuals exhibited three-component swallowing problems. The most frequent combination was reduced tongue control with a delayed pharyngeal swallow and reduced pharyngeal peristalsis (9%).

As seen in Table 11-2, of the 53 TBI persons, 20 individuals (38%) aspirated during VFG study. Aspiration before the swallow was the most common, due to an absent swallow, a delayed pharyngeal swallow, or the combination of reduced lingual control with delayed pharyngeal swallow. Only two individuals aspirated during the swallow because of reduced laryngeal closure. Aspiration after the swallow usually resulted from reduced pharyngeal peristalsis, as seen in four individuals. Only one person aspirated after the swallow because of cricopharyngeal dysfunction. No subject aspirated at more than one point in the swallowing sequence (i.e., a combination of before, during, or after the swallow).

Finally, the occurrence of aspiration with various food consistencies was examined (Table 11-3). Patients with delayed reflex with or without tongue control difficulty always aspirated on liquids, predominantly because the tongue could not control and hold the liquid cohesively and because the liquid splashed into the pharynx and into the airway in the time delay before the swallowing reflex triggered. Aspiration after the swallow occurred mainly on thicker consistencies (paste and masticated material) because there was a greater amount of residue in the pharynx with thicker foods.

Table 11-2. Etiology of aspiration, and its occurrence in relation to swallow in 20 traumatically brain-injured subjects

Etiology of aspiration	Relation to swallow		
	Before	*During*	*After*
Reduced tongue control and delayed reflex	7		
Delayed reflex	4		
Absent reflex	2		
Laryngeal closure		2	
Reduced peristalsis			4
Cricopharyngeal dysfunction			1
Total	13	2	5

Table 11-3. Frequency and co-occurrence of aspiration before, during, and after swallow as related to bolus consistency in 20 traumatically brain-injured subjects

Swallow disorder	Consistency of material				
	L	M	L,P	L,P,M	TOTAL
BEFORE SWALLOW					
Lingual control problems and delayed reflex	5		2	1	8
Delayed or absent reflex	4			1	5
DURING SWALLOW					
Reduced laryngeal elevation and closure	1	1			2
AFTER SWALLOW					
Reduced peristalsis		1	1	2	4
Cricopharyngeal dysfunction				1	1
Total	10	2	3	5	20

L = liquid; M = masticated; P = pureed.

TONGUE CONTROL FOR SWALLOWING

The type of lingual impairment seen in the TBI population differs from that seen in other neurologically impaired groups. Lazarus and Logemann (1986) examined the types and patterns of tongue movement observed during swallowing in 20 TBI subjects. These subjects were identified as having lingual control problems on VFG evaluation of swallow. All subjects were undergoing swallow therapy before their VFG study. Patient age ranged from 6 to 50, with a mean of 29. The time from head injury until the VFG study varied from 2 weeks to 3 years, 4 months in these subjects. The length of time between head injury and VFG study was examined, and no relationship was apparent between severity of lingual dysfunction and length of time after trauma when the VFG study was performed.

Severity of tongue dysfunction during swallowing was defined by measuring oral transit time. Delays in oral transit of 10 to 15 seconds or more were rated severe lingual dysfunction; delays of 10 to 15 seconds were rated as moderate lingual dysfunction; and delays of 1–5 seconds were rated as mild lingual dysfunction. Oral transit times of 1 second or less constituted normal lingual functioning. In addition to the measures of oral transit times, the types and patterns of tongue movement exhibited by each subject were noted. The following observations were made: (1) number of repetitive tongue movements required to initiate the swallow reflex, (2) range of movement of the base of tongue relative to the posterior pharyngeal wall, and (3) range of vertical movement of the tongue tip, mid-tongue, and back tongue relative to the hard and soft palate. Lingual range was quantified by percentage, specifically, less than 25 percent of total range, 50 percent of total range, 75 percent of total range, or 100 percent of total range (implying complete linguopalatal or linguoposterior pharyngeal wall contact).

Results of this study showed that severity of lingual dysfunction correlated with differences in vertical tongue movement by portion of the tongue. Specifically, tongue tip function remained fairly intact across severity groups. However, greater severity of lingual control correlated with reduced ability to elevate the posterior portion of the tongue and reduced ability to move the base of the tongue to the posterior pharyngeal wall during swallow attempts.

When examining the average number of discrete tongue movements required to propel the bolus into the pharynx by each lingual control group, fewer movements were required to propel the bolus within the mild group compared with the moderate and severe groups, although there was a fairly wide range in each group, particularly within the severe group.

TONGUE CONTROL FOR SPEECH AND SWALLOWING

When examining the relationship between a specific portion of the tongue and the severity of lingual dysfunction for swallowing and speech, a similar trend was found in tongue functioning for swallowing as seen in the previously mentioned study. Lazarus and Logemann (1987a) examined the relationship between the severity of lingual dysfunction for swallowing and for speech, by specific portion of tongue, in 20 TBI subjects. These subjects were identified as having lingual control problems on VFG evaluation of deglutition. Severity of tongue dysfunction for swallowing was defined as discussed in the previous study (by measuring oral transit time). All subjects had been undergoing speech and swallow therapy before their VFG study.

Severity of tongue dysfunction during speech was defined by the ability to produce linguopalatal contacts for the tip-alveolar, blade-palatal, and back-velar consonant phonemes /t, tʃ, k/ in consonant-vowel-consonant (CVC) words. If the individual was unable to produce speech, ability to elevate specific portions of the tongue (i.e., tip, mid, and back) or resist against a tongue blade placed on the tip, mid, or back portion of the tongue was examined. Subjects were given ample time to respond, since many demonstrated speech or lingual initiation problems. Linguopalatal contact for speech was labeled *complete* (+) or *absent* (−), since VFG was not used for this portion of the examination and finer gradations of tongue elevation could not be precisely determined by observation.

The relationship between length of coma, if present, and severity of the lingual control deficit for swallowing was also examined. Approximately half the subjects had been in coma after onset of injury. In these individuals, there was increased severity of lingual dysfunction for swallow as length of coma increased. The relationship between severity of lingual dysfunction for swallow and severity of dysarthria was examined (Table 11-4). There appeared to be greater severity of dysarthria across all lingual dysfunction groups for swallowing. However, those subjects demonstrating normal speech or mild or moderate dysarthrias (only 25% of the subjects) showed similar mild or moderate tongue dysfunction for swallowing.

When examining the relationship between tongue tip range of movement for swallow and overall dysfunction for deglutition, all three severity groups demonstrated intact tongue tip to palate contact during swallow. When examining the relationship between mid-tongue to palate range of motion during swallow and overall severity of lingual dysfunction for deglutition, most of the subjects with mild and moderate lingual dysfunction were able to maintain a complete mid-tongue to palate seal during swallow attempts. However, few subjects with severe lingual dysfunction for deglutition could achieve a complete seal. An even greater disparity in range could be seen when examining range of back tongue movement for swallow as related to severity of the lingual control problem for deglutition. Four of the seven subjects with severe lingual control problems were unable to elevate the posterior tongue more than half way to the palate.

When examining the range of tongue movement to the posterior pharyngeal wall as related to severity of lingual control during swallow, there was more variability of tongue range within the mildly impaired lingual control category. However, both the moderate and severe lingual control groups demonstrated minimal base of tongue to posterior pharyngeal wall movement during swallow attempts.

Table 11-4. Severity of lingual dysfunction for swallow as related to severity of dysarthria for 20 traumatically brain-injured subjects

Degree of tongue dysfunction for swallow	Degree of dysarthria			
	Normal	Mild	Moderate	Severe
Mild	2	1	—	4
Moderate	—	1	—	5
Severe	—	—	1	6

Table 11-5. Number of discrete tongue movements required to initiate swallow according to lingual dysfunction group

Number of tongue movements

	2	4	6	8		10	12	14	16	18	20	22	24	26	28	30

MILD
Liquid ⊢—X—————————⊣
Paste ⊢———X—————————⊣
Masticated ⊢———X—————⊣

MODERATE
Liquid ⊢—————————X——————————⊣
Paste ⊢—————————————X—————⊣
Masticated ⱶXⱳ

SEVERE
Liquid ⊢—————————————————X————————————————————————⊣
Paste ⊢—X—⊣
Masticated ⱶXⱳ

Table 11-6. Ability to elevate tongue (tip, middle, back) for speech according to dysarthria severity as observed in 20 traumatically brain-injured subjects

	Degree of dysarthria (%)		
Tongue portion	*Mild*	*Moderate*	*Severe*
Tip	100	100	40
Mid	100	100	13
Back	100	100	20

As seen in Table 11-5, when examining the mean number of discrete tongue movements required to propel the bolus into the pharynx by each lingual control group, fewer movements were required to propel the bolus within the mild and moderate groups compared with the severe group, although there was a fairly wide range within the severe group.

The ability to elevate the tongue (tip, mid, and back) for speech according to severity of dysarthria was examined (Table 11-6). Almost all subjects in the mild and moderate dysarthria groups were able to elevate all portions of the tongue to the palate for speech. Forty percent of the subjects in the severe dysarthria category could elevate the tongue tip; however, few subjects could elevate the middle and back portions of the tongue.

Table 11-7 shows the relationship between tongue function for speech

Table 11-7. Relationship between tongue function disorders for speech and for swallowing according to portion of the tongue involved in 20 traumatically brain-injured subjects

Tongue function disorder	Tip	Middle	Back
+ Speech + Swallow	11	6	6
− Speech + Swallow	08	9	8
− Speech − Swallow	01	4	6
+ Speech − Swallow	—	1	—

and swallowing according to portion of the tongue involved. A large percentage of subjects in each group demonstrated intact lingual function for swallow but not for speech. The highest correlation between speech and swallow functioning occurred within the tongue tip category, although almost as many subjects had intact tongue tip function for swallow but not for speech. When examining these relationships of speech and swallowing for the mid and back portions of the tongue, the majority of subjects had intact tongue functioning for swallowing but not for speech. A small percentage had reduced tongue functioning for both speech and swallow.

In summary, severity of lingual dysfunction during deglutition in these TBI individuals appears to relate to a reduction in lingual range of movement in specific portions of the tongue and the number of movements required to propel a bolus into the pharynx. When examining tongue dysfunction for swallow according to each severity group, those subjects with mildly impaired lingual dysfunction for swallow varied in the extent of their intact lingual functioning for speech. In the moderate lingual dysfunction for swallow group, fewer subjects demonstrated intact functioning for speech. The group with severely impaired lingual function demonstrated the greatest number of subjects with severe lingual dysfunction for speech. However, it was difficult to determine whether neuromotor involvement or cognitive-initiation deficits played greater roles in subjects' performance on speech and nonspeech voluntary tongue gestures.

Interestingly, some of the subjects in the severe lingual dysfunction for swallow category were able to maintain complete lingual-palatal contacts during swallow attempts. However, these subjects exhibited reduced anteroposterior tongue movements. Specifically, there was minimal or absent rolling, squeezing, or backward motion of the tongue. Often the pharyngeal swallow would be triggered while the majority or all of the bolus remained in the oral cavity after the swallow. Swallowing efficiency in these subjects was very reduced. In general, severity of tongue dysfunction for speech did not appear to correlate with severity of tongue dysfunction for swallowing. The majority of subjects across lingual severity groups for swallow demonstrated severe lingual dysfunction for speech. These data support the hypothesis that neuromotor control of the tongue for speech may be distinct and separate from the neuromotor control needed for swallowing.

RECOVERY OF SWALLOW FUNCTIONING

Lazarus and Logemann (1985) examined the patterns and degree of recovery of swallow function in 15 TBI subjects referred for VFG evaluation of a swallowing disorder. At the time of their initial radiographic study, three subjects were eating orally (one on a general diet and two on pureed diets). Seven subjects had tracheostomy tubes at the time of their swallow evaluations. None of these subjects with tracheostomy tubes demonstrated swallowing problems directly related to the presence of their tracheostomy tubes. All subjects in this study were reevaluated by VFG examination at least once to assess improvement in swallowing from 5 days to 22 months following their initial swallow examination. All subjects were undergoing swallow therapy.

The degree of severity of each subject's swallowing problem was defined using three parameters: (1) increase in oral transit times, (2) length of delay in triggering of the pharyngeal swallow, and (3) severity of aspiration. If any subject demonstrated at least one rating of severe in any of the three categories delineated above, the swallowing problem was labeled severe. If two of the three ratings were moderate, the subject's swallowing problem was labeled moderate. If two or all three ratings were mild, the subject was labeled as having a mild swallowing problem. All subjects had been undergoing speech and swallowing therapy before and after their initial VFG evaluation. Table 11-8, based on the initial VFG study, shows the severity of dysarthria, swallowing problems, and aspiration for the 15 subjects as related to presence and duration of coma. Severity of speech impairment generally coincided with swallowing severity. There was a strong tendency toward greater severity of swallowing problems in subjects who had been comatose. Duration of coma, however, did not appear to correlate with severity of swallowing problems. Nor did there appear to be any significant relationship between duration of gastrostomy or nasogastric tube placement and initial severity of swallowing problem. Five of the subjects who demonstrated severe swallowing problems did not aspirate, probably because they were given only very small amounts of material per bolus.

When examining the mean oral transit times of liquid swallows for all subjects on all VFG studies, it was found that oral transit times improved in 12 of the 15 subjects. When examining pharyngeal transit times, it was found that there was variability in the triggering of the pharyngeal swal-

Table 11-8. Coma duration, severity of dysarthria, severity of dysphagia, and presence of aspiration for 15 traumatically brain-injured subjects

Subject	Dysarthria	Coma duration	Dysphagia	Aspiration
1	No speech	—	Severe	
2	Moderate	—	Mild	
3	Moderate	—	Moderate	
4	—	Moderate		
5	Normal speech	—	Mild	
6	Moderate	0.4 week	Mild	+ (Mild)
7	No meaningful communica-tion	0.7 week	Moderate	+ (Moderate)
8	No meaningful communica-tion	3.0 weeks	Severe	+ (Mild)
9	Severe	8.0 weeks	Severe	+ (Mild)
10	No meaningful communica-tion	8.0 weeks	Severe	
11	Severe	8.0 weeks	Severe	
12	No meaningful communica-tion	12.0 weeks	Moderate	
13	Moderate	16.0 weeks	Severe	
14	Moderate	20.0 weeks	Mild	
15	No speech	Chronic vegetative state	Severe	

low within VFG studies. Some subjects demonstrated slight delays in triggering of the swallow on their first liquid swallow and normalized on their subsequent swallow. Only two subjects did not demonstrate any delay in triggering of the pharyngeal swallow on their initial and subsequent studies. Of the remaining 13 who did demonstrate delays, nine subjects improved in triggering of the swallow over subsequent studies. Five of the nine recovered normal triggering of the swallow. Four of these subjects normalized on their second study, and one subject normalized on his third study. The other four subjects demonstrated shorter delays but did not return to normal.

On paste consistencies, eight of 12 subjects who could tolerate this consistency improved on oral transit measures. Only one subject demonstrated normal triggering of the pharyngeal swallow on paste swallows in the initial VFG study. The same intrasubject variability in triggering of the pharyngeal swallow seen on liquid swallows was observed on paste swallows within each VFG study, with the first paste swallow being slower. Of the 12 subjects who swallowed a paste consistency, seven improved in triggering of the swallow. Three of the seven exhibited normal triggering on subsequent VFG studies.

Only two of the 15 subjects were able to take a masticated consistency on two successive VFG studies. Both these subjects improved in swallow functioning.

Table 11-9 shows the improvement in swallow function according to consistencies tested, aspiration, change in diet, and swallowing severity from the first to the final VFG study for the 15 subjects. Six subjects were able to tolerate new consistencies on subsequent VFG studies. Five subjects who aspirated on their initial study showed no aspiration on their final study. Two subjects who did not aspirate on their initial study aspirated in small amounts on subsequent studies. Nine of the 12 subjects receiving nonoral feeding were able to tolerate some type of oral diet at the time of their final VFG study. Eight subjects improved in their overall swallowing severity rating; one worsened; and six remained the same. All those whose severity remained the same had mild to moderate problems. Table 11-10 shows the improvement in swallow function from the initial to the final VFG study by specific motility disorder. Lingual control and triggering of the pharyngeal swallow improved in severity on subsequent swallows in all but one subject, who exhibited neither of these problems on his first study. All these subjects had received tongue exercises and thermal stimulation of the pharyngeal swallow. Pharyngeal peristalsis, if impaired on initial studies, appeared to improve the least over time. Only two subjects with reduced pharyngeal peristalsis demonstrated normal functioning at their final VFG study. Two subjects with lingual control problems and a delayed triggering of the pharyngeal swallow improved in both of these areas, but, with the improvement, a cricopharyngeal disorder was uncovered.

In summary, improved swallow function in these TBI subjects was characterized by improvement in oral and pharyngeal transit times, reduction or elimination of aspiration, reduction or elimination of residue in the pharynx, and ability to tolerate new food consistencies. Overall improvement in swallow functioning also included (1) increase in the amount of food swallowed per bolus, (2) presence of spontaneous

Table 11-9. Improvement in swallow function according to consistency of material, aspiration, change in diet, and dysphagia severity from first to last videofluroscopic study in 15 traumatically brain-injured subjects

	Number of consistencies presented at VFG			Presence of aspiration	Number of Subjects receiving oral intake	Dysphagia severity		
Study	L	P	M			+	−	Same
First	15	10	04	6	03			
Final	15	12	06	3	12	7	2	6

L = liquid; P = pureed; M = masticated.

Table 11-10. **Improvement in swallow function from
initial to final videofluoroscopic study by specific
motility disorder in 15 traumatically brain-injured subjects**

Disorder	Number of Subjects	Improved	Normal-ized	No change	New problem
Reduced lingual control	11	(6) 55%	(4) 36%	(1) 9%	0
Delayed triggering of reflex	12	(9) 75%	(3) 36%	0	0
Reduced pharyngeal peristalsis	9	(4) 44%	(2) 22%	(2) 22%	(1) 11%
Cricopharyngeal dysfunction	5	(2) 40%	(1) 20%	0	(2) 40%

reswallowing to clear residue from the oral cavity or pharynx, (3) presence of spontaneous coughing in response to aspiration, and (4) reduction in the number of nonproductive tongue movements to manipulate and propel the bolus into the pharynx.

None of the subjects in this study exhibited a normal swallow on the final VFG study. However, subjects with slightly slower than normal swallow were receiving some type of oral diet and were not aspirating. The length of time required for recovery of swallow function after trauma varied widely within the subjects studied. For example, in subjects who normalized in at least one motility disorder, length of time until normalization varied from 1 week to 9 months. It is evident that TBI individuals continue to improve in swallow function over fairly long periods. Spontaneous recovery and swallow therapy can have a positive impact for a number of months after trauma. The author has seen recovery of swallow functioning occur in a dysphagic individual over a 9-month period.

ASSESSMENT OF SWALLOWING

Various procedures are used to examine the oropharyngeal stages of the swallow. *Cinefluoroscopy* has been used in the past to examine deglutition (Donner and Silbiger, 1966; Mandelstam and Lieber, 1970). Cinefluoroscopy defines the swallowing physiology and etiology of the dysphagia; however, since there are 60 frames per second, the radiation exposure is a contraindication to routine use of this procedure. *Ultrasound* is another technique used to examine the anatomy and physiology of the tongue during the oral preparatory and oral phases of the swallow. However, its use is limited to study of the oral cavity, since ultrasound cannot visualize the pharynx (Shawker and colleagues, 1983, 1984). *Scintigraphy* is useful to examine bolus passage through the pharynx (Muz and colleagues, 1987); however, adjacent structures cannot be visualized using this technique. Scintigraphy records the passage of a radionuclide bolus through the upper digestive tract. Bolus flow measures and presence and percentage of aspiration down to the level of the lower bronchi can be determined using this technique (Muz and colleagues, 1987). *Manometry* has been used to assess esophaegeal peristalsis and upper and lower esophageal sphincter functioning (Fyke and Code, 1955). Manometry can also be used to examine pressures generated within the pharynx, cricopharyngeus muscle, and upper esophagus. However, aspiration cannot be assessed using this techinque. The *modified barium swallow* uses videofluoroscopy (VFG) to examine the oral and pharyngeal stages of the swallow (Logemann, 1983). This procedure provides excellent visualization of the structures within the oral cavity and pharynx. The speed of the swallow is well visualized, so that both oral and pharyngeal transit times and motility disorders can be determined. It also defines the etiology and precise amount of aspiration. In addition, residue within the oral cavity and pharynx can be visualized. The effects of therapy techniques can be examined during the VFG procedure. Manometry has recently been combined with fluoroscopy to examine oropharyngeal swallow functioning (Kahrilas and colleagues, 1988; McConnel and colleagues, 1986, 1987, 1988). Simultaneous manometric and VFG swallow studies provide additional information concerning pressures generated within the hyopharynx during the swallow. This technique is presently being used primarily for research purposes. However, current clinical practice with the TBI population utilizes VFG to evaluate swallow function.

THE MODIFIED BARIUM SWALLOW

The Lateral View

During the modified barium swallow procedure, the dysphagic individual is initially situated upright in the lateral plane. As seen in Figure 11-1, the fluoroscopic tube is focused on the lips anteriorly, the palate superiorly, the vertebral spine posteriorly, and the seventh cervical vertebra inferiorly (Logemann, 1983, 1986a). Since many wheelchairs are too wide to fit within the space between the fluoroscopic tube and table, several chairs have been devised to fit between this space. These chairs can easily accommodate nonambulatory individuals. Often, the fluoroscopic tube does not move low enough for the oral cavity and pharynx to be visualized. A ramp can be constructed, approximately 8 to 10 inches high, so that the individual can be wheeled up high enough for adequate visualization of the oropharynx. Individuals with TBI who are sent for their swallow studies on hospital carts can undergo dysphagia examina-

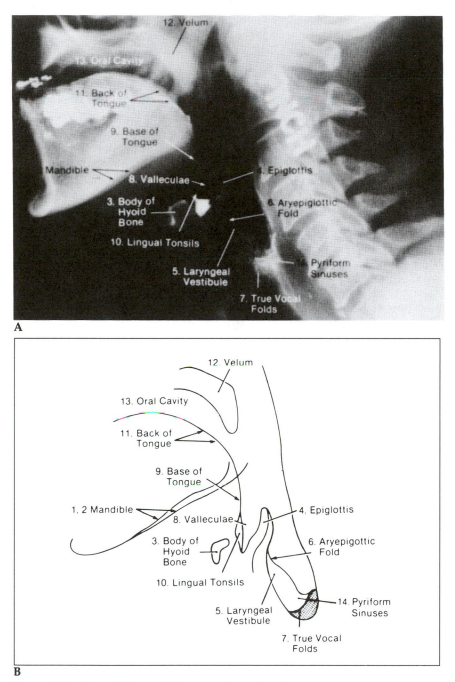

Figure 11-1. Lateral view of the upper aerodigestive tract as seen on x-ray film. (From Logemann, J. A. (1986a) *Manual for the videofluorographic study of swallowing*. Boston: College-Hill Press.)

tions, provided that the cart is narrow enough to fit between the tube and the table. The author has seen several individuals for VFG examinations sent from hospital intensive care units in their hospital beds. The VFG study can be attempted as long as the head of the bed or cart can be elevated to at least 30 degrees. For VFG studies on infants and small children, parents are asked to bring their children's car seats or strollers. Strollers can be wheeled up on ramps. However, if the stroller is situated too low to view the oropharynx, it can be placed atop a cart, with weights next to the wheels to act as anchors. Car seats or tumbleform chairs can also be placed atop carts and weighted for safety. Ventilator-dependent individuals can undergo VFG studies if they can be hooked up to portable ventilators or if a respiratory therapist can accompany the individual and periodically ventilate the individual during the VFG study.

Substances

During the VFG procedure, substances of various consistencies are typically presented. For example, two swallows each of one third to one fourth teaspoon of liquid barium, barium paste, and one fourth of a cookie coated with barium are presented in our clinical practice. The etiology of the dysphagia should be defined. Oral and pharyngeal transit times, motility disorders, and presence of aspiration should be determined for each swallow. If the individual aspirates, the clinician should determine what therapy techniques might eliminate this aspiration and whether the individual could tolerate a firmer consistency. Individuals are initially given liquids to swallow, since liquids define the etiology of aspiration without occluding the airway. If the individual does not aspirate on liquids, or if the motility disorder would not preclude giving the individual another consistency, he or she is then given two swallows each of one fourth teaspoon of a paste consistency, such as a pudding mixed with barium paste. Esophatrast is a widely used paste. If the individual can chew or does well enough with the paste consistency to attempt the masticated swallow, he or she is then given two swallows of one fourth of a cookie coated with a barium paste.

Persons with severe TBI are often unable to initiate any oral movements for a swallow when given liquids or even pastes. There appears to be a reduced sensory awareness and recognition of the bolus. Therefore, a very small piece (one eighth teaspoon) of a cookie coated with barium paste should be introduced, since the cookie often provides adequate sensory input to facilitate oral movements for chewing. The liquid and paste consistencies can then be introduced. Care should be given when introducing a spoon, since the TBI individual may have a strong bite reflex. Spoons constructed of a molded hard plastic are useful, since they will not break when bitten. Often, tongue functioning is so severely reduced that the person is unable to propel the bolus into the pharynx. Thus, it is difficult to establish the presence of a pharyngeal swallow. Therefore, a 1-ml syringe may be introduced into the posterior oral cavity so that liquid can be placed into the pharynx, bypassing the oral phase, to determine whether a pharyngeal swallow is present (Dobie, 1978). In this case, the dysphagic individual should continue with nonoral feeding because of the severity of lingual dysfunction, even if he or she demonstrates a pharyngeal swallow. The information gained during this swallow study will be helpful concerning overall level of swallow functioning and therapy needs.

Bolus Size

For those individuals already receiving oral diets who have been referred for evaluation to confirm appropriateness of diet, or for those with whom there is a question of aspiration, bolus size should be examined. Providing calibrated bolus sizes is useful even for individuals who are not yet taking anything orally but who appear to be swallowing functionally during their swallow study. Varying the size of the bolus has been found to alter the timing and movement patterns of the neuromuscular components of the swallow in normal subjects (Dodds and colleagues, 1988; Kahrilas and colleagues, 1988; Tracy and Logemann, 1987) as well as in the neurologically impaired population, including the TBI population (Rasley and Logemann, 1987). If tongue functioning and timely triggering of the pharyngeal swallow occur during a one-fourth-teaspoon swallow of liquids, with no aspiration, calibrated larger amounts of liquids are presented to stress the swallowing mechanism and to determine whether larger amounts prove to be more difficult or easier to handle.

Calibrated liquid boluses usually are introduced using a syringe. A 1-ml liquid bolus is syringed onto a spoon and presented twice. If the individual tolerates this size bolus, two swallows of a 3-ml bolus are syringed directly into the individual's mouth. If lip closure is reduced, the 3-ml bolus can be syringed onto a spoon and presented. Oftentimes, a 1-ml bolus does not provide adequate sensory input to elicit voluntary initiation of the swallow and a timely triggering of the pharyngeal swallow, and a 3- or 5-ml bolus must be introduced (Rasley and Logemann, 1987). If lip closure is adequate to maintain a seal around the syringe and the individual tolerates the 3-ml bolus, two swallows of a 5-ml bolus are introduced. If this amount is tolerated without aspiration, and if the clinician feels that it is safe for the individual to take a larger bolus (based on previous swallows), a 10-ml bolus is presented. The 10-ml bolus is the amount a person might swallow if taking a gulp of liquid from a cup. Using calibrated bolus sizes stresses the swallowing mechanism so that the clinician can determine the amount the patient can swallow per bolus without being placed at risk for aspiration. If bolus size is not examined, the person might resume eating at meals and try guzzling a cup of liquid if merely told that he or she "*passed*" his swallow test, only having been examined on swallows of one fourth teaspoon of liquid. One should be cautioned, however, that calibrated bolus studies are warranted only if swallowing functioning is such that the system could tolerate larger amounts of liquids. The individual is given two swallows each of a quarter teaspoon of barium paste. If tongue functioning appears adequate to attempt a masticated consistency, the individual is given two swallows each of a quarter cookie coated with barium paste. Calibrated bolus studies are not indicated on paste and masticated consistences, unless a person who had "*passed*" the swallow study was found to be aspirating during meals. An additional examination would then be useful to determine whether larger amounts of foods per swallow could be causing the person to aspirate. It is also important to observe the person during mealtime to determine how large a bolus is being taken per swallow. Some persons with TBI have difficulty with inhibition and tend to take too large an amount per swallow or to eat their food too quickly, without reswallowing to clear residue that may be present within the pharynx.

Anteroposterior View

Following the initial swallows in the lateral plane, dysphagic persons can be seated in the anteroposterior view, facing the VFG tube. This view allows for visualization of the symmetry of residue within the oral cavity and pharynx (Donner 1974; Donner and Silbiger, 1966; Logemann, 1983). Specifically, one can determine whether there is residue in one or both pyriform sinuses, one or both lower lateral sulci, the hard and soft palate, and on the dorsum of the tongue. The anteroposterior view also provides information concerning vocal fold functioning. If the person can phonate, an examination of the true vocal cords during productions of /a/ can identify a unilateral or bilateral vocal cord paresis or paralysis. The person's head should be tilted back slightly during phonation to move the mandible from view and allow for better visualization of the true vocal cords. Uneven heights of vocal cords during adduction can also be detected, particularly if an individual has sustained laryngeal trauma or laryngeal reconstruction. One might only want to examine the residue within the oropharynx in the anteroposterior view, having determined the etiology of the dysphagia in the lateral view. The anteroposterior view is also useful to try compensatory postural techniques during the swallow study to determine whether these techniques might assist the passage of food through the oral cavity and pharynx. The clinician should not use the anteroposterior view to establish the etiology of the swallowing disorder or to determine whether an individual is aspirating. The dysphagia is much more clearly defined in the lateral plane (Logemann, 1983).

Aspiration

Aspiration is defined as the entrance of food or liquid into the larynx below the level of the true vocal cords. Aspiration may be accompanied by coughing, which is a reflexive attempt to expectorate material that has been aspirated (Linden and Siebens, 1983). It has been found that silent aspiration occurs in approximately 40 percent of hospital patients with neurologic disorders seen bedside for swallow evaluations, as confirmed by VFG study (Splaingard and colleagues, 1988; Jenkins and colleagues, 1984). Aspiration can occur at different times during the swallow, specifically, *before, during,* or *after* the swallow (Logemann, 1983). For example, a dysphagic individual can have a delayed triggering of the swallow, with aspiration before the swallow, and reduced pharyngeal peristalsis resulting in residue within the pharynx, causing aspiration after the swallow. Therefore, it is important to identify when the aspiration is occurring and the etiology of the aspiration to ensure that therapy recommendations are appropriate.

Aspiration Before the Swallow. Aspiration before the swallow can occur when the bolus enters the pharynx before triggering the pharyngeal swallow. At this point in the swallow sequence, the airway is wide open. Aspiration before the swallow occurs because of reduced tongue control or a delayed or absent pharyngeal swallow or both. If tongue control is poor, material can slip over the tongue base into the pharynx and into the open airway. This can occur during swallows of any consistency; however, loss of liquid over the tongue base is common if tongue control is poor, since liquid is less viscous than paste and masticated consistencies and can quickly spill over into the pharynx and the airway. Masticated material, however, can also be aspirated before the swallow if tongue control is reduced. The dysphagic individual can be chewing the bolus during the oral preparatory phase of the swallow, and portions of the bolus may slip over the tongue base and into the pharynx while the person is chewing.

A delayed pharyngeal swallow can also cause aspiration before the swallow (Curtis and Hudson, 1983; Logemann, 1983, 1986b). In this case, the tongue propels the bolus posteriorly into the pharynx, but there is a delay in the onset of the pharyngeal swallow. The bolus may fall into the valleculae, may slip down along the aryepiglottic folds and into the pyriform sinuses, or may fall directly into the airway. The bolus can sometimes be seen entering the laryngeal vestibule and being squeezed out as the larynx elevates and closes. This is not aspiration. However, if bolus size were to increase, there is a greater likelihood that aspiration might occur. A pharyngeal swallow is defined as absent if it takes longer than 30 seconds for all components of the pharyngeal swallow to occur once material has been propelled into the pharynx (Logemann, 1983).

Aspiration During the Swallow. Aspiration during the swallow can occur when there is reduced laryngeal closure. This can occur with a unilateral or bilateral vocal cord paresis or paralysis. Impaired vocal cord closure can result from laryngeal trauma, chest trauma, or prolonged endotracheal intubation. Also, vocal cord paresis and paralysis can be the result of surgical procedures designed to stabilize the cervical spine following spinal cord injury in the TBI population (Capen and colleagues, 1986). Reduced laryngeal closure can be accompanied by reduced laryngeal elevation (Ekberg and Schultz, 1986; Logemann, 1983).

Aspiration After the Swallow. Aspiration after the swallow can occur when residue in the pharynx is aspirated after the pharyngeal swallow is completed, at which time the airway is wide open. Aspiration after the swallow can occur for several reasons. A generalized reduction in pharyngeal peristalsis results in residue within the pharynx. This residue can coat the posterior pharyngeal walls, epiglottis, valleculae, aryepiglottic folds, pyriform sinuses, and laryngeal vestibule. Material can then slip downward by gravity into the airway. A unilateral pharyngeal paresis or paralysis can also result in residue within the pharynx. This occurs because the pharyngeal constrictor musculature cannot effectively clear the bolus through the pharynx. There is typically more residue within the pharynx and pyriform sinus on the affected side of the pharynx (Kirchner, 1967). Reduced laryneal elevation can also cause residue in the pharynx, since the constrictor musculature cannot clear the bolus through the pharynx when the larynx does not elevate and tuck itself out of the way under the tongue base.

Cricopharyngeal dysfunction can also contribute to aspiration after the swallow. It has been found that relaxation and opening are two components of cricopharyngeal functioning during swallowing, with relaxation occuring just before opening (Kahrilas and colleagues, 1988). If the cricopharyngeus muscle does not relax or open during the pharyngeal swallow, all or part of the bolus can remain above the esophagus within the pyriform sinuses. This material might then slip anteriorly over the arytenoid cartilage into the airway. Aspiration might not necessarily occur on the first swallow of material. There is often a buildup of residue within the pharynx that eventually is aspirated after three or four swallows (Hurwitz and colleagues, 1975; Kilman and Goyal, 1976; Logemann, 1983; Schultz and colleagues, 1979).

EVALUATING SWALLOWING EFFICIENCY DURING THE VFG EXAMINATION

Once the clinician has defined the etiology of the dysphagia, swallow therapy maneuvers and compensatory postural techniques can be evaluated during VFG to determine whether swallow functioning can be improved. Postural techniques are useful to compensate for a swallowing problem. It is not the swallowing physiology that is changed, but the flow of food and liquid. Head posturing can be utilized for most individuals other than those functioning at a very low level who cannot follow simple commands. Level of alertness, cognitive functioning, and memory skills in the individual with TBI and dysphagia must be determined prior to the introduction and implementation of actual therapy techniques. Certain swallow therapy techniques that require good auditory comprehension and ability to follow a two- or three-step command (such as the supraglottic swallow and the Mendelsohn maneuver) cannot be taught and implemented with the lower level functioning TBI individual.

POSTURES

Head Forward

Tilting the head forward widens the vallecular space (the space between the tongue base and epiglottis). This is useful for those individuals who demonstrate delays in the onset of the pharyngeal swallow. The widened vallecular space will hold material safely above and out of the airway until the pharyngeal swallow occurs (Ekberg, 1986; Logemann, 1983; Weber, 1974). If palatal functioning is reduced, there may be nasal regurgitation of liquids and foods into the nasopharynx. This can occur when there is residue within the pharynx that builds up and gets squeezed upward into the nasopharynx. If the individual rapidly swallows successively from a cup, liquids can leak upward into the nasal cavity. Taking small amounts per sip or bite, with care to feed slowly, and slightly tilting the head down eliminates this problem (Logemann, 1983).

Head Back

Head-back posture is useful for those individuals who have difficulty propelling material through the oral cavity due to tongue dysfunction.

Tilting the head back facilitates oral transit of material. However, this therapy technique should be used only with those individuals who demonstrate adequate airway closure and a timely triggering of the pharyngeal swallow. Otherwise, material that is propelled rather quickly into the pharynx (using this technique) could easily be aspirated before the swallow. To prevent this from occurring, the individual can be taught the supraglottic sequence, a voluntary airway closure technique, in combination with the head-back posture (Logemann, 1983). A more detailed description of the supraglottic swallow sequence can be found under the section **Swallow Maneuvers.**

Head Turn

The head-turn technique is useful for those individuals in whom residue is localized primarily on one side of the pharynx, specifically, within one pyriform sinus. This can easily be seen in the anterior-posterior view on VFG and is typical of individuals with unilateral pharyngeal dysfunction. Turning the head ninety degrees towards the affected side (the side with the greater residue) helps channel the bolus down the pyriform sinus on the side where the pharyngeal constrictor musculature is functioning. Head turning obliterates the pyriform sinus on the affected side, preventing additional residue from collecting within the pharynx. The head-turn posture has been found to be useful in individuals with cricopharyngeal dysfunction. Simultaneous videofluoroscopic and manometric examination revealed lower pressures to be found during cricopharyngeus opening with head turned ninety degrees (Logemann, Kahrilas, & Kobara, in press).

Head Tilt

The head-tilt posture is useful for unilateral pharyngeal disorders. The head is tilted towards the unaffected side of the pharynx, channeling the bolus through the same side. This technique is also useful for unilateral oral problems. If pocketing of food due to lingual weakness or reduced lingual control is a problem, tilting the head towards the unaffected side will prevent build-up of residue within the oral cavity and will aid in oral transit of material. The head-tilt posture can be combined with head-back posturing, if airway protection and triggering of the pharyngeal swallow are intact (Logemann, 1983).

Laying the Individual Down

Laying the dysphagic individual down on his side can improve swallow functioning when there is residue that is being aspirated after the swallow. This posture eliminates the effects of gravity, so that residue remains on the pharyngeal wall, rather than falling into the airway after the swallow. This residue is often cleared on subsequent bolus swallows and repeat dry swallows, eliminating aspiration. The dysphagic individual should always be lying on his better side if there is a unilateral oral or pharyngeal dysfunction.

SWALLOW MANEUVERS

Supraglottic Swallow

The supraglottic swallow is a technique to improve airway closure before and during the swallow. The dysphagic individual is instructed to take a sip or bite, hold his breath tightly, swallow, and finally, to cough (while still holding his breath). This technique requires a fairly intact memory and ability to sequence three steps. The supraglottic swallow sequence is useful for those individuals who are at risk for aspiration before the swallow, and who have residue in the pharynx after the swallow that might be aspirated after the swallow.

Thermal Sensitization

Thermal sensitization is a technique used when the onset of the pharyngeal swallow is delayed or absent. Pommerenke (1928) found that stimulation to the region within the base of the anterior faucial arches appeared to elicit a pharyngeal swallow. Providing cold sensation to this area has been shown effective in improving oral awareness and sensation such that there is quicker triggering of the pharyngeal swallow when the swallow is volitionally initiated (Lazzara, Lazarus, & Logemann, 1986). A size 00 laryngeal mirror is dipped in ice and then bilaterally stroked to the base of the anterior faucial arches. The dysphagic individual is then instructed to initiate a dry swallow, or swallow a bolus of food or liquid. Thermal sensitization has proven to improve the speed of the triggering of the pharyngeal response in several neurologically impaired populations, including CVA, TBI and surgically treated brain tumors (Lazzara and colleagues, 1986). This technique may require several trials before an improvement in triggering of the pharyngeal swallow can be seen.

Mendelsohn Maneuver

The Mendelsohn maneuver facilitates opening of the cricopharyngeus muscle during the swallow if there is known cricopharyngeal dysfunc-

tion (Logemann, 1987). The dysphagic individual is instructed to prolong the elevation of his larynx when he feels the larynx elevate and the
back of the throat closing during the swallow. The person is also told to
pull his tongue far back within the oral cavity, in order to prolong laryngeal elevation. This technique is designed to create greater superior and
anterior movement of the larynx in order to provide anterior stretch on
the cricopharyngeus for improved opening (Logemann, 1987).

DETERMINATION OF SWALLOW EFFICIENCY

After a VFG examination has established the etiology of the individual's
dysphagia, extent of aspiration (if present) and effects of therapy techniques, the clinician should determine the overall efficiency of the person's swallow before recommending a specific therapy or diet. It has
been found, in the oral cancer population, that a dysphagic individual
who takes longer than 10 seconds to swallow a bolus of food or liquid
will usually avoid that consistency at mealtime. In addition, within this
same cancer population, a dysphagic person who aspirates 10 percent of
a bolus (or more) will discontinue that consistency of food or liquid at
meals (Logemann, 1983; Wheeler and colleagues, 1980). Therefore, elimination of these food consistencies would be a good clinical recommendation if oral transit times are greater than 10 seconds or if an individual is
aspirating 10 percent or more of a bolus. Clinicians might even counsel
elimination of a food consistency if an individual aspirates 5 percent of a
bolus.

The fact that a dysphagic individual has not aspirated during the VFG
study does not necessarily indicate that he or she is ready for oral nutrition. The TBI individual is often unaware of either the presence of aspiration or the risks of aspiration when eating. These individuals may be at
great risk for aspiration, particularly if swallow efficiency is impaired.
Several measures of swallowing efficiency can be used.

Oral Efficiency

The oral efficiency measure is defined as 100 minus the percentage of the
bolus cleared from the oral cavity divided by the oral transit time (Meyer
and Logemann, 1986). The clinician need not mathematically calculate
this measure for each swallow. However, the clinician should note how
long it takes the dysphagic individual to clear the bolus from the oral
cavity and how much residue remains within the oral cavity. Oral efficiency is considered very reduced if more than 10 seconds are required
to propel the bolus into the pharynx or if the majority of the bolus
remains in the oral cavity after the swallow.

Overall Swallowing Efficiency

The swallowing efficiency measure is defined as 100 minus the percentage of oral residue and pharyngeal residue plus the percentage aspirated divided by the combined oral and pharyngeal transit times (Meyer and Logemann, 1986). Again, the clinician need not calculate this measure for each swallow. Reduced swallowing efficiency in the individual with long oral and pharyngeal transit times (indicating difficulty propelling the bolus through the pharynx and a delayed pharyngeal swallow) who also has a large percentage of the bolus remaining in the pharynx should preclude safe oral nutrition.

Following the VFG study, the clinician and radiologist either jointly or separately write up the results of the study. The VFG report should include oral and pharyngeal transit times, any motility disorders seen within the oral cavity and pharynx, presence and timing of aspiration (e.g., before, during and after), etiology of aspiration, changes in swallow functioning when utilizing therapy techniques, and swallow therapy recommendations and diet recommendations.

THE BEDSIDE SWALLOW EVALUATION

The bedside or *"clinical"* swallow evaluation plays an integral part in the assessment of dysphagia in the TBI individual. Optimally, the bedside and VFG evaluations should both be performed on all individuals with dysphagia, since both provide valuable information concerning the person's ability to sustain oral nutrition. The bedside swallow evaluation provides information about the dysphagic person as a whole, not just his swallowing mechanism. Specifically, information is gathered concerning level of alertness, mentation, memory, motivation, oromotor skills, and family support.

History

It is crucial to obtain a thorough history of the dysphagic individual, including all swallowing complaints. If the person is unable to provide this information, the hospital chart should be read thoroughly. In addition, information should be gathered from a family member, if possible, before the swallow evaluation. The onset and the exact nature of the injury should be documented, as well as accompanying injuries. Within the spinal cord-injured population, specific types and patterns of dysphagia have been reported (Lazzara and colleagues, 1986). In addition, it is not uncommon for dysphagia to occur postoperatively in those individuals who have undergone surgical stabilization of the cervical spine that incorporated anterior approaches to spinal fusion (Capen and colleagues, 1986; Capen and colleagues, 1987). Dysphagia was reported to be temporary in all cases. In this author's experience, dysphagia following cervical spine stabilization using the anterior approach typically occurs within the pharyngeal phase. Specifically, individuals typically exhibit reduced pharyngeal constrictor functioning and cricopharyngeal dysfunctioning, as seen by a generalized residue remaining in the pharynx or residue within the pyriform sinus area after the swallow. It is this author's experience that recovery of function usually occurs spontaneously over a 1- to 3-month period.

Facial trauma may affect lip closure and tongue and jaw functioning, thus interfering with the oral preparatory and oral stages of the swallow. Following facial trauma, the mandible and maxilla may be fractured, often requiring wiring, so that the jaw must be tightly closed for an extended length of time. This would interfere with jaw opening and ability to chew. Laryngeal trauma may alter elevation and closure of the larynx, impairing the pharyngeal stage of the swallow. Chest trauma can create pressure or damage to the recurrent laryngeal nerve, causing a vocal cord paralysis, which could contribute to aspiration during the swallow. Damage to the chest or laryngeal area can reduce the individual's ability to cough effectively and clear the airway. The exact nature of laryngeal damage and type of laryngeal reconstruction should be ascertained to determine the precise physiologic changes that might be interfering with normal swallow functioning. Presence of a t-e fistula should always be considered as a possible cause of aspiration in the presence of laryngeal or chest trauma.

What are the dysphagic individual's symptoms of dysphagia? Avoidance of certain or all foods is an obvious sign that the person is having difficulty swallowing. However, more subtle signs include avoidance of certain foods by specific consistency (i.e., liquids or foods requiring mastication), pocketing of food within the mouth, spitting out of food, increased time to complete a meal, spiked temperatures (indicating probable pneumonias), and expectoration of food and liquid out through the mouth, nares, or tracheostomy tubes. Complaints of choking and of food sticking in the throat are common with dysphagia. What is the frequency with which the dysphagia occurs? Is there difficulty every meal, every few days, etc.? Has the dysphagic individual tried anything to improve swallow functioning, such as taking smaller sips or bites or chewing on "the better" side of the mouth? If the individual is taking food orally, is it by self-feeding or feeding by a nurse or a family member? This is a consideration when making recommendations regarding oral nutrition.

The impulsive TBI person will likely not exhibit the same restraint in speed of eating and in gauging the appropriate amount per bolus that a caregiver would demonstrate. What is the individual's cognitive status and level of alertness? Is he or she alert enough to complete an entire meal? Is he or she able to remember a specific therapy technique to be used on every swallow or when swallowing a specific consistency? This author does not recommend attempting a bedside swallow evaluation on individuals who are crying, drowsy, combative, severely agitated, or totally unresponsive. The person who exhibits any of these behaviors would not be able voluntarily to initiate and follow through with a swallow without great risk for aspiration. Ventilator-dependent individuals should be seen for bedside swallow examinations to determine overall cognitive and oromotor functioning. However, it is not recommended that ventilator-dependent individuals be given anything to swallow, since voice quality on phonation, which is a good indicator of aspiration, cannot be assessed.

Presence and Duration of Coma

Coma is another factor to be considered, although to date few data exist correlating these factors to severity of swallow dysfunction in the TBI individual (Lazarus and Logemann, 1985). Information concerning CT and magnetic resonance imaging (MRI) results can be useful. Intracranial pressure (ICP) ratings after injury, as well as any surgeries required to reduce these pressures, should be noted. ICP ratings after injury are believed to be accurate prognostic indicators for recovery in head injury (Langfitt and Gennarelli, 1982; Lobato and colleagues, 1979). However, it is not crucial to obtain this information before evaluating an individual's swallowing. Any previous medical diagnoses should be noted, such as a history of Parkinson's disease, cerebrovascular accident, multiple sclerosis, amyotrophic lateral sclerosis, or other neurologic disorders, since these disorders demonstrate characteristic dysphagic patterns (Blonsky and colleagues, 1975; Donner and Silbeger, 1966; Dworkin and Hartman, 1979; Fabiszak, 1986; Kobara and Logemann, 1987; Meyer and Logemann, 1986; Robbins and colleagues, 1986; Veis and Logemann, 1985).

Pulmonary Status

Before examining the swallow of a person with TBI the clinician should inquire of the physician, nurse, or pulmonary specialist whether the dysphagic person would be able to tolerate the small amounts of aspiration that might occur on bedside evaluation of swallowing. This is especially important in the TBI individual with concomitant spinal cord injury who has a history of pneumonia or who requires frequent suctioning of copious secretions. Such a person is likely to be chronically aspirating and should be given fewer swallows of food or liquid during the bedside swallow evaluation.

Tracheostomy Tubes

It is not uncommon for persons with swallowing problems to have a tracheotomy. The presence of a tracheotomy tube and its type will affect the swallow evaluation. If the dysphagic individual is tracheostomized, the clinician should determine what type of tracheostomy tube is present within the tracheostomy site. The tracheostomy tube may be cuffed, uncuffed, fenestrated, unfenestrated, plugged, or unplugged. If the tracheostomy tube is cuffed, the clinician should determine whether the cuff is inflated or deflated. If the cuff is inflated, the dysphagic individual should not aspirate his or her own secretions. However, the clinician should always check to see whether an individual is able to produce voice while the cuff is inflated. In some individuals, inflated cuffs do not abut the entire circumference of the tracheal wall, and there may be leakage around the cuff with aspiration of materials (Pinkus, 1973). This is not routinely seen, however. If the cuff is deflated, aspirated material can slip around the cuff, below the tracheostomy tube, and into the lower trachea. The clinician should inquire from the managing nurse, physician, or respiratory therapist whether the cuff can be deflated during the swallow evaluation. The clinician, as the consulting professional with expertise in dysphagia management, must verify the presence of aspiration. Thus, cuffed tubes should be deflated whenever possible during bedside examinations. Plugged tracheostomy tubes should be unplugged after the swallow so that aspirated materials can be visualized when expectorated through the tracheostomy tube. Fenestrated tracheostomy tubes should have inner cannulas removed during the swallow study so that aspirated material will slip through the fenestration and continue on below the tracheostomy tube into the trachea, to be visualized, one hopes, when expectorated through the tracheostomy tube.

Neurologic Evaluation

Results of neurologic evaluations provide information concerning cranial nerve functioning and presence of preexisting neurologic conditions, chronic or progressive. Otolaryngologic evaluations provide information concerning vocal cord functioning and possible presence of pooled secretions within the pharynx, the latter being a good indicator of reduced pharyngeal sensation or an infrequent spontaneous swallow of one's secretions. Unilateral pooling of secretions can also indicate unilateral paresis of the constrictor musculature (Kirchner, 1967). The clinician should note what medications are being given, particularly those that tend to cause drowsiness and reduced levels of alertness. The drowsy individual is not a good candidate for a swallow evaluation, either bedside or VFG study.

The Oromotor Evaluation

An oromotor evaluation should be performed before food and liquid are presented. Movement rate, range, strength, precision, and coordination during isolated and rapidly repeated-alternated nonspeech and speech movements of the vocal tract musculature should be examined. Isolated nonspeech gestures should include (1) labial protrusion, retraction, and closure; (2) lingual lateralization protrusion; and (3) lingual tip elevation inside to the upper alveolar ridge and outside of the mouth, lingual depression, and back tongue elevation. Rapidly repeated-alternated nonspeech labial movements should include rapid protrusion and retraction of the lips. Rapidly repeated-alternated nonspeech lingual movements should include rapid tongue lateralization. Isolated speech movements of the lips include articulation of /pa/, /u/, and /i/ and of the tongue include /ta/, t ʃ a/, and /ka/. Rapidly alternated-repeated speech movements of the lips and tongue should include repetition of /pa/, /u-i/, /ta/, /ka/, and the sequence /pataka/. Labial strength testing should examine resistance to a tongue blade placed between the lips along the left and right margins and midline. Lingual strength testing should examine resistance to a tongue blade placed along the lateral margins, on the mid-dorsum (with the instruction to push up with the tongue) and against the tongue tip (with the instruction to protrude the tongue against the blade). The velum should be examined at rest and during sustained phonation of /a/. Symmetry of movement, ability to elevate and retract the palate, and presence of any fatiguing should be noted.

A careful examination of voice quality on phonation is crucial, since voice quality can indicate presence of secretions within the pharynx. In addition, voice quality before and after having given the person food or liquid may greatly differ, being much less clear after the swallow. A wet, gurgly voice quality heard on phonation or during quiet breathing after a swallow can indicate presence of secretions or residue sitting above the airway within the pharynx (Linden and Siebens, 1983; Logemann, 1983). A weak, breathy voice can indicate a unilateral or bilateral vocal cord paralysis. A harsh, rough, or diplophonic voice might also indicate a unilateral voice cord paralysis (Aaronson, 1980). Maximum pitch range should be ascertained by having the person slide up the pitch scale on an /i/ and slide down on an /a/. Breath support should be examined during sustained phonation of /o/ following normal and deep breaths. The ability to produce three distinct loudness levels, indicating the extent of voluntary control of respiration, should be determined. What is the nature of the dysphagic person's speech in conversation? The presence and severity of dysarthria and apraxia should be noted. What is the overall intelligibility? Are the linguopalatal contacts during consonant productions precise and complete? If not, there may be reduced lingual elevation for the oral preparatory and oral stages of the swallow.

Evaluation of Reflexes. The oromotor examination should include evaluation of all three reflexes, including the palatal, gag, and cough. The palatal reflex can be elicited by lightly touching the palate at the juncture of the hard and soft palate with an iced size 00 laryngeal mirror. This stimulation should elicit elevation of the soft palate similar to that seen during phonation (Logemann, 1983). The presence of a gag reflex should be tested by applying firm pressure to the posterior dorsum of the tongue on both sides, touching the faucial arches and, if no response has occurred, contacting the posterior pharyngeal wall. A sphincteric-type movement, with elevation of the palate and medialward movement of the faucial arches and lateral pharyngeal walls, can be observed on elicitation of a full gag reflex.

The absence of any or all of these reflexes does not preclude the absence of a pharyngeal swallow (Jenkins and colleagues, 1984; Logemann and Lazarus, 1987). There is a common misconception that the absence of a gag reflex indicates a reduced ability to effect a pharyngeal swallow. The presence or absence of the gag reflex does not necessarily coexist with the presence or absence of a pharyngeal swallow. Different neurophysiologic pathways are involved in elicitation of the gag and the swallow (Kahrilas and colleagues, 1987). In addition, the gag is not a protective mechanism for swallowing. The function of the gag reflex is to prevent noxious stimuli, such as vomitus and refluxed gastric contents, from entering the airway. Food is not a noxious stimulus and so would not elicit a gag. The protective mechanism for the swallow is not the gag reflex but the cough reflex, designed to expectorate food and liquids from the airway.

Evaluation of Oral Sensation. The oromotor examination should also include an oral sensation examination. This can be done with cotton swabs, presenting light and firm pressure to the lips, tongue, and cheeks. Two-point discrimination should also be tested, if possible. However, this is infrequently achieved within the TBI population, since many of these individuals are hypersensitive, hypertonic, or hyperreflexive to stimuli presented near or in the oral cavity. Reactions to other stimuli presented within the region of the oral cavity should be noted. Stimuli can include cold versus warm and salty versus sweet. The clinician should determine which regions within the oral cavity are most sensitive. During the swallow evaluation, food or liquid might need to be placed within these areas.

Evaluation of the Pharyngeal Swallow

Triggering of the pharyngeal swallow should initially be evaluated on a swallow of saliva. The timing of the oral and pharyngeal stages of the swallow should be examined by manually feeling for laryngeal elevation and tongue movement using a four-finger technique (Logemann, 1983). Two fingers are placed on the thyroid cartilage, one finger is placed on the neck at the approximate location of the hyoid bone, and the last finger is placed under the jaw at the level of the mental symphysis. The dysphagic individual is instructed to swallow. The clinician then notes the time from when tongue movement is felt (indicating onset of tongue movement to initiate the swallow) until the larynx elevates and returns to rest (indicating triggering of the pharyngeal swallow). It should take 1 second from the time that tongue movement is felt until the pharyngeal swallow occurs. If the onset of the pharyngeal swallow occurs after 1 second, this is defined as a delayed pharyngeal swallow. The presence of very mild delays in the onset of the pharyngeal swallow can be missed using the four-finger technique. This is the reason that VFG studies are crucial, particularly when the dysphagic individual demonstrates a very mild delay in the pharyngeal swallow and is silently aspirating before the swallow. However, slightly longer delays are easily detected using this technique. The presence of lingual problems, specifically, lack of lingual initiation or lingual control problems, can also be easily detected using this technique.

Often, saliva does not provide adequate sensory and proprioceptive input to effect a pharyngeal swallow. Therefore, it is recommended to introduce a food or liquid bolus, even if there is no pharyngeal swallow or a very delayed swallow on saliva swallows. The easiest consistency that is reported by the dysphagic individual or family member should be introduced first. This is done to reduce the person's anxiety level, which may already be quite high, particularly if eating has not been a pleasant experience. Very small amounts (one third to one fourth teaspoon) should be given per bolus. Liquids should be given on a spoon, since the amount can be measured more precisely than if the person took a sip from a cup. If the individual has poor tongue functioning, a 1-ml bolus from a syringe can be introduced into the posterior oral cavity to determine whether a pharyngeal swallow is present. Or one fourth teaspoon of pureed food (such as applesauce, pudding, or yogurt) can be placed in the posterior oral cavity with a tongue blade to bypass the oral phase and determine whether a pharyngeal swallow is present. If tongue functioning is very reduced, as seen on oromotor examination, as evidenced during pureed swallows by very increased oral transit times (oral transit is normally 1 second) and presence of residue within the oral cavity after the swallow, masticated consistencies (e.g., one eighth to one quarter of a plain butter cookie or cracker) should not be introduced. The individual should be asked to phonate *"ah"* after every swallow to evaluate voice quality. A *"wet"* and gurgly voice indicates the presence of residue above the airway that could be aspirated after the swallow. The clinician should have the individual rapidly pant in and out to assess voice quality on inspiration and exhalation. The clinician should then ask the person to turn the head from side to side and up and down and then phonate an *"ah"* again. If there is residue within the pharynx, changes in head posture may dislodge this material, directing it toward the airway, where presence of this material may be identifiable by voice quality or audible cough.

If the individual's jaw is wired shut secondary to facial trauma, the clinician must ascertain that the individual has a good triggering of the pharyngeal swallow. Thus, a catheter attached to a syringe can be placed within the oral cavity. Liquid can be syringed into the oral cavity with care to give small amounts per bolus. If lip closure can be accomplished and the individual is able to create adequate intraoral pressures to suck inward, a straw can be used instead of the catheter.

Evaluation of Aspiration. It is crucial to ascertain whether an individual is aspirating on bedside swallow evaluation when there is no access to VFG study to confirm aspiration. The oral cavity should be examined for residue after each pureed and masticated swallow. Presence of residue within the oral cavity indicates reduced tongue functioning during the oral preparatory and oral stages. Material can adhere to the hard and soft palate (if lingual elevation is reduced), the lateral lower sulci (if lingual lateralization is reduced), and the anterior lower sulcus (if lingual protrusion and depression are reduced). In addition, material may adhere to the dorsum of the tongue if linguopalatal contact (vertical range of motion), anteroposterior tongue range, and fine tongue control for cupping and shaping are reduced. Reduced lip closure, due to reduced range of motion or strength, would result in drooling out the front of the mouth. It is important to note whether the person responds to aspiration. An individual who coughs or attempts to clear the throat or "dry swallows" repeatedly (to clear residue from his pharynx) has some degree of pharyngeal and laryngeal sensation and some awareness of residue within the pharynx.

When the clinician has assessed oral functioning and has determined whether the pharyngeal swallow appears to be triggering on time (by the completion of the bedside swallow examination), the clinician should have a good sense of tongue functioning and oral transit of the bolus, the patient's ability to trigger the pharyngeal swallow, the presence of any delay, and the presence of any aspiration. The clinician should also have a sense of what specific consistencies the individual can tolerate. If the bedside swallow evaluation indicates what appears to be an adequate swallowing mechanism, the clinician might allow self-feeding for the TBI individual. This often identifies behaviors that may lead to problems not seen when small, calibrated amounts are being presented at a slow pace, as in a VFG examination. TBI patients often impulsively shovel food into their mouths, frequently pocketing the food, without pausing to swallow or reswallow if there is residue in the oral cavity and pharynx. Individuals might guzzle liquids from a cup or straw and take very large portions on their spoon or fork. Following a bedside swallow examination as described, recommendations can be made regarding size of bolus per swallow, pacing of swallows during meals, and the need for supervision at mealtime.

THERAPY

POSITIONING AND ENVIRONMENT

When beginning swallow therapy, the clinician should initially determine the best head and trunk positioning to facilitate the most normal tone and inhibit abnormal reflexes, such as the tonic jaw jerk, jaw opening reflex, and bite reflex (Alexander, 1987; Morris, 1985; Mueller, 1975). Extraneous stimuli should be eliminated when providing swallow therapy. A quiet setting with low lights is helpful to reduce excess sensory input that may trigger abnormal reflexes. Extraneous sensory input can also distract and interfere with therapy sessions in the TBI individual who exhibits impulsivity and distractibility. Instructions to the dysphagic individual should be kept simple and clear. The clinician should present therapy exercises at a slow, even pace to create a less threatening and less negative therapy environment. In addition, this will provide time for the clinician to assess the person's reactions to the stimuli being presented (Hargrove, 1980).

HYPERTONICITY, HYPERREFLEXIA, HYPERSENSITIVITY

The person with TBI who demonstrates hypertonicity, hyperreflexia, and hypersensitivity poses a particular challenge to the clinician. This individual must be desensitized to the presence of tactile stimuli in the mouth area and within the oral cavity. The clinician should carefully work toward the individual's mouth, initially by stroking downward across the cheeks towards the corners of the mouth. Light touch and stroking of the lips and chin area will help desensitize the person to tactile stimuli within the lip area. Once this has been achieved, the clinician should introduce stimuli of varying textures, temperatures, and degrees of tactile pressure. A spoon can serve as a *"smooth"* stimuli and can be lightly touched along all margins of the lips. A metal spoon or one constructed of moulded plastic should be used to reduce the chances of breakage within the oral cavity if the individual has an active bite reflex. A rolled-up piece of gauze can serve as a *"rough"* texture. The gauze can then be moistened with liquid and stroked along the lips to desensitize the individual to a *"wet"* sensation. The gauze can also be chilled and warmed up in warm water and placed around the mouth and on the lips to assess the effects of, and desensitize the individual to, varying temperatures. Light and firm pressure should then be introduced along the lip margins, using different textures (rough and smooth), different temperatures (warm, room temperature, and cold), and wet and dry. Different tastes should be tried in therapy, including salty, sweet, and sour, Gauze can be dipped into salty, sweet, and sour solutions and lightly touched along the lip margins (Griffin, 1974).

When moving into the oral cavity, the clinician should begin with the least noxious stimuli, as determined by the aforementioned tasks. The clinician can begin along the inner margins of the lips, working inward until the tongue can be touched. A similar procedure using different textures, temperatures, and pressures should be used to desensitize the individual to stimuli presented on the tongue. The clinician should lightly touch and then stroke the lateral margins and the mid-dorsum of the tongue with a gloved finger, tongue blade, rolled-up gauze, or end of a spoon. Touching and stroking should begin at the anterior margins of the tongue and cautiously worked posteriorly on the tongue. Firm pressure on the tongue should then be introduced with a gloved finger or whatever stimuli is the least noxious to the individual. Light touch and stroking should be employed along the buccal mucosa, moving from the corners of the mouth back toward the faucial arch area. This last task is useful for desensitization when thermal sensitization of the pharyngeal swallow is necessary. To provide thermal sensitization, a laryngeal mirror, size 00, must be introduced into the posterior oral cavity at the base of the anterior faucial arches. Once the person with TBI has become desensitized to stimuli presented around and within the oral cavity, therapy techniques can be implemented to improve labial and lingual functioning and to improve triggering of the pharyngeal swallow.

HYPOTONICITY, HYPOREFLEXIA, HYPOSENSITIVITY

Traumatically brain injured persons who exhibit hypotonicity, hyporeflexia and hyposensitivity require therapy that is designed to improve responsiveness, increase sensitivity and increase tone within the vocal tract musculature. Therapy tasks should incorporate a variety of stimuli, including different temperatures, pressures, textures and tastes, as discussed in the hyperfunctioning group. However, therapy should initially focus on determining which stimuli (e.g. taste, temperature, texture or pressure) elicit the most consistent positive responses from the individual. Those stimuli that cause maximum responsiveness should then be incorporated into therapy tasks. The use of touching, stroking and pressure is crucial with the hypofunctioning individual to improve tone and sensitivity. Within this population, it is unlikely that the clinician will inadvertently trigger abnormal reflexes.

ORAL AND ORAL PREPARATORY STAGES

Improving Lip Closure

Exercises to improve lip closure focus on improving range and strength of closure to seal the bolus within the mouth and to prevent drooling during the oral preparatory and oral phases of swallow. Stimulation to the lip area, as previously discussed, can facilitate lip closure movements. If partial lip closure is present, tongue blades can be placed between the lips and can be successively removed as lip closure improves. Rolled up gauze can also be used in this fashion, beginning with a large piece of gauze, and reducing the size of the gauze as lip closure improves. The clinician should also work on lip closure around a cup and spoon. If range of motion is reduced on protrusion and retraction, therapy should focus on increasing range, providing visual models and tactile cues, and employing speech exercises, using oo and ee, if the individual is able to vocalize. Lip closure exercises should also incorporate speech production exercises using the bilabials (p,b,m) if the dysphagic individual can vocalize.

Increasing Lip Strength

To increase strength of labial closure, a tongue blade can be placed between the lips midline and along the lateral margins, with instructions to purse the lips tightly. The clinician then provides resistance by lightly pulling outward on the blade. A candy lifesaver or button with a string running through it can be placed between the lips. The clinician then pulls lightly on the string to offer resistance while the individual attempts to maintain firm lip closure on the button or lifesaver.

Improving Buccal Tone

Stimulation of the buccal mucosa within the mouth can improve buccal tone. In addition, the dysphagic person can be instructed to puff out the cheeks, while the clinician simultaneously offers resistance, with light pressure of the hand applied inward on the cheek. If buccal tone is very reduced, as seen in a unilateral facial paralysis, the clinician or dysphagic person can place a hand firmly against the cheek during the oral prepara- tory stages of the swallow and instruct the person to tilt the head toward the unaffected side. This technique effectively occludes the lower lateral sulcus, where food and liquid could collect, and channels the food and liquid down the unaffected side of the oral cavity during oral transit, thus achieving a quicker oral transit (Logemann, 1983).

Redirecting Bolus Flow

The head back posture, previously mentioned as a useful compensatory posture, can facilitate oral transit if tongue functioning is very impaired. Gravity will help drain material through the oral cavity and into the pharynx. The dysphagic individual must have good airway protection and good triggering of the pharyngeal swallow for this technique to be safely used and to prevent aspiration before the swallow.

The head tilt posture redirects the flow of food within the oral cavity. In addition, the speech pathologist can work with the maxillofacial prosthodontist to construct a maxillary reshaping prosthesis. This pros- thesis can redirect the flow of food or saliva to the better-functioning side of the oral cavity. In addition, the palate can be effectively lowered with the prosthesis to improve linguopalatal contacts for swallowing if vertical tongue range is very reduced (Davis and colleagues, 1987; Wheeler and colleagues, 1980).

Improving Tongue Range of Motion

In general, tongue exercises are designed to improve the speed, range, precision, and coordination of movement for manipulation and propul- sion of food and liquid into the pharynx. Tongue range of motion exer- cises should be employed to improve elevation of the tip, middle, and back tongue, comprising the vertical element of tongue range. In addi- tion, range of motion exercises should also include lingual protrusion and backward movement of the tongue, comprising the anteroposterior element of tongue range. Exercises should also include lateralization of the tongue, required for placement and retrieval of food from the teeth. The clinician can place small amounts of food on the lips or lightly brush the lips with liquid. Instructions are given to retrieve the food with the tongue. This exercise can improve lingual range for protrusion, elevation, and lateralization and can also improve lingual control (Logemann, 1983; Morris, 1977). Small amounts of food such as peanut butter can be placed on the hard palate with instructions to retrieve the food. This activity improves vertical lingual range of motion, giving the individual the linguopalatal contacts necessary for mashing food and initiating and propelling the bolus.

Improving Lingual Control

Gauze manipulation exercises are used to improve fine lingual control. The clinician rolls up a piece of gauze and places it on the mid-dorsum of the tongue. The dysphagic individual then attempts to maneuver the gauze over to the teeth on both lateral margins. The individual is then instructed to try and move the gauze backward in the mouth, as if he or she were going to swallow it. The person should be instructed to stop just before gaging feels imminent. This exercise is designed to improve the up and backward movement of the tongue, which is necessary to initiate the swallow. The clinician holds the outer edge of the gauze at all times so that the person does not choke on it or lose it within the oropharynx. Gauze can be exchanged for licorice sticks, beef jerkies, popsicles, and suckers. However, the clinician should be cautious when using food, since the dysphagic person might bite down and subsequently choke on the piece of food. To ensure that this does not happen, the clinician can place food within a piece of gauze. The dysphagic individual can then get the taste and tactile sensation and pleasure from the food but will not be put at risk for aspiration. Fine tongue shaping and cupping, which is necessary for holding the bolus and sealing it against the hard palate, can be accomplished by placing a spoon on the dorsum of the tongue. This technique often results in elevation of the lateral tongue margins.

Increasing Lingual Strength

Lingual resistance exercises are used to increase lingual strength, particularly for chewing, control of the bolus of food, and propulsion of food into the pharynx. The clinician can use a tongue blade, finger, or spoon to lightly resist the tip, lateral margins, and dorsum of the tongue while the dysphagic individual is instructed to try and push forward, laterally, and up against the object or finger.

Speech exercises should be incorporated into the dysphagic person's swallowing therapy program whenever possible (Logemann, 1983; Robbins, 1985). Improving precision of labial closure for bilabial consonants, lingual shaping for vowels, glides, and fricatives, and linguopalatal contacts for tip-alveolar, blade-palatal, and back-velar plosive consonant phonemes can improve range, rate, precision, and coordination of nonspeech movements for swallowing.

PHARYNGEAL STAGE

The TBI population often demonstrates delays in triggering the pharyngeal swallow. Therefore, therapy focuses on improving the speed of onset of the pharyngeal swallow.

Thermal Sensitization

Thermal sensitization is used to improve triggering of the pharyngeal swallow when the onset of the swallow is delayed or absent. A size 00 laryngeal mirror is chilled in ice for 10 seconds and then placed in the oral cavity at the base of the anterior faucial arches. The TBI individual often must be desensitized to the presence of the laryngeal mirror near or within the oral cavity. Desensitization may take several weeks. Once this is achieved, the clinician strokes three to four times using the metal portion of the mirror, removes the mirror, and instructs the dysphagic person to swallow. This technique can be used with swallows of saliva, liquids, and foods. It can be done before or during meals if the dysphagic individual is currently taking an oral diet. If the individual is just practicing with liquids, the clinician fills a straw (used as a pipet) with a ¼ inch of liquid and places it in the area being sensitized. After providing the thermal sensitization, the liquid is presented with the instruction to swallow. Small amounts of food can also be introduced in the same fashion if the dysphagic individual is at this stage in therapy. The clinician should be assessing improvement in triggering of the pharyngeal swallow on all swallow attempts, using the four-finger technique described earlier in the bedside evaluation section.

   When providing thermal sensitization, the clinician should attempt to elicit ten to 12 swallows, since triggering of the pharyngeal swallow often fatigues after this point. This therapy technique should be done at least three to five times per day, as the individual can tolerate. It should be attempted for at least 1 to 2 months before a decision is made to discontinue usage, when no significant improvement has been made in triggering of the pharyngeal response. Helfrich-Miller and colleagues (1986) provided thermal sensitization with profoundly retarded cerebral palsied individuals who demonstrated delays in triggering of the pharyngeal swallow. Thermal sensitization was provided for 4-month intervals and was found to improve triggering of the pharyngeal swallow in all subjects, as documented by baseline and followup VFG study.

The Suck-Swallow

Elicitation of the suck-swallow has also been used to improve triggering of the pharyngeal swallow (Heimlich and Connor, 1979; Ramsey, 1986). This technique incorporates use of a nipple attached to a feeding line. The sucking action of the tongue is reported to elicit a pharyngeal swallow (Ramsey, 1986). This technique can also be used with popsicles, since they tend to be less infantilizing than the nipple.*

Dry Swallows, Liquid Wash

Reduced pharyngeal peristalsis contributes to residue within the pharynx after the swallow. If the residue is generalized throughout the pharynx, indicating a bilateral weakness, the residue can often be cleared with one or two repeat dry swallows. In addition, a liquid swallow following swallows of thicker consistencies can clear residue from the pharynx. The clinician should make sure that the dysphagic individual can handle liquids and should monitor the amount of liquid being swallowed per bolus.

Changing Food Consistency

Changing the consistency of food can eliminate residue problems. The dysphagic person may do better if the diet consists of soft food rather than a general diet. If the residue problem is more pronounced, the patient may be able to handle only liquids and pureed foods. If the residue problem is severe, the dysphagic person might be able to handle only thin and thick liquids.

Postural and Swallow Therapy Maneuvers

The various postural techniques described earlier, as used during VFG study, can reduce dysphagia associated with residue in the pharynx. These postures include head turn, head tilt, and lying down. These are techniques designed to change the flow of food and liquid, not the swallowing physiology. The Mendelsohn maneuver, as described previously, can be used when there is a cricopharyngeal dysfunction and posturing does not significantly improve passage of food through the cricopharyngeus. Postural techniques can be combined with techniques to improve swallowing physiology, such as head forward and turned or head back and supraglottic swallow. Thermal sensitization and the Men-

---

*J. Logemann, personal communication, 1988.

delsohn maneuver can be combined with any of the above-mentioned techniques.

Myotomy

Myotomy, involving sectioning of the pharyngeal constrictor musculature, has been used to improve cricopharyngeal functioning (Blakely and colleagues, 1968; Gay and colleagues, 1984). However, long-term effects on cricopharyngeal functioning are questionable. In addition, cricopharyngeal functioning has often been found to improve spontaneously over time (Hurwitz and colleagues, 1975; Kilman and Goyal, 1976; Logemann, 1983; Schultz and colleagues, 1979).

Improving Laryngeal Adduction

Laryngeal adduction exercises can improve vocal cord functioning if a unilateral true vocal cord paresis or paralysis is present. The dysphagic individual who is able to vocalize is instructed to produce vowels with a hard glottal attack. Pulling and pushing exercises with simultaneous phonation can increase cervical and laryngeal tension and result in improved glottic closure. If the individual is quadriplegic, the clinician can instruct the person to push with the forehead against the clinician's hand, while phonating with a hard glottal attack. This may increase laryngeal tension and improve glottic closure. If the person is unable to vocalize secondary to being tracheostomized or due to a severe dysarthria, he or she can be instructed to hold the breath tightly and bear down with the abdominal muscles to effect glottic closure. Turning the head to the affected side in a unilateral vocal cord paresis or paralysis can also improve swallow functioning. Using this maneuver, the functioning vocal cord will cross midline and effectively close the glottis during the swallow. Teflon injection into the affected vocal cord has also been used to improve glottic competency (Dobie, 1978).

Increasing Laryngeal Elevation

Therapy to improve reduced laryngeal elevation can include having the dysphagic person slide up into falsetto if he or she is able to vocalize. This technique should cause an upward movement of the larynx. Often this is not a feasible technique, since many TBI individuals are unable to phonate. Also, many of them do not have adequate laryngeal control to slide up in pitch. Pulling the tongue far back in the mouth can also effect better elevation of the larynx, since the backward movement of the tongue causes upward stretch on the larynx from the suprahyoid musculature (Bosma, 1980). The individual must demonstrate fairly fine voluntary lingual control (impossible for many TBI individuals) as well as a high level of cognitive functioning to achieve this task. The clinician should instruct the dysphagic person to use the supraglottic swallow technique, if the person has the cognitive capacity, to clear residue from above the airway. The dysphagic individual can also be instructed to clear the throat and reswallow to clear residue if fairly good laryngeal control and functioning exist.

ALTERNATE NUTRITION

Despite aggressive swallow intervention, some dysphagic individuals require alternate nutritional means for primary nutrition. In these individuals, nasogastric tubes, gastrostomies, pharyngostomies, and jeujunostomies should be maintained during the course of swallow therapy. Supplemental feedings ensure that the dysphagic individual is receiving adequate nutrition. In addition, the presence of nonoral nutritional support can reduce anxiety levels associated with eating and swallow therapy. Those individuals who tend to take a long time to complete their meals, or who are only practicing their swallowing exercises with food, will not feel compelled to eat seven or eight times a day to maintain their caloric intake. Swallow functioning is not typically compromised with the presence of tracheostomy tubes. In addition, maintenance of tracheostomy tubes can often reduce anxiety levels in the dysphagic individual, since it is often easier to expectorate material out through the tube than out through the mouth.

REPEAT VIDEOFLUOROSCOPIC

VFG studies should be repeated to assess improvement in swallow functioning and to facilitate decision making regarding diet changes and changes to be made in swallow therapy. Criteria for repeating a VFG study should include improvement in overall oral motor functioning and specific improvement in swallow functioning (e.g., improvement in triggering of the pharyngeal swallow). Decisions concerning improvement in oromotor and swallow functioning should be based on the clinician's judgment, with additional input from the managing nursing staff, dietician, and other involved professionals. Diet and swallow therapy recommendations should then be made by the clinician performing the repeat VFG study. The clinician and managing team should then closely monitor the TBI individual's ability to tolerate the new diet and swallow exercises. It is the managing physician's role to make the final decision concerning nutrition in the dysphagic patient with TBI.

THE TEAM APPROACH

Management of the dysphagic individual with TBI is a team effort. Involved staff can include the speech pathologist, occupational therapist, radiologist, rehabilitation medicine physician, pulmonary specialist, gastroenterologist, otolaryngologist, neurologist, maxillofacial prosthodontist, nurse, and dietician. Frequent communication among the staff should be maintained throughout the dysphagic individual's course of treatment to improve swallowing. Family members are also important members of the team. They can ensure that swallow therapy recommendations are followed at home during meals and that swallow exercises are completed during the day. The family can often identify signs of improvement or deterioration in swallow functioning.

Not all dysphagic TBI individuals will regain sufficient swallow functioning to allow for oral nutrition. Although recovery of swallow functioning can occur long after the onset of injury, the clinician and the dysphagia team must acknowledge when a dysphagic person has reached maximum potential in swallow functioning. The length of time and degree of improvement in swallow therapy, results of repeat VFG studies over time, and status in overall oromotor and swallow functioning must be considered in decisions regarding permanent nonoral nutrition. Some dysphagic individuals may have impaired oropharyngeal functioning such that they would not be able to receive adequate oral nutrition due to reduced swallow efficiency. In this case, the individuals may be able to take food or liquids orally in small amounts for pleasure, receiving their primary nutrition through gastrostomy or jejeunostomy. Others, however, may demonstrate such severe impairment in swallow functioning that even the smallest amount of food or liquid taken orally would put them at risk for aspiration. A decision must be made to maintain this latter group on nonoral nutrition only. Quality of life issues must always be addressed. The potential for recurrent aspiration pneumonia does not contribute to quality of life for those severely dysphagic individuals who are allowed to take nutrition orally.

REFERENCES

Alexander, R. (1987). Oral-motor treatment for infants and young children with cerebral palsy. *Seminars in Speech and Language, 8,* 87–100.

Aronson, A. (1980). *Clinical voice disorders: An inter-disciplinary approach.* New York: Thieme-Stratton.

Blakely, W., Garety, B., and Smith, D. (1968). Section of the cricopharyngeus muscle for dysphagia. *Archives of Surgery, 96,* 745–760.

Blonsky, E., Logemann, J., Boshes, B., and Fisher, H. (1975). Comparison of speech and swallowing function in patients with tremor disorders and in normal geriatric patients: A cinefluoroscopic study. *Journal of Gerontology, 30,* 299–303.

Bosma, J. (1980). Physiology of the mouth, pharynx and esophagus. In M. Paparella and D. Shumrick (Eds.), *Otolaryngology* (ed 2.). (pp.319–345). Philadelphia: Saunders.

Capen, D., Garland, D., and Waters, R. (1986). Surgical stabilization of the cervical spine—a comparative analysis of anterior and posterior spine fusions. *Clinical Orthopaedics and Related Research, 196,* 229–237.

Capen, D., Nelson, R., Zigler, J., Waters, R., and Garland, D. (1987). Surgical stabilization of the cervical spine: A comparative analysis of anterior and posterior spine fusions. *Paraplegia, 25,* 111–119.

Curtis, D., and Hudson, T. (1983). Laryngeotracheal aspiration: Analysis of specific neuromuscular factors. *Radiology, 149,* 517–522.

Curtis, D., Cruess, D., and Dachman, A. (1985). Normal erect swallowing—normal functioning and incidence of variations. *Investigative Radiology, 20,* 717–726.

Daly, D., Code, C., and Andersen, H. (1962). Disturbances of swallowing and esophageal motility in patients with multiple sclerosis. *Neurology, 12,* 250–256.

Davis, J., Lazarus, C., Logemann, J., and Hurst, P. (1987). Effect of a maxillary glossectomy prosthesis on articulation and swallowing. *Journal of Prosthetic Dentistry, 57,* 715–719.

Dobie, R. (1978). Rehabilitation of swallowing disorders. *American Family Physician, 27,* 84–95.

Dodds, W. Man, K., Cook, I. Kahrilas, P. Steward, S., and Kern, M. (1988). Influence of bolus volume on swallow induced hyoid movement in normal subjects. *American Journal of Radiology, 150,* 1202–1209.

Donner, M. (1974). Swallowing mechanism and neuromuscular disorders. *Seminars in Roentgenology, 9,* 273–282.

Donner, M., and Silbiger, M. (1966). Cinefluorographic analysis of pharyngeal swallowing in neuromuscular disorders. *American Journal of Medical Sciences, 251,* 600–616.

Dworkin, J., and Hartman, D. (1979). Progressive speech deterioration and dysphagia in amyotrophic lateral sclerosis: Case report. *Archives of Physical Medicine and Rehabilitation, 60,* 423–425.

Ekberg, O. (1986). The posture of the head and pharyngeal swallowing. *Acta Radiologica (Diag.) 27,* 691–696.

Ekberg, O., and Schultze, T. (1986). Pharyngeal swallowing in patients with paresis of the recurrent nerve. *Acta Radiologica Diagnostica, 27,* 697–700.

Ekedahl, C., Mansson, I., and Sandberg, N. (1974). Swallowing dysfunction in the brain damaged with drooling. *Acta Otolaryngologica, 78,* 141–149.

Fabiszak, A. (1986). *An investigation of swallowing patterns in subgroups with multiple sclerosis and normal subjects using objective temporal measures.* PhD dissertation, Northwestern University, Evanston, IL.

Fyke, F., and Code, C. (1955). Resting and deglutition pressures in the pharyngoesophageal region. *Gastroenterology, 29,* 24–34.

Gay, I., Chisin, R., and Elidan, J. (1984). Myotomy of the cricopharyngeal muscle—a treatment for dysphagia and aspiration in neurologic disorders. *Laryngologie, 105,* 271–274.

Griffin, K. (1974). Swallowing training for dysphagic patients. *Archives of Physical Medicine and Rehabilitation, 55,* 467–470.

Groher, M. (1986). The prevalence of swallowing disorders in two teaching hospitals. *Dysphagia, 1,* 3–6.

Hargrove, R. (1980). Feeding the severely dysphagic patient. *Journal of Neurosurgical Nursing, 12,* 102–107.

Helfrich-Miller, K., Rector, K., and Straka, J. (1986). Dysphagia: Its treatment in the profoundly retarded patient with cerebral palsy. *Archives of Physical Medicine and Rehabilitation, 67,* 520–525.

Heimlich, H., and O'Connor, T. (1979). Relearning the swallowing process. *Annals of Otology, Rhinology and Laryngology, 88,* 794–797.

Hurwitz, A., Nelson, J., and Haddad, J. (1975). Oropharyngeal dysphagia— manometric and cine-esophagraphic findings. *Digestive Diseases, 20,* 313– 323.

Jenkins, P., Lazarus, C., and Logemann, J. (1984). *The co-occurrence of oropharyngeal reflexes.* Paper presented at the American Speech-Language-Hearing Association annual meeting, San Francisco.

Kahrilas, P., Dodds, W., Dent, J., Logemann, J., and Shaker, R. (1988). Upper esophageal sphincter function during deglutition. *Gastroenterology, 95,* 52–62.

Kahrilas, P., Logemann, J., Bakil, N., Dodds, W., Dent, J., and Tarbis, S. (1987). The dynamics of the swallow reflex with and without topical oropharyngeal anesthesia. *Abstracts Digestive Diseases and Sciences, 32,* 916.

Kilman, W., and Goyal, R. (1976). Disorders of pharyngeal and upper esophageal sphincter motor function. *Archives of Internal Medicine, 136,* 592–600.

Kirchner, J. (1967). Pharyngeal and esophageal dysfunction: The diagnosis. *Minnesota Journal of Medicine, 50,* 921–924.

Kobara, M., and Logemann, J. (1987). *Comparative analysis of dysphagia following left and right cortical infarcts and brainstem infarcts.* Paper presented at the American Speech-Language-Hearing Convention, New Orleans.

Langfitt, T., and Gennarelli, T. (1982). Can outcome from head injury be improved? *Journal of Neurosurgery, 56,* 19–25.

Lazarus, C., and Logemann, J. (1985). *Recovery of swallowing function in closed head trauma patients.* Paper presented at the American Speech-Language-Hearing Association, Washington, DC.

Lazarus, C., and Logemann, J. (1986). *Lingual control in closed head trauma patients.* Paper presented at the American Speech-Language-Hearing Association, Detroit.

Lazarus, C., and Logemann, J. (1987a). *Lingual control for speech and swallowing in head trauma.* Paper presented at the American Speech-Language-Hearing Association, New Orleans.

Lazarus, C., and Logemann, J. (1987b). Swallowing disorders in closed head trauma patients. *Archives of Physical Medicine and Rehabilitation, 68,* 79–84.

Lazzara, G., Lazarus, C., and Logemann, J. (1984). *Swallowing disorders in spinal cord injury.* Paper presented at the American Speech-Language-Hearing Association, San Francisco.

Lazzara, G., Lazarus, C., and Logemann, J. (1986). Impact of thermal stimulation on the triggering of the swallowing reflex. *Dysphagia, 1,* 73–77.

Linden, P., and Siebens, A. (1983). Dysphagia: Predicting laryngeal penetration. *Archives of Physical Medicine and Rehabilitation, 64,* 281–284.

Lobato, R., Rivas, J., Portillo, J. Velasco, L., Cordobes, F., Esparza, J., and Lamas, E. (1979). Prognostic value of intracranial pressure levels during acute phase of severe head injuries. *Acta Neurochirugie (Suppl) 28,* 70–73.

Logemann, J. (1983). *Evaluation and treatment of swallowing disorders.* Boston: College-Hill Press.

Logemann, J. (1986a). *Manual for the videofluorographic study of swallowing.* Boston: College-Hill Press.

Logemann, J. (1986b). Treatment of aspiration related to dysphagia: An overview. *Dysphagia, 1,* 34–38.

Logemann, J. (1987). *Control of cricopharyngeal opening with the Mendelsohn maneuver.* Paper presented at the American Speech-Language-Hearing Association, New Orleans.

Logemann, J., and Lazarus, C. (1987). Authors' response to Tanya Warms. *Dysphagia, 2,* 56–58.

Logemann, J., Kahrilas, P., and Kobara, M. (in press). Benefit of head rotation on pharyngoesophageal dysphagia. *Archives of Physical Medicine and Rehabilitation.*

Logemann, J., Lazarus, C., and Jenkins, P. (1982). *The relationship between clinical judgment and radiographic assessment of aspiration.* Paper presented at the American Speech-Language-Hearing Association, Toronto.

Mandelstam, P., and Lieber, A. (1970). Cineradiographic evaluation of the esophagus in normal adults. *Gastroenterology, 58,* 29–32.

Mannson, I., and Sandberg, N. (1975). Salivary stimulus and swallowing reflex in man. *Acta Otolaryngologica, 79,* 445–450.

McConnel, F. (1988). Analysis of pressure generation and bolus transit during pharyngeal swallowing. *Laryngoscope, 98,* 71–78.

McConnel, F., Mendelsohn, M., and Logemann, J. (1986). Examination of swallowing after total laryngectomy using manofluorography. *Head and Neck Surgery, 9,* 3–12.

McConnel, F., Mendelsohn, M., and Logemann, J. (1987). Manofluorography of deglutition after supraglottic laryngectomy. *Head and Neck Surgery, Jan/Feb,* 142–150.

McConnel, F., Mendelsohn, M., and Logemann, J. (1988). Manofluorography of deglutition after total laryngopharyngectomy. *Plastic and Reconstructive Surgery, 81,* 346–351.

Meyer, T., and Logemann, J. (1986). *An analysis of tongue strength and swallowing efficiency in amyotrophic lateral sclerosis.* PhD dissertation, Northwestern University, Evanston, IL.

Miller, A. (1986). Neurophysiologic basis of swallowing. *Dysphagia, 1,* 91–100.

Morris, S. (1977). *Program guidelines for children with feeding problems.* Edison, NJ: Childcraft.

Morris, S. (1985). Developmental implications for the management of feeding problems in neurologically impaired infants. In J. Logemann (Ed.), *Seminars in speech and language* (pp. 193–314). New York: Thieme-Stratton.

Mueller, H. (1975). Feeding. In N. Finnie (Ed.), *Handling the young cerebral palsy child at home.* New York: Dutton.

Muz, I., Mathog, R., Miller, P., Rosen, R., and Borrero, J. (1987). Detection and quantification of laryngotracheopulmonary aspiration with scintography. *Laryngoscope, 97,* 1180–1185.

Pinkus, N. (1973). The dangers of oral feeding in the presence of cuffed tracheostomy tubes. *Medical Journal of Australia, 1,* 1238–1240.

Pommerenke, W. (1928). A study of the sensory areas eliciting the swallowing reflex. *American Journal of Physiology, 84,* 36–41.

Ramsey, G. (1986). Suckle facilitation of feeding in selected adult dysphagic patients. *Dysphagia, 1,* 7–12.

Rasley, A., and Logemann, J. (1987). *Effect of bolus size on oropharyngeal swallowing in dysphagic patients.* Paper presented at the American Speech-Language-Hearing Association, New Orleans.

Reines, H., and Harris, R. (1987). Pulmonary complications of acute spinal cord injuries. *Neurosurgery, 21,* 193–196.

Robbins, J. (1985). Swallowing and speech production in the neurologically impaired adult. In J. Logemann (Ed.), *Seminars in speech and language* (pp. 293–314). New York: Thieme-Stratton.

Robbins, J. (1987). Swallowing in ALS and motor neuron disease. In R. Brooks (Ed.), *Neurologic clinics: Amyotrophic lateral sclerosis 2* (pp. 213–229). Philadelphia: Saunders.

Robbins, J., Logemann, J., and Kirchner, H. (1986). Swallowing and speech production in Parkinson's disease. *Annals of Neurology*, 283–287.

Schultz, A., Niemtzow, P., Jacobs, S., and Naso, F. (1979). Dysphagia associated with cricopharyngeal dysfunction. *Archives of Physical Medicine and Rehabilitation*, 60, 381–384.

Shawker, T., Sonies, B., Stone, M., and Baum, B. (1983). Real-time ultrasound visualization of tongue movement during swallowing. *Journal of Clinical Ultrasound*, 11, 485–494.

Shawker, T., Sonies, B., Hall, T., and Baum, B. (1984). Ultrasound analysis of tongue, hyoid, and larynx activity during swallowing. *Investigative Radiology*, 19, 82–86.

Sochaniwskyj, A., Koheil, R., Bablich, K., Milner, M., and Kenny, D. (1986). Oral motor functioning, frequency of swallowing and drooling in normal children and in children with cerebral palsy. *Archives of Physical Medicine and Rehabilitation*, 67, 866–874.

Splaingard, M., Hutchins, B., Sulton, L., and Chaudhuri, G. (1988). Aspiration in rehabilitation patients: Videofluoroscopy versus bedside clinical assessment. *Archives of Physical Medicine and Rehabilitation*, 69, 637–640.

Tracy, J., and Logemann, J. (1987). *The effects of bolus size on oropharyngeal deglutition.* Paper presented at the American Speech-Language-Hearing Association, New Orleans.

Veis, S., and Logemann, J. (1985). The nature of swallowing in CVA patients. *Archives of Physical Medicine and Rehabilitation*, 66, 372–375.

Weber, B. (1974). Eating with a trach. *American Journal of Nursing*, 74, 1439.

Wheeler, R., Logemann, J., and Rosen, M. (1980). Maxillary reshaping prostheses: Effectiveness in improving speech and swallowing of post-surgical oral cancer patients. *Journal of Prosthetic Dentistry*, 43, 313–319.

Winstein, C. (1983). Neurogenic dysphagia—frequency, progression and outcome in adults following head injury. *Physical Therapy*, 63, 1992–1996.

BIBLIOGRAPHY

Ardran, G., and Kemp, F. (1967). The mechanism of the larynx. II. The epiglottis and closure of the larynx. *British Journal of Radiology*, 40, 372–389.
   This article gives a detailed description of the mechanism involved in closure of the larynx during normal deglutition.

Donner, M., and Silbiger, M. (1966). Cinefluorographic analysis of pharyngeal swallowing in neuromuscular disorders. *American Journal of Medical Sciences*, 251, 600–616.
   This article examines the types of pharyngeal swallowing problems associated with a variety of neuromuscular diseases, using cinefluoroscopy.

Lazarus, C., and Logemann, J. (1987). The nature of swallowing disorders in closed head trauma patients. *Archives of Physical Medicine and Rehabilitation*, 68, 79–84.

This article gives a detailed description of the types of swallowing problems seen in a group of 53 brain-injured subjects. Frequency, co-occurrence of swallowing problems, and occurrence of aspiration are examined.

Logemann, J. (1983). *Evaluation and treatment of swallowing disorders.* Boston: College-Hill Press.

This book gives an overview of normal swallowing and types of dysphagia and a detailed description of the modified barium swallow procedure. Specific types of swallowing disorders as seen in a variety of neurologically impaired head and neck cancer surgical populations are defined. Treatment strategies and overall management issues are discussed.

Miller, A. (1986). Neurophysiologic basis of swallowing. *Dysphagia, 1,* 91–100.

This article details the neurophysiology of normal deglutition, defining the neural pathways and musculature involved in swallowing. The effects of sensory input and feedback on swallow elicitation are discussed.

Index

Index